REPRODUCTION IN NEW WORLD PRIMATES

REPRODUCTION IN NEW WORLD PRIMATES

New Models in Medical Science

Edited by
Professor John Hearn
Director, The Institute of Zoology,
The Zoological Society of London

MTP PRESS LIMITED
International Medical Publishers
LANCASTER · BOSTON · THE HAGUE

Published in the UK and Europe by

MTP Press Limited

Falcon House

Lancaster, England

British Library Cataloguing in Publication Data

Reproduction in new world primates.
1. Monkeys---South America
2. Reproduction
I. Hearn, John
591.4'6 QL876
ISBN-13: 978-94-009-7324-4 e-ISBN-13: 978-94-009-7322-0
DOI: 10.107/978-94-009-7322-0

Published in the USA by

MTP Press

A division of Kluwer Boston Inc.

190 Old Derby Street

Hingham, MA 02043, USA

Library of Congress Cataloging in Publication Data

Main entry under title:

Reproduction in new world primates.

Bibliography: p.
Includes index.
1. Primates--Reproduction. 2. Primates--Latin America--Reproduction. 3. Mammals--Reproduction.
I. Hearn, John, 1943- .
QL737.P9R35 1982 599.8'2 82-12682

Contents

LIST OF CONTRIBUTORS

A.F. COIMBRA-FILHO

Centro de Primatologia de
Rio de Janeiro (CRPJ),
DECAM-FEEMA,
Rio de Janeiro, Brazil.

J.H. DENARI

Instituto Latinoamericana de
Investigaciones Médicas de la
Universidad del Salvador
(ILAIMUS ex ILAFIR),
Galván 4102 (1431),
Buenos Aires, Argentina.

A.F. DIXSON

The Institute of Zoology,
The Zoological Society of London,
Regent's Park,
London NW1 4RY, England.

W.R. DUKELOW

Endocrine Research Unit,
Michigan State University,
East Lansing, MI 48824, USA.

G. EPPLE

Monell Chemical Senses Center,
3500 Market Street,
Philadelphia, PA 19104, USA.

J.P. HEARN

The Institute of Zoology,
The Zoological Society of London,
Regent's Park,
London NW1 4RY, England.

Y. KATZ

Monell Chemical Senses Center,
3500 Market Street,
Philadelphia, PA 19104, USA.

R.A. MITTERMEIER

World Wildlife Fund-US,
1601 Connecticut Avenue NW,
Washington DC 20009, USA

and

Department of Anatomical Sciences,
Health Sciences Center,
State University of New York,
Stony Brook, NY 11794, USA.

C.A. NAGLE

Instituto Latinoamericana de
Investigaciones Médicas de la
Universidad del Salvador
(ILAIMUS ex ILAFIR),
Galván 4102 (1431),
Buenos Aires, Argentina.

PREFACE

The New World primates are becoming widely used in scientific and medical work in fields from anthropology to zoology, behaviour to urology. They have unique attributes for studies in cancer, infectious diseases, genetics, virology and reproduction. However, it is only now that their reproductive physiology is being clarified in any depth and this book is a first synthesis of that knowledge.

The nine authors involved in this project have presented an up to date account of the major New World species used in biological and medical science. In addition to their distribution and conservation in the wild, essential biological data from laboratory studies are presented on reproductive cycles, gestation length, seasonal breeding, puberty and other factors. The major applications of these species in research are explored.

Whenever possible, research workers should steer away from using endangered species in their studies. The New World monkeys used in research in any numbers are still fairly common in the wild, yet their greatest advantages are in their smalle size and high fecundity. This makes possible the establishment of self sustaining captive breeding colonies at a fraction of the time and cost necessary for the more conventional Old World laboratory primates. Consequently the drain on wild stocks need not be extensive as only breeding nuclei should be necessary. Complacency is out of order, however, as the destruction of their natural habitats will undoubtedly place more species on the endangered list before long. It is the management and conservation of these primates in the future, both in the wild and in captivity, that will depend on a sound knowledge of their reproductive physiology.

This book is aimed at primatologists and research workers in biomedical science whose studies depend on an understanding of the physiology of their animals. It will also be of value to students and perhaps to those who administer research and to whom questions of research planning and funding are of interest.

I am most grateful to my friends, who have served as authors on this project, for their hard work and observance of deadlines. My thanks in full measure go to Connie Nutkins, for without her assistance this volume would not have been completed. I acknowledge too the quiet yet persistent encouragement and support of David Bloomer and Phil Johnstone of MTP Press.

John Hearn

London, October 1982

Chapter 1

Distribution and Conservation of New World Primate Species used in Biomedical Research

R. A. Mittermeier & A. F. Coimbra-Filho

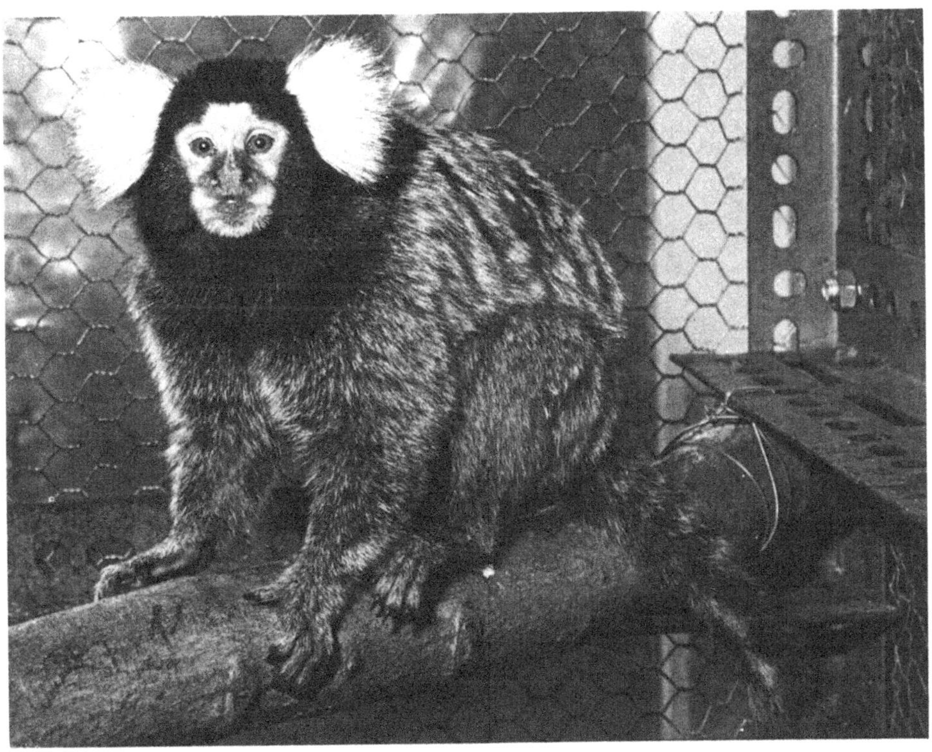

The Common marmoset, Callithrix jacchus, a primate that is bred to the fifth generation in captivity.

DISTRIBUTION AND CONSERVATION OF NEW WORLD PRIMATE SPECIES USED IN BIOMEDICAL RESEARCH

Russell A. Mittermeier*

Adelmar F. Coimbra-Filho**

* World Wildlife Fund-US, 1601 Connecticut Avenue NW, Washington DC 20009; AND Department of Anatomical Sciences, Health Sciences Center, State University of New York, Stony Brook, NY11794, USA.

**Centro de Primatologia de Rio de Janeiro (CRPJ), DECAM-FEEMA, Rio de Janeiro, Brazil.

INTRODUCTION

The New World monkeys have achieved a position of considerable importance in biomedical research over the past two decades. One species, the squirrel monkey, is second only to the rhesus monkey in frequency of use in the laboratory; several others, notably the night monkey and several species of tamarins, are the preferred animal models for certain kinds of research; and still another, the common marmoset, possesses characteristics that, in all probability, will make it a valuable general laboratory primate of the future.

However, it is important to note that the habitat available for New World monkeys, all of which are arboreal, forest-dwelling animals, is fast decreasing over almost all of South and Central America. The burgeoning human population is penetrating into every corner of the continent, destroying or drastically modifying previously undisturbed forest areas, and large scale development programs, such as those currently under way in various parts of Amazonia, often include widespread clear-cutting of prime primate habitat.

In addition, primates have always been an important source of food for man in South America, especially in the Amazonian region[1]. Hunting of monkeys continues to be a serious factor today, and has been exacerbated by the human population increase, the arrival of more sophisticated weapons, the disappearance of other larger game species, and the decrease of available forest habitat.

Although rarely the major factor in the decline of a species, the demand for New World monkeys as laboratory animals has added to these other pressures and has certainly been a more conspicuous and quantifiable threat than either habitat destruction or hunting. Tens of thousands of New World monkeys were exported during the 1960's and early 1970's, mainly through the major trading centers of Leticia, Colombia, Iquitos, Peru and Barranquilla, Colombia, but also from a number of other dealers scattered across South and Central America. Mortality was often high in this trade, and exploitation of wild populations was carried out without the barest minimum of demographic data or other ecological information.

This trade made it clear to the governments of exporting countries that non-human primates were an important natural resource. At the same time, however, the extent of the trade and the absence of demographic data on the animals being exploited became a source of considerable concern, both to conservationists and to the governments of the countries involved. Another problem was that much of the profit in the primate trade seemed to be accruing to foreign-based dealers, with minimal benefit to the countries from which the animals originated. Eventually, the combination of these factors led to the declaration of export bans in the principal source countries. Brazil was first with its 1967 Fauna Protection Law, but the most important bans were by the major primate exporters, Colombia and Peru, in 1973. At present, only one South American country, Bolivia, still permits large-scale export of wild-caught primates.

The controversy over the trade that eventually led to the export bans had been growing in the late 1960's and early 1970's, and it gradually brought with it an increased awareness of the need for more data on wild populations of New World monkeys. The biomedical community, which was losing an abundant source of inexpensive laboratory animals, began to support status surveys and censuses - ostensibly in the hopes of providing the data base required for rational sustained yield exploitation and also to convince governments that the primates used in research were not endangered.

At about the same time, wildlife conservationists, who had been concerned about the effects of the trade all along, began to realize that there was little in the way of solid, quantitative data on either the effects of the trade or on any other aspect of New World monkey conservation. They were also becoming increasingly alarmed by the apparent downward trends in primate populations all over South America, particularly those associated with the ambitious new development programs like Brazil's Transamazonian highway. Again, more detailed investigation of Neotropical primate populations was clearly necessary.

As a result, the early to mid 1970's saw a surge of field work on New World monkeys, both in the former exporting countries and also in countries where little or no trade had ever existed. Noteworthy among these early efforts were investigations funded by the National Institutes of Health (NIH) of the United States, in conjunction with the US National Academy of Sciences and the Pan American Health Organization (PAHO), and carried out in Peru, Colombia, Bolivia, Guyana and northern Argentina (eg.[2-12]), and by the New York Zoological Society, the World Wildlide Fund-US, the US Peace Corps and other organizations in Peru, Colombia, Brazil, Surinam, French Guiana and Panama (eg.[13-26]). Interest in these important animals has continued to grwo since the mid 1970's and new field projects are being initiated every year.

The purpose of this chapter is to review what these studies have told us about the conservation status of the New World monkey species currently considered important in biomedical research and discussed in greater detail in the following chapters of this book. The information in this chapter hopefully will assist researchers in understanding the conservation problems faced by the various New World monkey species, and should help to steer them away from species (eg.

Saguinus oedipus) that, though important, are already so depleted in the wild that future exploitation of natural populations is no longer feasible. A brief review of taxonomy and distribution is provided as well, since these topics are basic to understanding the current conservation situation of each species.

THE TUFTED CAPUCHIN MONKEY (Cebus apella)

Taxonomy and Distribution

Most recent authors (eg.[27-32]) have recognized four species of capuchin monkeys. The last major taxonomic investigation of this genus was carried out by Hershkovitz[28] over 30 years ago, but Kinzey[33] recently has initiated studies on the subspecies of Cebus apella in eastern Brazil. In his 1949 paper, Hershkovitz divides the four capuchin species into two groups based on the presence or absence of distinct frontal tufts of hair on the heads of both sexes. His "untufted group" includes Cebus capucinus, Cebus albifrons and Cebus nigrivittatus, and his "tufted group" only Cebus apella and its various subspecies.

Cebus apella is the capuchin species of greatest importance in biomedical research. A medium-sized monkey and the largest of the New World monkeys widely used in research, the tufted capuchin wieghs 3 to 5 kg[22], with males often exceeding females by 1 to 2 kg. This species has the largest range of any South American monkey, extending from the llanos or plains of Colombia (where it inhabits gallery forests), through almost all of Amazonia and the Guianas, south and east to the Mato Grosso of central Brazil, the Atlantic forests of eastern Brazil, and the subtropical forests of northern Argentina[31,33,34]. Only one subspecies, Cebus apella apella, is currently recognized from Amazonia[35], but more subspeciation has occurred in the south and east. Kinzey[33] recognizes three subspecies from the Atlantic forests of eastern Brazil, and one from adjacent parts of the cerrado (savanna) formations of central Brazil. The eastern subspecies include Cebus apella xanthosternos, which is found only in the southern part of the state of Bahia, north of the Rio Jequitinhonha[32], Cebus apella robustus, which occurs to the south of C. a. xanthosternos in southern Bahia, eastern Minas Gerais and northern Espírito Santo north of the Rio Doce, and Cebus apella nigritus, which lives south of the Rio Doce in Espírito Santo and southeastern Minas Gerais and extends further south to Rio de Janeiro, São Paulo, Paraná, Santa Catarina and Rio Grande do Sul[33]. The wide-ranging Cebus apella libidinosus (which, according to Kinzey includes the previously recognized subspecies Cebus apella cay) occurs from northeastern Brazil, through the cerrado formations of central Brazil, and presumably also into Paraguay, Bolivia and northern Argentina. However, the subspecific status of C. apella in these countries is still not clear since they were not covered in Kinzey's[33] investigation.

A rough map of the distribution of C. apella is given in Fig. 1. Hill[36] provides a map for this species, but it is out-of-date, incomplete and replete with errors. Hernandez-Camacho and Cooper[35] give a detailed map of C. apella distribution in Colombia, and Kinzey's[33] paper maps the distribution of the eastern Brazilian subspecies.

Ecology and Conservation Status

C. apella is a very adaptable animal capable of utilizing a wide range of food items and living in many different forest types. It is omniverous, and feeds mainly on fruits of many species, on seeds, and on arthropods, supplemented by flowers, young leaves, other plant parts, and an occasional small vertebrate[22,34,37]. It is also very flexible in choice of habitat, and has been reported from almost every kind of natural forest formation within its range, at altitudes ranging from sea level to 2700 m[1,34,35]. It adapts well to the presence of man, utilizing secondary forests in the vicinity of human habitations and also raiding plantations to feed on corn and cultivated fruits[5,6,22,35,38,39,40].

The conservation status of wild populations of *C. apella* varies considerably from region to region, depending on the extent of habitat destruction and the degree to which primates are hunted locally as a food item. In the Guianas, for example, and especially in Surinam and French Guiana, *C. apella* is still a quite common animal, and habitat destruction is not yet a major factor because of the sparse human population. *C. apella* is a popular food item in the interior of these two countries, but again the level of exploitation is so low that it does not yet pose a serious threat to wild populations.

The status of *C. apella* in the Amazon drainage basin is much more variable. In parts of Brazilian Amazonia, where extensive clear-cutting of forest has occurred, *C. apella* and all other arboreal species have disappeared. In other parts of the same region, where only minimum habitat modification through shifting slash-and-burn agriculture has taken place, *C. apella* usually survives well provided hunting pressure is not too heavy.

Although large scale habitat destruction is usually the major factor in the decline of *Cebus* populations and in spite of the fact that the animals adapt well to low level hunting pressure, heavy hunting pressure can be a serious factor even in areas where little or no habitat destruction is taking place. In some parts of Peruvian Amazon (eg. in the vicinity of Iquitos, the largest city) hunting pressure and especially commercial hunting to serve local meat markets, has resulted in the disappearance of *C. apella* from many areas of perfectly suitable habitat[2]. Castro *et al*[7] found that some 280 capuchin monkeys (150 *C. albifrons* and 130 *C. apella*) were sold for food in the Iquitos market in a period of just 160 days from February to August, 1973, and this is undoubtedly only a very small portion of the animals killed for local use in the region.

In the ecologically devastated Atlantic forest region of eastern Brazil, *C. apella* usually does far better than almost all other nonhuman primates, with the possible exception of a few of the more adaptable *Callithrix* species. *C. a. nigritus*, for example, is still found in almost every forest over 500 ha in size that has been afforded the slightest degree of protection, mainly because hunting pressure is not a serious factor throughout most of its range. C. a. robustus also survives well in remnant forest patches, but very little of its habitat still exists. C. a. xanthosternos, in contrast, is now very rare and endangered within its highly restricted range. Its southern Bahian distribution is in the major cocoa-growing region of Brazil, where considerable habitat modification has taken place, and lumbering activities are destroying most of the forest not suitable for cocoa-growing. In addition, there is a strong tradition of primate hunting in southern Bahia. Indeed, the two largest primate species in this area, the northern brown howler monkey (Alouatta fusca fusca) and the woolly spider monkey (Brachyteles arachnoides), are either already extinct or very nearly so[41].

The effects of live capture and the trade on C. apella are difficult to evaluate. The international trade was significant, though never of the magnitude of that involving the squirrel monkey and some of the tamarins. During the 1960's and early 1970's, several thousand C. apella were exported annually from the major Amazonian trading centers of Iquitos, Peru and Leticia, Colombia (eg. Castro[42] reports annual exports of 1200-2600 for the period 1964-1973), and this certainly may have contributed to the local rarity of the species in the vicinity of these towns. However, it is unlikely to have had a major effect over the whole of Amazonia, and was almost certainly less than the number killed annually for food.

All things considered, the status of the currently recognized subspecies of C. apella can be summarized as follows:

- C. apella apella - still common in most of Amazonia, but locally rare or extinct in areas of heavy hunting and/or forest clearance.
- C. apella nigritus - still common in remaining forests within its range and one of the most abundant eastern Brazilian monkeys; nonetheless, only a fraction of its original habitat still exists.
- C. apella robustus - a vulnerable subspecies; still occurs in some of the forest patches remaining within its small range, but much of its habitat has already been destroyed.
- C. apella xanthosternos - an endangered subspecies; very rare or already locally extinct throughout its very small range.
- C. apella libidinosus - status unknown.

THE NIGHT MONKEY (Aotus spp.)

Taxonomy and Distribution

The status of the many distinct populations of this widespread and variable genus presents one of the major problems in New World monkey systematics. Most authors of the past three decades (eg.[28,29,30,31,43,44]) have recognized a single, wide-ranging, variable species, with five to nine subspecies or phenotypes. However, recent cytogenetic research has demonstrated that several Aotus populations differ in chromosome number and morphology, and these may represent distinct species.

DeBoer[45-47], Brumback[48,49], and Willenborg and Brumback[50], for instance, discussed three different karyotypes from three major areas, whereas Ma *et al*[51] described nine from five major areas. Brumback[48], somewhat prematurely, assigned specific names to the three karyotypes he investigated, calling them *Aotus trivirgatus*, *Aotus azarae* and *Aotus griseimembra*, but Thorington[52] recommends caution in interpreting *Aotus* chromosome numbers. He states that:

"some populations are apparently polymorphic for chromosome number, and the accumulating data are suggestive that chromosome number may vary clinally, which is quite consistent with the hypothesis that there is only one species."

Thorington and Vorek[44] have also studied coat color and pattern, craniometry, permanent tooth eruption, and sequence of epiphyseal union. They describe three basically different phenotypes, each with several variations, but continue to recognize only one species.

Much more detailed laboratory and field data are required before any further conclusions on *Aotus* systematics can be drawn. Hershkovitz (pers.comm.), in conjunction with N. Ma of the New England Regional Primate Center, is currently carrying out such an investigation and will hopefully clarify much of the confusion surrounding this genus. It is urgent that we have a clear picture of *Aotus* systematics, since this kind of information is essential for captive breeding projects involving this biomedically-important species. As noted by Elliott *et al*[53], previous attempts at laboratory breeding of *Aotus* were frequently unsuccessful because animals with different karyotypes were paired.

The genus *Aotus* has a large range that extends from about 81°W in Panama, through northern Colombia and adjacent parts of Venezuela, into upper Amazonia and as far south as the *Chaco* region of Paraguay and Bolivia and the Chaco and Formosa provinces of northern Argentina[12,31,35]. However, it is absent from the Guianas and the adjacent northeastern portion of Brazilian Amazonia, although it has been recorded from several localities on the south bank of the Rio Amazonas near its mouth[44]. It is also absent from the entire Atlantic forest region of eastern Brazil.

A rough distribution map for *Aotus* is provided in Fig. 2. Thorington and Vorek[44] also include a map for the genus, and Hernandez-Camacho and Cooper[35] give a detailed map for Colombia. Hill's[36] map is out-of-date and includes many errors.

Ecology and Conservation Status

Aotus is the world's only nocturnal monkey and it has rarely been studied in the wild. Most of the field data on the animal come from investigations by Wright[54,55] in Peruvian Amazonia, by Soini and Moya[56] on Isla Iquitos near Iquitos, Peru, and by Rathbun and Gache[10,12] in northern Argentina. Moynihan[57] published a detailed behavioral study of the species, based mainly on captive observations but also including some field data, Thorington *et al*[58] radio-tracked a single individual released on Barro Colorado Island in Panama, and Heltne[59] conducted a

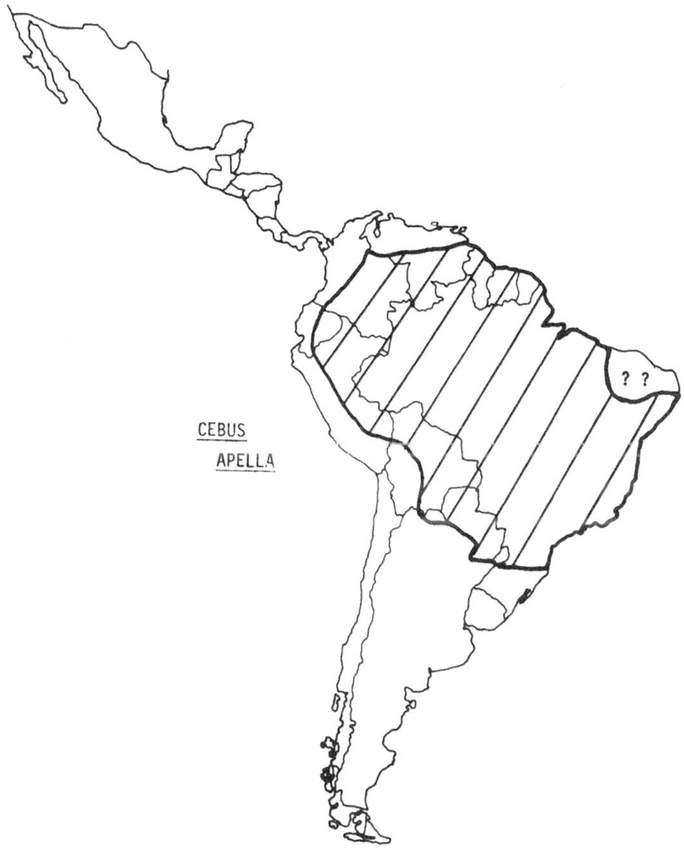

FIGURE 1

Distribution of *Cebus apella*

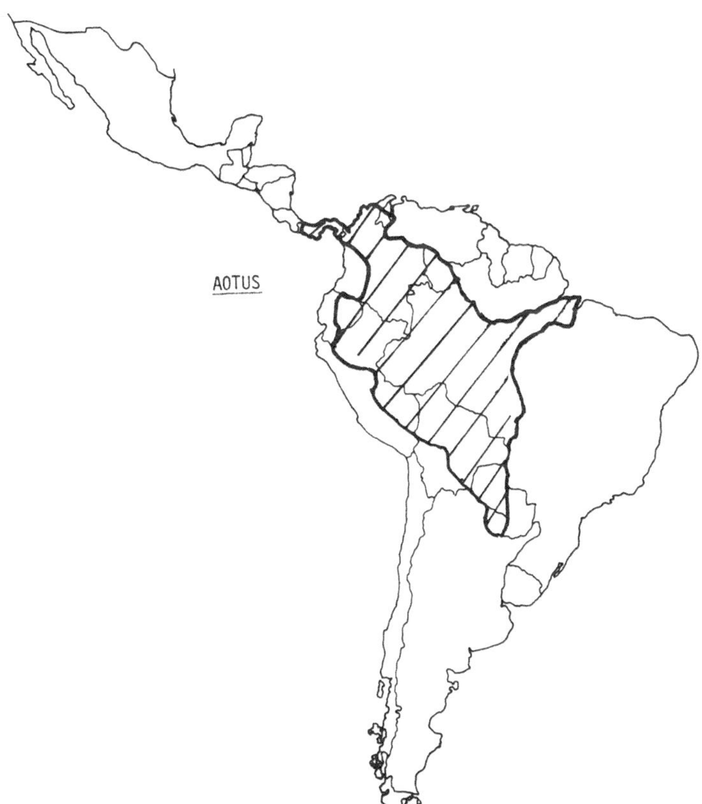

FIGURE 2

Distribution of *Aotus* sp.

brief survey of Aotus in northern Colombia.

These studies and various anecdotal reports indicate that Aotus is a very adaptable animal that feeds mainly on fruit, together with some arthropods, flowers and leaves, and that it occurs in a wide variety of habitats from sea level to 3,200 m[35]. It sometimes lives in tree holes, but vine tangles and other sleeping sites are also used[10,12,54,55]. Although it is active only at night in most parts of its range, Rathbun and Gache[10,12] note that Aotus in northern Argentina is also active during the day.

The conservation status of Aotus varies considerably from region to region. In northern Colombia, it is clear that the animals are already endangered (Hernandez-Camacho, pers. comm., 1981). Habitat destruction in recent years has drastically reduced the habitat available to this and other northern Colombian monkeys, and the trade in these animals, that are the preferred night monkeys for malarial research (eg.[60,61]) has been heavier than that in Amazonia (eg. Green[16] gives figures of 1,213 exported and 1,580 "transported" in the northern Colombian coastal region in 1971, and a major portion of the Aotus entering the US during the peak years of exploitation originated in northern Colombia). The situation becomes even more serious when one realizes that several taxa cocur in northern Colombia. Hernandez-Camacho and Cooper[35] believe that there are three subspecies in this area, each of them with quite small ranges. Exploitation of these animals should end immediately, and a comprehensive habitat survey (preferably using Landsat satellite imagery), together with several ecological field studies, should be initiated as soon as possible. The same should be done with adjacent Aotus populations in Panama.

Rathbun and Gache's[10,12] data from northern Argentina indicate that Aotus is found at low densities throughout this part of its range. Although they do not consider these populations to be endangered, they advise against any exploitation without a solid ecological data base already in hand.

The situation appears to be somewhat better in Amazonia. The little information available suggests that Aotus is still relatively abundant in most of this region. It occurs in close proximity to human habitations and, being nocturnal and small, is rarely hunted as a food item. Nonetheless, some Indian tribes do eat it (eg.[63]), and it is occasionally captured as a pet by local people[1].

The trade in Amazonian Aotus was of small scale compared to that in species like Saimiri and Saguinus. Castro[42] and Soini[64], for instance, cite annual export figures ranging from 150 to 850 for the Iquitos trade in the 1960's and early 1970's and, judging from total imports of Colombian Aotus (eg.[65]), the figures from Leticia were similar. Whether the comparatively low numbers exported indicate low species density, difficulty in trapping, or minimal demand for Amazonian Aotus is not certain.

In the period 1976-1979, roughly 400-700 Aotus were imported annually into the US from Bolivia, Panama and Paraguay combined (D. Mack, pers. comm.); there are indications that the trade is ending in Panama and Paraquay, but Bolivia continues to export.

Although the subjective impression is that Amazonian Aotus are holding their own, a clear knowledge of the number of taxa must await Hershkovitz's revision of the genus. Without this basic information, together with much more detailed census work and ecological investigation, further exploitation of Aotus populations in Amazonia is not to be recommended. If the Amazonian animals are divided into a number of different species or subspecies, it may be that some (eg. in northern Bolivia) are already under dangerous pressure and that current trapping activities are threatening the future of a very valuable biomedical resource. A temporary ban on all trapping and export of Aotus, at least until further data on ecology, taxonomy and distribution become available, would seem advisable.

THE COTTON-TOP (Saguinus oedipus) AND OTHER TAMARINS

Taxonomy and Distribution

Saguinus is the most diverse New World monkey genus, with 10-11 species and 32 taxa currently recognized[32,66]. This genus was formerly one of the most confusing in the Order Primates, but Hershkovitz[66,67] has done an outstanding job clarifying its taxonomy. Of the species now recognized, four are considered important for biomedical research: the cotton-top tamarin (Saguinus oedipus, or Saguinus oedipus oedipus according to Hershkovitz[66]), Spix's moustached tamarin (Saguinus mystax mystax), several subspecies of the saddleback tamarin (Saguinus fuscicollis) and Geoffroy's moustached tamarin or, as it is sometimes called, the red-bellied or "rufiventer" tamarin (Saguinus labiatus labiatus).

The genus Saguinus is primarily upper Amazonian in distribution, with six species and 24 subspecies being found in the vast region to the west of the Rio Negro and the Rio Madeira. Two other species, S. midas and S. bicolor are found in lower Amazonia, east of the Rio Negro; two, S. oedipus and S. leucopus, occur in northern Colombia; and one, S. geoffroyi, ranges from extreme northwestern Colombia into Panama and a corner of Costa Rica[31,32,66].

S. oedipus is found only in a small area in northwestern Colombia (Fig. 3), between the Río Atrato and the lower Río Cauca-Magdalena in the Departments of Atlántico, Bolivar, Córdoba, northwestern Antióquia, and possibly northeastern Chocó on the east bank of the Río Atrato. Struhsaker et al[3] obtained reports that the species may once have occurred to the east of the Rio Magdalena and they suggest that the original distribution coincided with that of the dry forests of northwestern Colombia. Hershkovitz[66], on the other hand, believes that the cotton-top tamarin never existed east of the Magdalena. In any case, any suitable habitat that may once have existed in this area has now been replaced by agriculture.

The southern limit of S. oedipus in the Andean foothills is poorly defined, but Hernandez-Camacho and Cooper[35] believe that it extends at least as far south as the Río León. The species was previously thought to have a continuous distribution in the upper Río Sinú region, but Neyman's[68] interviews with local Indians along the upper Sinú (above the Río Verde) indicated that the animal does not occur there.

According to Hershkovitz[66], the altitudinal limit for S. oedipus is 1,500 m. Hernandez-Camacho and Cooper[35], however, state that the highest reported localities are about 400 m and Neyman[68] believes the range to be 50-300 m.

Hershkovitz[66] considers the closely related S. geoffroyi from extreme northwestern Colombia and tropical forest zones of Panama and the bordering Coto region of southeastern Costa Rica to be nothing more than a subspecies of S. oedipus. Hernandez-Camacho and Cooper[35] and Mittermeier and Coimbra-Filho[32], however, believe it to be a distinct species. This species has not been used in biomedical research.

The second biomedically-important species, Saguinus mystax mystax, is found in upper Amazonia, between the Rio Juruá in Brazil and the Río Tapiche (a tributary of the Río Ucayali) in Peru ([66]; P. Soini, pers. comm.; Fig. 4). Two other subspecies, Saguinus mystax pileatus and Saguinus mystax pluto, range to the east of S. m. mystax in Brazilian Amazonia, and have never been used in biomedical research.

The next important species, Saguinus fuscicollis, has a large range in upper Amazonia (Fig. 5), being found from the foothills of the Andes in Colombia, Ecuador, Peru and Bolivia, east to the Rio Madeira in Brazil and the Río Mamoré in Bolivia and north to the south bank of the Rio Solimões (= upper Rio Amazonas in Brazil) and its north bank tributary, the Rio Japurá-Caquetá-Caguán. Of the 14 subspecies recognized by Hershkovitz[66], six have been used to varying extent in biomedical research. The most important apparently has been Illiger's saddleback tamarin (Saguinus fuscicollis illigeri) from Peruvian Amazonia. Others used include the red-mantled saddleback tamarin (Saguinus fuscicollis lagonotus) from Peruvian and Ecuadorian Amazonia, Geoffroy's saddleback tamarin (Saguinus fuscicollis nigrifrons) and the Andean saddleback tamarin (Saguinus fuscicollis leucogenys) from Peruvian Amazonia, Spix's saddleback tamarin (Saguinus fuscicollis fuscicollis) from Brazilian and Peruvian Amazonia, and Weddell's saddleback tamarin (Saguinus fuscicollis weddelli) from Peru, Bolivia and Brazil[64,69,70.71]. Soini[64] reports that another subspecies, Saguinus fuscicollis tripartitus, was also exported from time to time, but we have never seen specimens of this animal in the trade. For more details on the distribution of Saguinus fuscicollis subspecies, the reader is referred to Hershkovitz[66].

Geoffroy's moustached tamarin (Saguinus labiatus labiatus) has become important in biomedical research in the past few years. It occurs between the Rio Madeira and the Rio Purus in the Brazilian states of Amazonas and Acre, and extends southward into the lowlands of Pando, Bolivia and Madre de Dios, Peru, between the upper Río Madre de Dios and the Río Purus[4,66,72] (Fig. 4). A second subspecies, Saguinus labiatus thomasi, is thus far known only from the type locality, the Rio Tonantins on the north bank of the Rio Solimões in Brazil[66].

The last tamarin species used to any extent in biomedical research is Spix's black-mantle tamarin, Saguinus nigricollis nigricollis. This animal is closely related to S. fuscicollis and is found in upper Amazonia, Brazil, Colombia and Peru, between the Rio Solimões and the Río Putumayo and west through Leticia, Colombia to the mouth of the Río Napo in Peru[66] (Fig. 4). A second subspecies, Saguinus nigricollis graellsi, ranges to the east of S. n. nigricollis, between the Río Putumayo-Guamués in Colombia, south into Ecuador and Peru as far as the Río Marañon, and then west to the Río Pastaza[66].

Ecology and Conservation Status

All species of Saguinus thus far investigated have proven to be very adaptable animals. They show a strong preference for edge habitats, and survive well in (and may even prefer) secondary forest situations resulting from human activities like slash-and-burn agriculture and small-scale selective hand-logging, eg.[9,11,21,22,37]. This is undoubtedly related to their diet which, in addition to fruits and a variety of other plant foods, includes a high proportion of insects and other arthropods that abound in such ecotone environments. Saguinus populations living in proximity to human habitations also benefit to some extent from the presence of man because he hunts out both potential predators (eg. eagles, hawks, tayras, small cats) and larger primate competitors. Tamarins themselves, however, are rarely hunted for food because of their small size (eg.[2,22]). Consequently, these monkeys often occur at higher densities in secondary forests near villages than in undisturbed rain forest (eg.[22,73]).

This adaptability, together with the fact that these animals give birth to twins, breed at least once (and sometimes twice) a year, and reach maturity in less than two years, means that they are able to withstand the effects of limited exploitation. However, like all other forest-dwelling primates, they cannot adapt to large-scale clear-cutting of forest, and disappear quickly in the face of forest clearance for agriculture, cattle-raising or industry.

Unfortunately, the latter is the case within the range of Saguinus oedipus, which is without a doubt the most endangered Neotropical monkey species used widely in biomedical research. The endangered status of S. oedipus was recognized by the Colombians as far back as the late 1960's, and was mentioned by a number of other researchers (eg.[62,74]). However the status of this animal was finally brought to the general attention of the international primatological community at the August 1975 Conference on the Biology and Conservation of the Callitrichidae in Front Royal, Virginia. A report by Patricia Neyman, the only primatologist with extensive field experience with this species, indicated that only a fraction of its original habitat remained, and that ongoing trade activities were contributing to its rapid decline. Her plea led to the inclusion of S. oedipus in the IUCN Red Data Book, and to its eventual placement on the US

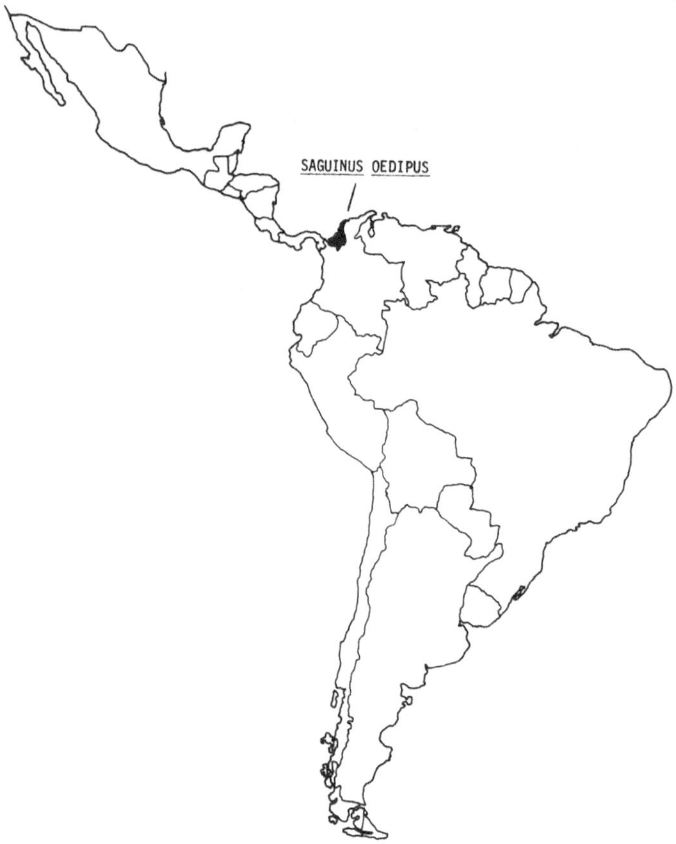

FIGURE 3

Distribution of
Saguinus oedipus

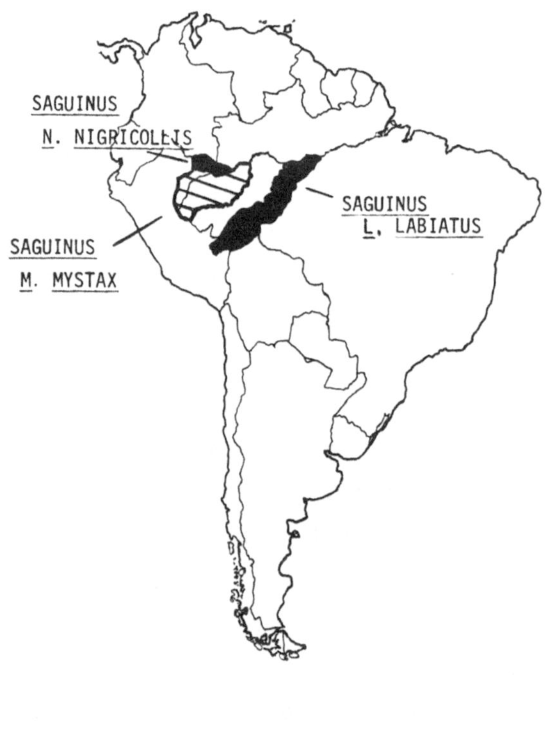

FIGURE 4

Distribution of
Saguinus sp.

Endangered Species List.

In her report, Neyman showed that at least 70% of the forest cover in the range of *S. oedipus* had already been replaced with pasture and farmland by 1966, and that the densely-inhabited northern three-quarters of its distribution included only about 5% of the remaining forest habitat. This small area was further divided into isolated patches of secondary forest, not all of which contained tamarins. She pointed out that most of these patches were probably not large enough to ensure the long-term survival of tamarin populations, even in the unlikely event that they could be fully protected.

Many of these patches undoubtedly have disappeared in the interim. Both wood and wildlife were continually being extracted during the time that Neyman was there. Furthermore, forested land in Colombia that is not yielding timber is considered unexploited and by law and custom is open to squatters, even if privately-owned.

The southern quarter of the species' range still had fairly extensive tracts of primary forest as of 1966 (the date of the last vegetation map), but 1973 satellite photographs and low-altitude flights carried out in 1974[3] indicated that considerable deforestation had taken place since 1966. Since this area was being opened up to colonization at the time of Neyman's report, even more deforestation is sure to have taken place in the interim[26,68].

Needless to say, trade activities, which were concentrated in the ecologically devastated northern part of the species' range, added greatly to the problems, and undoubtedly helped contribute to local extinctions. Numbers exported in the years of peak exploitation certainly exceeded the replacement rate in the dispersed forest fragments that made up most of the cotton-top tamarin's range. Green[16], for instance, cites US import figures of 3,098, 3,753 and 2,068 cotton-tops for 1968, 1969 and 1970, and this does not include animals lost during capture, transport and holding. Hernandez-Camacho and Cooper[35] further estimated that as many as 30,000-40,000 cotton-tops were exported during the 10-15 years of peak exploitation (the 1960's and early 1970's).

The trade in the late 1960's and early 1970's took place in spite of the fact that the Colombian government had instituted a total ban on cotton-top export from 1969-1972, and had included the animal on its endangered species list. In 1973, the Colombian government (INDERENA Resolution no. 392) ended all legal export of primates (although exceptions were made for scientific use until 1974). In the same year, the cotton-top was placed on Appendix I of CITES, the Convention on International Trade in Endangered Species. In spite of this, several hundred cotton-tops per year continued to be imported into the US and Europe. Many of them came via Panama, where they were provided with false export documents, and some went through Bolivia and Paraguay as well. This illegal trade continued to flourish and found a ready market in the US until *S. oedipus* was finally placed on the US Endangered Species List in 1976.

One still hears occasional reports of illegal shipments of S. oedipus to Europe, but the bulk of the trade appears to have ended when the US, which always provided the largest market for this species, finally instituted effective protection.

Fortunately, the prospects for the other tamarin species are somewhat better. Saguinus fuscicollis appears to be an especially adaptable species, and all the surveys and studies conducted within its range (eg.[2,5,35,95]) have shown it to be one of the more abundant and adaptable primate species. During the peak years of the Amazonian primate trade, some 1,000-4,000 Saguinus of several species were exported annually from Iquitos (eg.[42,64]), and similar numbers went out from Leticia. A substantial portion of these were S. fuscicollis sspp., although records at the time did not distinguish among the different tamarin species. All commercial trade from these two ports ended with the Colombian and Peruvian export bans, but S. fuscicollis (probably the subspecies weddelli) is still being exported from Bolivia. In addition, 450 S. fuscicollis were exported to the US in 1977-1979 through a special agreement between the Peruvian government and the Pan-American Health Organization-sponsored Peruvian Primate Project, and small shipments of this kind are expected to continue.

Saguinus mystax mystax is not quite as common as S. fuscicollis, with which it sometimes travel in polyspecific associations (eg.[75]), but it too is relatively abundant and adaptable (P. Soini, pers. comm.). Dawson[73], for instance, found it to be common along the edges of fields in terra firme habitat around Fonte Boa in Brazilian Amazonia, and members of the Peruvian Primate Project have also found it to be common in several river basins in Peruvian Amazonia (eg.[76]). As with S. fuscicollis, all commercial export of S. m. mystax ended with the Colombian and Peruvian export bans, but approximately 200 were exported through an arrangement with the Brazilian government in 1975[73], and a total of 1,300 were exported to the US by the Peruvian Primate Project between 1976 and 1979. As with S. fuscicollis, the latter arrangement is expected to continue.

Saguinus labiatus labiatus only began to enter the trade in the mid-1970's after the Colombian and Peruvian bans, and is now becoming more important in research. It is closely related to S. mystax and may prove useful for many of the same kinds of studies. It also seems to be hardier in captivity (G. Epple, pers. comm.). All S. labiatus appear to be coming out of Bolivia, with numbers imported into the US ranging from 300-1,600 per year in the period 1976-1979 (D. Mack, pers. comm.). Since Bolivia also ships to other countries, the total exported may, in fact, be much higher. The only data available on wild populations of S. labiatus come from a survey conducted in 1975 by Heltne et al[5] in Bolivia; from studies by Pook and co-workers[77-79] in Bolivia; and from a brief survey by the Peruvian Primate Project in southern Peru[72]. These investigations indicate that the species is relatively abundant, but certainly more detailed long-term ecological studies should be conducted to determine to what extent further exploitation of wild populations is possible. The current trade in Bolivia should be restricted until such data become available.

Finally, we have Saguinus nigricollis nigricollis, which was sometimes used in biomedical research when the Leticia trade was still active (eg.[80,81,82]). Most of these tamarins originated from Leticia, although some were also exported from Iquitos[64]. When Colombia and Peru instituted export bans, all trade in S. nigricollis seems to have ended and it no longer appears to be used in biomedical research. It is also not among the species handled by the PAHO-psonsored Peruvian Primate Project. In any case, it too seems to be a highly adaptable species. Hernandez-Camacho and Cooper[35] report that it was the most frequently encountered primate species in a survey conducted upriver from Leticia, in spite of the fact that this was one of the areas in which the animal was trapped.

THE SQUIRREL MONKEY (Saimiri sciureus)

Taxonomy and Distribution

With the exception of Hill[36], who recognizes five species and 15 subspecies of Saimiri, most recent authors (eg.[27,29,30,31,32,52]) have listed either one or two species, depending on whether they consider the isolated Central American squirrel monkey a distinct species or merely a subspecies. Except for this Central American taxon (S. oerstedii), which is found only between 79°55' and 85°W in western Panama and southeastern Costa Rica, Saimiri is primarily an Amazonian genus. It is found in most of Amazonian Brazil, Colombia, Ecuador, Peru and Bolivia, in the three Guianas, and south of the Rio Orinoco in Venezuela (Fig. 6). It also crosses the eastern Cordillera of the Andes to enter Huila, Colombia, and extends as far south as Buenavista, Santa Cruz, and part of Chiquitos in Bolivia [31]. It may also occur in Paraguay, but it is defintely absent from the Atlantic forests of eastern Brazil.

Next to Aotus, Saimiri is the New World monkey genus most in need of revision. Although not as complex as Aotus, Saimiri is moderately variable in coat color and facial features, and several distinct taxa of either specific or subspecific status can be recognized within what is currently called Saimiri sciureus. Considering the importance of Saimiri in biomedical research, it is remarkable that no up-to-date revision has yet been carried out, in spite of warnings over a decade ago that: "without a workable taxonomy, we are hard put to organize, interpret and evaluate ..." the great body of literature that has accumulated on squirrel monkeys (Hershkovits, in[83], p.4). Lacking a modern revision, laboratory workers have had to refer to their animals by port of export (eg. S. sciureus Leticia; S. sciureus Iquitos) or by popular names based on the shape of the circumocular patch, ie. "Gothic arch" from Leticia, Colombia or "Roman arch" from Iquitos, Peru[84]. However, as pointed out by Hershkovitz (in[83], p.4):

"these characters are widely distributed individual variables. They are fully intergrading and both types may be present in the same troop. There may be a greater frequency of one over the other in some populations and either type

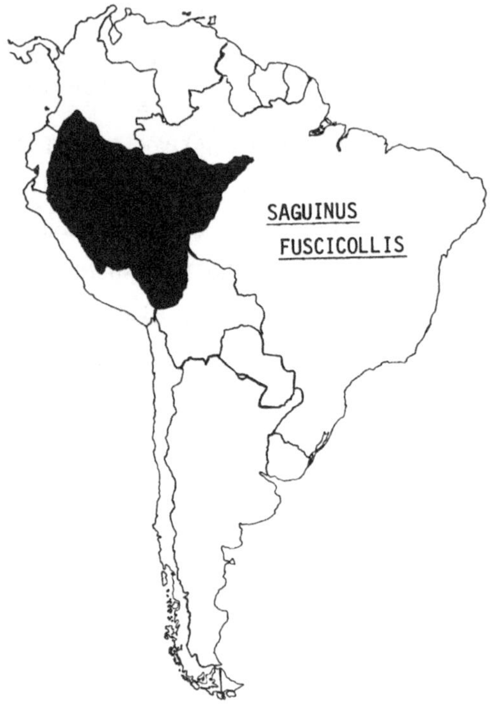

FIGURE 5

Distribution of
Saguinus fuscicollis

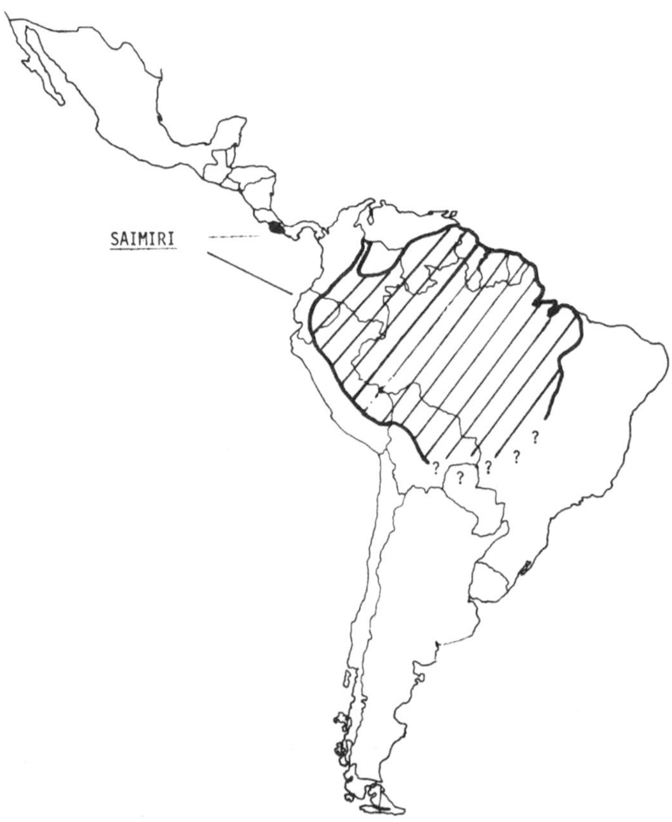

FIGURE 6

Distribution of
Saimiri sp.

may have a limited and qualified value of less than subspecific grade". Squirrel monkeys were also shipped from Georgetown, Guyana and, more recently, from Bolivia, and each of these countries has a different variety of squirrel monkey as well.

Thorington[52] believes that the most distinct Saimiri is found along the Rio Madeira in Brazil. He considers that there is no indication that this animal is intergrading with Bolivian Saimiri, and that there may be some evidence of sympatry with more typical S. sciureus along the Rio Amazonas.

The status of oerstedii from Central America remains uncertain, but most authors prefer to consider it nothing more than a subspecies. Thorington[52] sums up his opinion on the animal by stating that:

> "although oerstedii is unique in the genus, it does not differ from the Saimiri of Colombia by more than do the squirrel monkeys of Bolivia. Since there is a cline of intermediate forms between the Bolivian and Colombian Saimiri, demonstrating that they are conspecific, I argue by analogy that oerstedii should be considered a subspecies of Saimiri sciureus".

A study of Saimiri dentition by Orlosky[85] also supports subspecific status for oerstedii.

A revision of Saimiri is urgently needed, and Hershkovitz apparently also has plans for such a project. In 1968, he stated that "so far as my material permits me to judge there is but one species of Saimiri" (in[83], p.5). Data of karyotypic variation (eg.[86]) and the possibility of sympatry suggested by Thorington[52] may result in a reconsideration of this statement. However, even if only one species is finally recognized, clarification of Saimiri's subspecific variation and distribution would certainly be useful to biomedical researchers and conservationists alike.

Ecology and Conservation Status

Throughout most of Amazonia, Saimiri is the characteristic species of the densely overgrown river margins and the coastal swamp forests, and it is be far the most abundant species in these riverine habitats. Surprisingly, however, it is much rarer along the banks of the typical "black water" rivers (eg. the Rio Negro) than along the "white water" and "clear water" rivers such as the Rio Amazonas and the Rio Rapajos. Inland, it shows a strong preference for liane forest and secondary formations that are structurally similar to river edges, but it can be found at lower densities in many other forest types as well (eg.[1,37,87]). The preference for this kind of densely-vegetated habitat appears to be closely linked to Saimiri's diet, which includes high percentages of insects and other arthropods that abound in such formations. The other major component of Saimiri's diet is fruit, with flowers, buds, and an occasional small vertebrate playing a minor role[37,87].

Saimiri is almost exclusively an animal of the lowland forests, and rarely ranges higher than a few hundred meters in altitude[22,40]. Within its favored habitat, however, it is a very conspicuous animal, and is perhaps the most abundant monkey species in all of Amazonia. As with all other New World monkeys, it is threatened by widespread clear-cutting of forest, but it adapts well to the presence of man and is one of the few species that regularly can be seen in forests at the edge of villages and towns in Amazonia. Like the callitrichids, Saimiri makes use of and may even prefer the secondary formations resulting from slash-and-burn agriculture, which is still the most common form of agriculture in much of Amazonia. Since it is a small species (mean weight about 700 g[22,88]), it is far less persecuted as a food source than the larger monkeys (but more so than the callitrichids[22]). In the vicinity of villages, it may even benefit from the presence of man since he eliminates potential predators and larger primate competitors.

Saimiri is occasionally kept as a pet in Amazonia[1], but it is far less popular than Cebus or Lagothrix and total numbers involved are quite small. The international trade, however, was of major proportions, with Saimiri being by far the most important Neotropical species. Some 20,000-40,000 animals were exported annually during the 1960's just from Iquitos, Peru[64], and similar numbers went out from Leticia, Colombia. Several researchers[35,89] reported a decline of Saimiri populations in the immediate vicinity of Leticicia, Colombia, but the species still occurs in the Leticia and Iquitos regions, and is even abundant on Isla Iquitos, a large island right across from Iquitos itself[56].

It is difficult to assess the long-term effect of the Saimiri trade because appropriate demographic data were never collected. It does appear that upper Amazonian Saimiri populations were remarkably resistant even to the kind of heavy trapping pressure to which they were exposed during the peak years of the trade. Nonetheless, without adequate demographic data, it is impossible to determine how long such resistance and flexibility could have been maintained. If uncontrolled, large-scale exploitation such as once existed in Peru and Colombia were to continue over the long term, without any kind of ecological monitoring, it could possibly result in the serious decline and perhaps even the commercial extinction of this very important resource.

At the present time, the main source of supply for Saimiri is Bolivia, with between 600 and 3,300 exported annually to the US between 1976 and 1979 (D. Mack, pers. comm.). Figures are not available for exports to other countries. During the same period, the Peruvian Primate Project exported a total of 1,000 Saimiri to the US.

In contrast to Amazonian Saimiri, which cannot be considered threatened at the present time, the Central American squirrel monkey is already an endangered species. It has disappeared from much of its range in western Panama and Costa Rica because of widespread clear-cutting of forest. Fortunately, a good population appears to be under effective protection in the 36,00 ha Corcovado National Park on the Osa Peninsula in Costa Rica, but any commercial utilization of this taxon is clearly out of the question.

THE COMMON MARMOSET (*Callithrix jacchus*)

Taxonomy and Distribution

The genus *Callithrix* includes some dozen distinct taxa that are divided into three species by Hershkovitz[66] and seven by Coimbra-Filho and Mittermeier[32,90]. The disagreement involves the status of the eastern Brazilian *Callithrix* (*jacchus*, *penicillata*, *geoffroyi*, *flaviceps*, *aurita*), which Hershkovitz considers to be nothing more than subspecies of *C. jacchus*, but which Coimbra-Filho and Mittermeier maintain are distinct species. Recent investigations by Coimbra-Filho *et al*[41] also indicate that a sixth taxon, *Callithrix kuhlii* from southern Bahia, Brazil, is probably also a distinct species, although Hershkovitz[66] considers this animal only a hybrid population of *C. geoffroyi* and *C. penicillata*. A more detailed discussion of the eastern Brazilian *Callithrix* controversy is given in Mittermeier and Coimbra-Filho[32], and need not concern us further here.

In any case, the taxon *jacchus*, known as the common marmoset or the white-tufted-ear marmoset, is the best known member of the genus and the only *Callithrix* of importance in biomedical research. The natural range of *C. jacchus* is in northeastern Brazil and includes the scrub forests of the *caatinga* thorn bush formations in the states of Piauí and Ceará, and the Atlantic coastal forests of Paraiba, Pernambuco, Alagoas and Sergipe, south to the Bahia de Todos os Santos in eastern Bahia. Hershkovitz[66] also cites a record from western Bahia on the west bank of the Rio São Francisco, and two uncertain records from the eastern part of the state of Maranhão (Fig. 7).

Coimbra-Filho (in[90]; see also[91,92]) believes that the populations south of the Rio São Francisco and especially those in the Reconcavo da Bahia near Salvador, are the result of introduction by man (perhaps in aboriginal times), although Hershkovitz gives them as part of the natural range of the species. The origin of these particular Bahian populations is uncertain, but it is clear that *C. jacchus* has been introduced into a number of other areas south of its natural range. The best known populations are those in the city of Rio de Janeiro, where the species has been established since at least the turn of the century. It is especially abundant in the 2,700 ha Tijuca National Park in Rio, but can also be found in many other forest patches in the city.

In addition to the populations in Rio, *C. jacchus* apparently also occurs in forests in the city of Vitória, capital of the state of Espírito Santo, and is said to exist in Buenos Aires, Argentina, and in some parts of Paraguay, although the latter reports need to be confirmed.

Many of the new populations probably result from the release or escape of pets, since *C. jacchus* is commonly kept as a pet in eastern Brazil. However, at least part of the Rio population comes from a large-scale introduction around the turn of the century, carried out by a governor of Rio who released a variety of animals from his native northeast (H. Strang, pers. comm.).

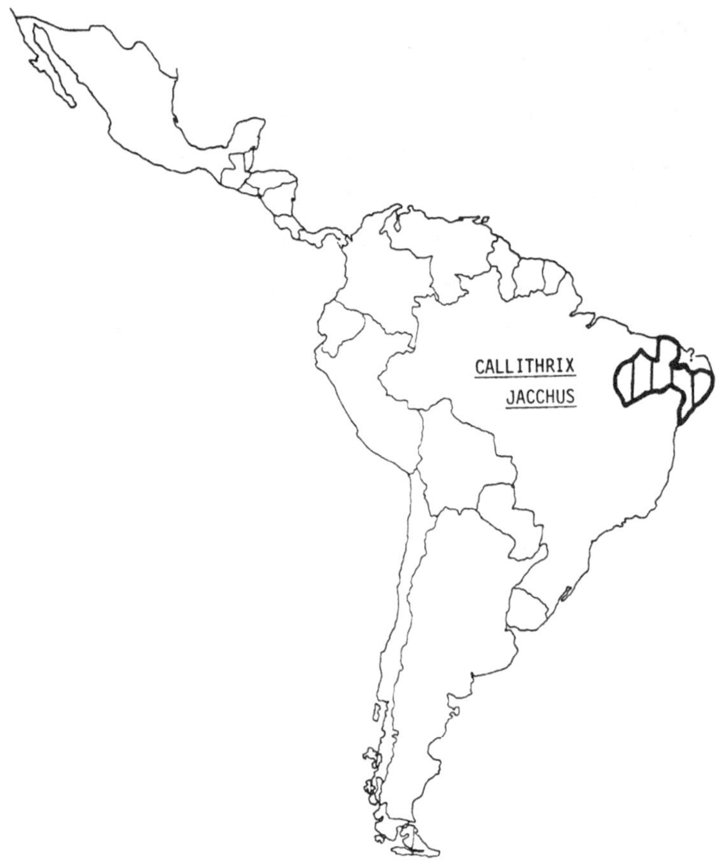

FIGURE 7. Distribution of Callithrix jacchus.

Ecology and Conservation Status

C. jacchus is a highly adaptable species and one of the few eastern Brazilian primate taxa not currently recognized as either endangered or vulnerable by the IUCN. Part of its success can probably be attributed to a dietary and dental specialization for exudate-eating[93]. All *Callithrix* species (and the pygmy marmoset, *Cebuella pygmaea*) have an unusual lower canine/incisor relationship which enables them to gouge holes into certain tree species and elicit the flow of gums, saps and other tree exudates. These substances are rich in carbohydrates and minerals and make up a major part of the marmoset diet, allowing the animal to live in areas where fruits, the usual source of carbohydrates for primates, may be in short supply. *C. jacchus* apparently depends heavily on exudates as a food source (Fig. 8), perhaps more so than the other eastern Brazilian *Callithrix*. This may have enabled it to adapt to the scrub forest environment of the *caatinga*, where few, if any, other primates are found, in addition to the richer Atlantic forests of the northeast. Consequently, when released into more southerly stretches of the Atlantic forest, it finds little difficulty in adapting.

Nonetheless, it is important to note that in spite of the common marmoset's success in adapting to new habitats, it may already be threatened in parts of its original range. Most of the habitat in the Atlantic forest portion of its range has already disappeared[94], and the destruction continues. Remaining populations of *C. jacchus* in this area are becoming more and more fragmented, increasing the danger of local extinctions, and the total population is certainly only a fraction of what it was in aboriginal times.

In addition, there is the threat posed by trade, this time mainly an internal trade. The legal international trade is no longer a factor, since it has been prohibited since the passage of the 1967 Brazilian Fauna Protection Law. However, there is still an illegal international trade and, more important, a large-scale local pet trade. Northeastern Brazil has a strong tradition of capturing monkeys, birds and other animals as pets, and *C. jacchus* has always been a favourite there and now also further to the south. Indeed, this monkey and the closely-related *Callithrix penicillata* from central Brazil are still sold openly, especially on the outskirts of Rio de Janeiro, in spite of the fact that this kind of internal trade was also prohibited by the 1967 Law. Such wasteful exploitation of this important wildlife resource should be ended as soon as possible.

The trade creates an additional problem, ie. what to do with confiscated marmosets. From time to time, large shipments of *C. jacchus* are confiscated by Brazilian authorities, and there is no established procedure for dealing with animals obtained in this manner. Many die while a decision is being made, and those remaining are sometimes released into the nearest available patch of forest. In one case in 1980, more than 100 animals were released in the municipality of

Silva Jardim in the state of Rio, quite close to the only existing reserve for the highly endangered golden lion tamarin (Leontopithecus r. rosalia).

Given the importance of C. jacchus and the fact that it may well turn out to be an important laboratory primate of the future, a special effort should be made to maintain the genetic variability of the species at several levels. One way to do this is to ensure that representative populations survive in protected areas within the natural range; another is to establish separate captive colonies using individuals from different parts of the natural range. Several parks and reserves in the northeast (eg. Ubajara National Park in Ceará) are already protecting some natural populations, but more protection is strongly recommended, even if it is necessary to set up small sanctuaries just for marmoset conservation. Captive colonies have already been initiated at the Rio de Janeiro Primate and several other Brazilian institutions.

DISCUSSION

From the material presented in this chapter, most of the New World monkey species currently of greatest importance to biomedical research are still among the least threatened. However, several taxa, notably the cotton-top tamarin and the northern Colombian night monkeys, are endangered, and may well become extinct before the turn of the century if present trends continue.

Recognizing the plight of endangered, vulnerable and rare primate species the world over, the IUCN Species Survival Commission (SCC), through its Primate Specialist Group, has recently formulated a policy statement on use of primates in biomedical research. Included in this statement is the following recommendation:

"A total of 54 primate taxa are currently considered endangered, vulnerable or rare by the IUCN. Since these taxa are either in serious decline or already at very low and precarious population levels, any exploitation of them threatens their continued survival. The IUCN therefore strongly recommends that:

1. endangered, vulnerable, and rare species not be considered for use in future biomedical research projects and that they be phased out of projects that are not already self-sustaining (ie. breeding all animals required in captivity, at least to the F_2 generation); and that
2. species categorized as status unknown or indeterminate also not be considered for use in such research projects until adequate data indicate that they are not endangered, vulnerable or rare."

This seems to be the wisest course of action, not only from the viewpoint of the conservationist or the protectionist, but also for the biomedical researcher. Indeed, there is little sense in investing time, effort or money in an endangered research model that simply will not be available in the very near future - even if small numbers of animals could be obtained for immediate use through special arrangements with the source countries.

For the convenience of readers interested in New World monkey conservation, Table 1 briefly reviews the status of all endangered, vulnerable, rare and indeterminate Neotropical primate taxa. This list is based mainly on the latest edition of the IUCN Red Data Book, Vol. I. Mammalia (1981), but also incorporates some information not yet included in the Red Data Book (eg.[41]).

Although the majority of New World monkeys of importance to biomedical research are in no immediate danger of extinction, there is certainly no cause for complacency. Trends all over the Neotropical region indicate that the tropical forest habitat of these arboreal animals will continue to be eroded year after year as the human population expands and as internationally-sponsored development programs work their way into the most remote corners of the continent. All primate populations, even of the most abundant species, will inevitably be affected by the changes now taking place in South and Central America, and everyone interested in ensuring the survival of these valuable animals must take an active role now in international conservation efforts on their behalf.

A Global Strategy for Primate Conservation, first developed by the IUCN/SSC Primate Specialist Group in 1978 and currently being updated, is designed to generate conservation action on behalf of primates wherever they occur. The Global Strategy includes some 45 projects in the Neotropical region, 12 of which are considered highest priority. Several of these are already under way, and a number of others will be initiated in the near future. They hopefully will provide the data bases needed for the establishment of new parks and reserves and for improved protection of existing areas. In addition, they should provide much behavioral and ecological information required for endangered species breeding programs such as the ones now in progress at the Rio de Janeiro Primate Center in Brazil.

While these efforts on behalf of endangered and vulnerable taxa continue, attempts are also under way to develop rational utilization programs for some of the more abundant species, the most obvious example to date being the PAHO-sponsored Peruvian Primate Project. This project, initiated in 1975 after the declaration of the Peruvian and Colombian export bans, is attempting to combine local captive breeding efforts, free-ranging island colonies, and cropping of wild populations in an attempt to develop a well-rounded program that will ensure a future supply of several biomedically-important species (mainly Saguinus m. mystax, Saguinus fuscicollis sspp., Saimiri sciureus and Aotus).

Although this project has a great deal of potential, it is still a long way from achieving its goals. Captive breeding has been small scale, and the breeding program for the most important species, Saguinus m. mystax, has thus far been almost totally unsuccessful. Most of the animals exported to date have been wild caught, and it is clear that utilization of wild populations is the most important aspect of the project. Considerable field work has already been conducted (eg.[56,72,75,76,80,96-98]), and this is certainly commendable. However, most of the field work to date has consisted of short-term surveys and experimentation with different trapping methods and, with few exceptions (eg.[95,99]), there has been little emphasis on long-term field studies. Indeed, as of 1980, long-term ecological studies of three of the four most important species in the program (Saguinus m. mystax, Saimiri sciureus, Aotus) had still not been initiated, and a study of the fourth (Saguinus fuscicollis) had only just began[93].

Surveys and censuses are, of course, essential, but it is equally important that programs of this kind include long-term field studies of the most important species. These investigations provide the demographic data base required for the development of sustained-yield trapping programs and special management areas, and also supply behavioral and dietary data that may hold the key to improving captive breeding programs.

It is also important that programs like this include some assistance to local governments in their efforts to establish and protect national parks, nature reserves, and wildlife sanctuaries, and that the programs do not concentrate only on the handfull of species of immediate interest. Species not currently considered important may be of great significance in the future, and it is essential that any program dealing with these animals incorporates measures to prevent further loss of genetic diversity in the Order Primates.

Finally, it is important not to make generalizations on the basis of results from one program or from a single species. The Peruvian Primate Program, for instance, is operating in an area with low human population density and relatively little habitat destruction. It also deals with abundant, highly adaptable species (eg. Saimiri, Saguinus fuscicollis) that survive well in many different forest types, including secondary forest, and have rapid breeding rates. Results from this project would have little applicability to ecologically-devastated areas like Colombia or southeastern Brazil, and information on Saguinus and Saimiri in Peruvian Amazonia would have minimal relevance when applied to Old World primates, to larger New World monkeys (eg. Ateles, Lagothrix), or even to other members of the same genera in parts of South America where habitat destruction is more of a problem.

In summary, we believe that:

1. primate utilization programs must be based on sound ecological data from long-term ecological studies and periodic surveys and censuses of key areas; that
2. such programs must be tailored specifically to local conditions and conservation problems and to the unique behavioral and ecological characteristics of the biomedically-important species in each region; and that
3. these programs should take an active role in the conservation of species not necessarily of immediate use to biomedical research, in recognition of the fact that maintenance of the total genetic diversity of the Order Primates is in the best interests of all concerned.

Table 1. New World monkeys considered endangered, vulnerable, rare or indeterminate by the IUCN. Columns 3 and 4 also provide information on specific national protection legislation (eg. endangered species lists) and status on CITES Appendices.

Species listed in the IUCN Red Data Book (Species recommended for listing)*	Red Data Book status (Recommended status)	CITES Appendix (I or II)***	Specific national protective legislation****
Callithrix argentata leucippe	Vulnerable	II	None
Callithrix humeralifer humeralifer Callithrix humeralifer chrysoleuca Callithrix humeralifer intermedius	Vulnerable	II	None
Callithrix aurita	Endangered	I	None
Callithrix flaviceps	Endangered	I	Brazilian Endangered Species List
(Callithrix geoffroyi)*	(Endangered)	II	None
Saguinus imperator imperator Saguinus imperator subgrisescens	Indeterminate	II	Peruvian Vulnerable Species List
Saguinus bicolor bicolor Saguinus bicolor martinsi Saguinus bicolor ochraceus	Endangered Indeterminate Indeterminate	I	US Endangered Species List
Saguinus oedipus	Endangered	I	Colombian Endangered Species List US Endangered Species List
(Saguinus geoffroyi)**	(Not yet listed in Red Data Book or recommended for inclusion)	I	None
Saguinus leucopus	Vulnerable	I	US Endangered Species List (Threatened Species)

Table 1 - continued

Leontopithecus rosalia	Endangered	I	Brazilian Endangered Species List US Endangered Species List
Leontopithecus chrysomelas	Endangered	I	Brazilian Endangered Species List US Endangered Species List
Leontopithecus chrysopygus	Endangered	I	Brazilian Endangered Species List US Endangered Species List
Callimico goeldii	Rare	I	Peruvian Rare Species List Brazilian Endangered Species List US Endangered Species List
(Aotus - northern Colombian and Panamanian species/subspecies)*	(Endangered)	II	None
Callicebus personatus personatus Callicebus personatus melanochir Callicebus personatus nigrifons	Vulnerable	II	None
(Pithecia albicans)*	(Vulnerable)	II	None
Chiropotes albinasus	Vulnerable	I	Brazilian Endangered Species List US Endangered Species List
Chiropotes satanas satanas	Endangered	II	None
Cacajao calvus calvus	Vulnerable (Endangered)	I	Brazilian Endangered Species List US Endangered Species List
Cacajao calvus rubicundus	Vulnerable	I	Brazilian Endangered Species List Peruvian Endangered Species List US Endangered Species List
Cacajao melanocephalus	Vulnerable	I	Brazilian Endangered Species List US Endangered Species List
Alouatta villosa (= pigra)	Indeterminate	II	US Endangered Species List (Threatened Species)

Table 1 - continued

(Alouatta palliata)**	(Not yet listed in Red Data Book or recommended for inclusion)	I	Peruvian Endangered Species List US Endangered Species List
Alouatta fusca	Indeterminate (Endangered)	II	Brazilian Endangered Species List
Ateles geoffroyi geoffroyi	Vulnerable	II	None
Ateles geoffroyi azuereusis		II	None
Ateles geoffroyi frontatus		I	US Endangered Species List
Ateles geoffroyi grisescens		II	None
Ateles geoffroyi orantus		II	None
Ateles geoffroyi pan		II	None
Ateles geoffroyi panamensis		I	US Endangered Species List
Ateles geoffroyi vellerosus		II	None
Ateles geoffroyi yucatensis		II	None
Ateles belzebuth belzebuth	Vulnerable	II	Peruvian Vulnerable Species List
Ateles belzebuth hybridus		II	None
Ateles belzebuth marginatus		II	None
Ateles fusciceps fusciceps	Vulnerable	II	None
Ateles fusciceps rufiventris (= robustus)		II	None
Ateles paniscus paniscus	Vulnerable	II	None
Ateles paniscus chamek		II	Peruvian Vulnerable Species List
Lagothrix lagotricha lagotricha	Vulnerable	II	Peruvian Vulnerable Species List
Lagothrix lagotricha cana			Peruvian Vulnerable Species List
Lagothrix lagotricha lugens			None
Lagothrix lagotricha poeppigii			Peruvian Vulnerable Species List
Lagotrhix flavicauda	Endangered	II	Peruvian Endangered Species List US Endangered Species List

Table 1 - continued

Brachyteles arachnoides	Endangered	I	Brazilian Endangered Species List US Endangered Species List

* Species in parentheses are not yet listed in the *Red Data Book*, but have been recommended for inclusion by the IUCN/SSC Primate Specialist Group. The source for the *Red Data Book* listings is *Red Date Book, Vol. I. Mammalia, Part I, Nearctic, Neotropical and Australasian Regions*, 1981, in prep.

** *Saguinus geoffroyi* and *Alouatta palliata* have not yet been listed or recommended for inclusion in the *Red Data Book*, but have been placed on this list because both are on Appendix I of CITES.

*** All primate species are listed on either Appendix I or Appendix II of the Convention on International Trade in Endangered Species (CITES).

**** In several countries (eg. Brazil, Colombia, Peru), all primates are officially protected under general wildlife laws. However, in column 4 we have noted only cases in which species receive additional protection through placement on national endangered species lists.

REFERENCES

1. Mittermeier, R. A. and Coimbra-Filho, A. F. (1977). Primate conservation in Brazilian Amazonia. In: Prince Rainier of Monaco and G. Bourne (eds.) Primate Conservation, pp. 117-166 (New York: Academic Press)
2. Freese, C. (1975). A census of non-human primates in Peru. In: Primate Censusing Studies in Peru and Colombia, pp. 17-42 (Washington, D. C.: Pan American Health Organization
3. Struhsaker, T. T., Glander, K., Chirivî, H. and Scott, N. J. (1975). A survey of primates and their habitats in northern Colombia. In: Primate Censusing Studies in Peru and Colombia, pp. 43-78 (Washington, D. C.: Pan American Health Organization)
4. Neville, M. (1975). Census of primates in Peru. In: Primate Censusing Studies in Peru and Colombia, pp. 3-15 (Washington, D. C.: Pan American Health Organization)
5. Heltne, P. G., Freese, C. and Whitesides, G. (1975). A field survey of nonhuman primate populations in Bolivia. Pan American Health Organization.
6. Muckenhirn, N. B., Mortensen, K, Vessey, S., Fraser, C. E. O. and Singh, B. (1975). Report on a primate survey in Guyana. Pan American Health Organization.
7. Castro, N., Revilla, J. and Neville, M. (1975/76). Carne de monte como una fuente de proteînas en Iquitos con referencia especial a monos. Rev. Forestal Peru, 6 (1-2), 19-32
8. Neville, M., Castro, N. and Revilla, J. (1976). Censusing primate populations in the reserved area of the Pacaya and Samiria Rivers, Dept. Loreto, Peru. Primates, 17 (2), 151-181
9. Bernstein, I. S., Balcaen, P., Dresdale, L., Gouzoules, H., Kavanagh, M., Patterson, T. and Neyman-Warner, P. (1976). Differential effects of forest degradation on primate populations. Primates, 17 (3), 401-411
10. Rathbun, G. B. and Gache, M. J. (1977). The status of Aotus trivirgatus in Argentina. Unpublished report, National Institutes of Health
11. Freese, C., Freese, M. A. and Castro, N. (1978). The status of callitrichids in Peru. In D. Kleiman (ed.), The Biology and Conservation of the Callitrichidae, pp. 121-130 (Washington, D. C.: Smithsonian Institution)
12. Rathbun, G. and Gache, M. J. (1980). Ecological survey of the night monkey, Aotus trivirgatus, in Formosa Province, Argentina. Primates, 21 (2), 211-219
13. Bailey, R. C., Brown, D. S., von Hildebrand, P., Mittermeier, R. A., Sponsel, L. E., and Wolf, K. E. (1974). Progress of a breeding project for non-human primates in Colombia. Nature, 248, 453-455
14. Sponsel, L. E., Brown, D. S., Bailey, R. C. and Mittermeier, R. A. (1974). Evaluation of squirrel monkey, Saimiri sciureus, ranching on Santa Sofia Island, Amazonas, Colombia. In: International Zoo Yearbook, 14, 233-240

15. Mittermeier, R.A., Macedo-Ruiz, H. de and Luscombe, B.A. (1975) A woolly monkey rediscovered in Peru. Oryx, 13 (1), 41-46
16. Green, K. (1976) The nonhuman primate trade in Colombia. In: R.W. Thorington, Jr. and P.G. Heltne (eds) Neotropical Primates: Field Studies and Conservation, pp.85-98. (Washington, DC: National Academy of Sciences)
17. Freese, C.H. (1976) Censusing Alouatta palliata, Ateles geoffroyi and Cebus capucinus in the Costa Rican dry forest. In: R.W. Thorington, Jr. and P.G. Heltne (eds) Neotropical Primates: Field Studies and Conservation, pp.4-9. (Washington, DC: National Academy of Sciences)
18. Baldwin, J.D. and Baldwin, J.I. (1976) Primate populations in Chiriqui, Panama. In: R.W. Thorington, Jr. and P.G. Heltne (eds) Neotropical Primates: Field Studies and Conservation, pp.20-31. (Washington, DC: National Academy of Sciences)
19. Mittermeier, R.A., Bailey, R.C., Sponsel, L.E. and Wolf, K.E. (1977) Primate ranching - results of an experiment. Oryx, 13 (5), 449-453
20. Mittermeier, R.A., Macedo-Ruiz, H. de, Luscombe, B.A. and Cassidy, J. (1977) Rediscovery and conservation of the Peruvian yellow-tailed woolly monkey. In: Prince Rainier of Monaco and G. Bourne (eds) Primate Conservation, pp.95-115. (New York: Academic Press)
21. Mittermeier, R.A., Coimbra-Filho, A.F. and van Roosmalen, M.G.M. (1978) Callitrichids in Brazil and the Guianas. Prim. Med., 10, 20-29
22. Mittermeier, R.A. (1977) Distribution, synecology and conservation of Surinam monkeys. Unpublished doctoral dissertation, Harvard University
23. Coimbra-Filho, A.F. and Mittermeier, R.A. (1977) Conservation of the Brazilian lion tamarins (Leontopithecus rosalia). In: Prince Rainier of Monaco and G. Bourne (eds) Primate Conservation, pp.59-94. (New York: Academic Press)
24. Mittermeier, R.A., Bailey, R.C. and Coimbra-Filho, A.F. (1978) Conservation status of the Callitrichidae in Brazilian Amazonia, Surinam and French Guiana. In: D.G. Kleiman (ed) The Biology and Conservation of the Callitrichidae, pp.137-146. (Washington, DC: Smithsonian Institution)
25. Mittermeier, R.A., van Roosmalen, M.G.M. and Coimbra-Filho, A.F. (1978) Conservation status of wild callitrichids. In: H. Rothe, H.J. Wolters and J.P. Hearn (eds) Biology and Behavior of Marmosets, pp.17-39. (Göttingen: Eigenverlag Hartmut Rothe).
26. Neyman, P.F. (1978) Aspects of the ecology and social organization of free-ranging cotton-top tamarins (Saguinus oedipus) and the conservation status of the species. In: D.G. Kleiman (ed) The Biology and Conservation of the Callitrichidae, pp.39-71. (Washington, DC: Smithsonian Institution)
27. Cabrera, A. (1958) Catálogo de los mamíferos de America del Sur. Rev. Mus. Argentino Cienc. Nat. "Bernardino Rivadavia", 4 (1), 307 pp.

28. Hershkovitz, P. (1949). Mammals of northern Colombia. Preliminary report no. 4: Monkeys (Primates), with taxonomic revisions of some forms. Proc. U. S. Nat. Mus., 98, 323-427

29. Hershkovitz, P. (1972). Notes on New World monkeys. International Zoo Yearbook, 12, 3-12

30. Napier, J. R. and Napier, P. H. (1967). A Handbook of Living Primates. (New York: Academic Press)

31. Napier, P. H. (1976). Catalogue of Primates in the British Museum (Natural History). Part I: Families Callitrichidae and Cebidae. (London: British Museum (Natural History)

32. Mittermeier, R. A. and Coimbra-Filho, A. F. (1981). Systematics: species and subspecies. In: A. F. Coimbra-Filho and R. A. Mittermeier (eds.) Ecology and Behavior of Neotropical Primates, Vol. 1, pp. 29-109. (Rio de Janeiro: Brazilian Academy of Sciences)

33. Kinzey, W. (1981). Distribution of some Neotropical primates and the model of Pleistocene forest refugia. In: G. T. Prance (ed.) The Biological Model of Diversification in the Tropics. (New York: Columbia University Press, in press)

34. Freese, C. and Oppenheimer, J. R. (1981). The capuchin monkeys, genus Cebus. In: A. F. Coimbra-Filho and R. A. Mittermeier (eds.) Ecology and Behavior of Neotropical Primates, Vol. I. (Rio de Janeiro: Brazilian Academy of Sciences)

35. Hernandez-Camacho, J. and Cooper, R. W. (1976). The nonhuman primates of Colombia. In: R. W. Thorington, Jr. and P. G. Heltne (eds.) Neotropical Primates: Field Studies and Conservation, pp. 35-69. (Washington, D. C.: National Academy of Sciences)

36. Hill, W. C. O. (1960). Primates. Comparative Anatomy and Taxonomy. IV. Cebidae, Part A. (New York: Wiley Interscience)

37. Mittermeier, R. A. and van Roosmalen, M. G. M. (1981). Preliminary observations on habitat utilization and diet in eight Surinam monkeys. Folia primat., in press.

38. Grimwood, I. (1969). Notes on the distribution and status of some Peruvian mammals, 1968. Special publ., no. 21, American Committee for International Wild Life Protection and New York Zoological Society.

39. Klein, L. L. and Klein, D. J. (1976). Neotropical primates: aspects of habitat usage, population density, and regional distribution in La Macarena, Colombia. In: R. W. Thorington, Jr. and P. G. Heltne (eds.) Neotropical Primates: Field Studies and Conservation, pp. 70-78. (Washington, D. C.: National Academy of Sciences)

40. Moynihan, M. H. (1976). The New World Primates. (Princeton, N. J.: Princeton Univ. Press).

41. Mittermeier, R. A., Coimbra-Filho, and Constable, I. (1981). Conservation

of eastern Brazilian primates. Unpublished report to the World Wildlife Fund.

42. Castro, N. (1978) Diagnóstico de la situación actual de los primates no humanos en el Peru y un plan nacional para su utilización racional. Ministerio de Agricultura y Alimentación, Dirección General Forestal y de Fauna, Dirección de Conservación, Lima, Peru

43. Cabrera, A. (1958) Catálogo de los mammiferos de America del Sur. Rev.Mus. Argentino Cienc. Nat. "Bernardino Rivadavia", 4 (1), 307 pp.

44. Thorington, R.W., Jr. and Vorek, R.E. (1976) Observations on the geographic variation and skeletal development of Aotus. Lab.Anim.Sci., 26(6), 1006-1021

45. DeBoer, L.E.M. (1971) A case of abnormal chromosome number in a female Aotus trivirgatus (Humboldt, 1811 - Cebidae, Primates). Genen.Phaenen., 14, 51-55

46. DeBoer, L.E.M. (1971) Chromosome studies in primates from zoological gardens in the Netherlands. Genen. Phaenen., 15 (2-3), 41-106

47. DeBoer, L.E.M. (1974) Cytotaxonomy of the Platyrrhini (Primates). Genen. Phaenen., 17, 1-115

48. Brumback, R.A. (1973) Two distinctive types of owl monkeys (Aotus). J. Med. Primatol., 2, 284-289

49. Brumback, R.A. (1974) A third species of the owl monkey (Aotus). J. Hered., 65, 321-323.

50. Brumback, R.A. and Willenborg, D.O. (1973) Serotaxonomy of Aotus: A preliminary study. Folia Primatol., 20, 106-111

51. Ma, N.S.F., Rossan, R.N., Kelley, S.T., Harper, J.S., Bedard, M.T. and Jones, T.C. (1978) Banding patterns of the chromosomes of two new karyotypes of the owl monkey, Aotus, captured in Panama. J. Med. Primatol., 7, 146-155

52. Thorington, R.W. Jr. (1976) The systematics of New World monkeys. First Inter-American Conference on Conservation and Utilization of American Nonhuman Primates in Biomedical Research, pp.8-18. (Washington, DC: Pan American Health Organization)

53. Elliott, M.W., Sehgal, P.K. and Chalifoux, L.C. (1976) Management and breeding of Aotus trivirgatus. Lab. Anim. Sci., 26 (6), 1037-1040

54. Wright, P. (1978) Home range, activity pattern and agonistic encounters of a group of night monkeys (Aotus trivirgatus) in Peru. Folia Primat., 29, 43-55

55. Wright, P. (1981) The night monkeys, genus Aotus. In: A.F. Coimbra-Filho and R.A. Mittermeier (eds) Ecology and Behavior of Neotropical Primates, Vol. 1, pp.211-240. (Rio de Janeiro: Brazilian Academy of Sciences)

56. Soini, P. and Moya, L. (1976) Informe sobre los resultados de los estudios primatólogicos en la Zona Norte de la Isla de Iquitos. Unpublished report to the Pan American Health Organization.

57. Moynihan, M.H. (1964) Some behavior patterns of platyrrhine monkeys. I. The night monkey (Aotus trivirgatus). Smithson.Misc.Publ., 146, 1-84

58. Thorington, R. W., Jr., Muckenhirn, N. A. and Montgomery, G. G. (1976). Movements of a wild night monkey (Aotus trivirgatus). In: R. W. Thorington, Jr. and P. G. Heltne (eds) Neotropical Primates: Field Studies and Conservation, pp. 32-34. (Washington, D. C.: National Adacemy of Sciences)
59. Heltne, P. G. (1977). Census of Aotus in the north of Colombia, 4 August - 30 September 1977. Unpublished report to the Pan American Health Organization
60. Young, M. D., Porter, J. A. and Johnson, C. M. (1966). Plasmodium vivax transmitted from man to monkey to man. Science, 154, 1006-1007
61. Wilson, R. J. and Voller, A. (1970). Malarial S-antigens from man and owl monkey infected with Plasmodium falciparum. Parasitol., 61, 461-464
62. Cooper, R. W. and Hernandez-Camacho, J. (1975). A current appraisal of Colombia's primate resources. In: G. Bermant and D. Lindburg (eds.) Primate Utilization and Conservation, pp. 37-66. (New York: John Wiley and Sons)
63. Mondolfi, E. (1976). Fauna silvestre de los bosques húmedos de Venezuela. In: Conservación de los Bosques Húmedos de Venezuela, pp. 113-181. (Caracas: Sierra Club - Consejo de Bienestar Rural)
64. Soini, P. (1972). The capture and commerce of live monkeys in the Amazonian region of Peru. Int. Zoo Yb., 12, 26-36
65. Muckenhirn, N. A. (1976). Addendum to the nonhuman primate trade in Colombia. In: R. W. Thorington, Jr. and P. G. Heltne (eds.) Neotropical Primates: Field Studies and Conservation, pp. 99-100. (Washington, D. C.: National Academy of Sciences)
66. Hershkovitz, P. (1977). Living New World Monkeys (Platyrrhini). (Chicago: Univ. of Chicago Press)
67. Hershkovitz, P. (1979). Races of the emperor tamarin, Saguinus imperator Goeldi (Callitrichidae, Primates). Primates, 20 (2), 277-287
68. Neyman, P. (1977). El titi cabeza-blanca (Saguinus oedipus Linnaeus, 1758) de la Costa Caribe de Colombia. Unpublished report to INDERENA and the New York Zoological Society
69. Gengozian, N. and Porter, R. P. (1971). Transplantation immunology in the marmoset. Med. Primat. 1970, 165-176
70. Gengozian, N., Batson, J. S. and Smith, T. A. (1978). Breeding of marmosets in a colony environment. Prim. Med., 10, 71-78
71. Provost, P. J., Villarejos, V. M. and Hilleman, M. R. (1978). Tests in rufiventer and other marmosets of susceptibility to human hepatitis A virus. Prim. Med., 10, 288-294
72. Encarnación, F. and Castro, N. (1978). Informe preliminar sobre censo de primates no humanos en el sur-oriente peruano: Iberia e Iñapari (Departamento de Madre de Dios), May 15 - June 14, 1978. Unpublished report to the Pan American Health Organization

73. Dawson, G. A. (1975). The Delta Regional Primate Research Center's Saguinus mystax trapping project: a field report. Unpublished report to the National Institutes of Health

74. Heltne, P. G. and Thorington, R. W., Jr. (1976). Problems and potentials for primate biology and conservation in the New World. In: R. W. Thorington, Jr. and P. G. Heltne (eds.) Neotropical Primates: Field Studies and Conservation, pp. 110-124. (Washington, D. C.: National Academy of Sciences)

75. Castro, R. and Soini, P. (1978). Field studies on Saguinus mystax and other callitrichids in Amazonian Peru. In: D. G. Kleiman (ed.) The Biology and Conservation of the Callitrichidae, pp. 73-78. (Washington, D. C.: Smithsonian Institution)

76. Moya, L., Olivares, L. V., Peralta, G. B. and Inga, J. E. R. (1979) Análisis poblacional de Saguinus mystax (Spix, 1823) (Callitrichidae) en la cuenca del Río Yarapa, Loreto, Peru. Bol. Comite Regional de Coordinación Proyecto Primates, 2 (1), 44 pp.

77. Pook, A. G. and Pook, J. (1979). The conservation status of the Goeldi's monkey, Callimico goeldii, in Bolivia. Dodo, 16, 40-45

78. Pook, A. G. and Pook, J. (1981). A field study of the socio-ecology of the goeldi's monkey (Callimico goeldii) in northern Bolivia. Folia primat., in press

79. Heltne, P. G., Wojcik, J. and Pook, A. G. (1981). Goeldi's monkey, genus Callimico. In: A. F. Coimbra-Filho and R. A. Mittermeier (eds.) Ecology and Behavior of Neotropical Primates, Vol. I, pp. 169-209. (Rio de Janeiro: Brazilian Academy of Sciences)

80. Ogden, J. D., Wolfe, L. G. and Deinhardt, F. W. (1978). Breeding Saguinus and Callithrix species of marmosets under laboratory conditions. Prim. Med., 10, 79-83

81. Hampton, S. H., Gross, M. J. and Hampton, J. K., Jr. (1978). A comparison of captive breeding performance and offspring survival in the family Callitrichidae. Prim. Med., 10, 88-95

82. Wolfe, L. G. and Deinhardt, F. (1978). Overview of viral oncology studies in Saguinus and Callithrix species. Prim. Med., 10, 96-118

83. Cooper, R. W. (1968). Squirrel monkey taxonomy and supply. In: L. A. Rosenblum and R. W. Cooper (eds.) The Squirrel Monkey, pp. 1-29. (New York: Academic Press)

84. MacLean, P. D. (1964). Mirror display in the squirrel monkey, Saimiri sciureus. Science, 146, 950-952

85. Orlosky, F. (1973). Comparative dental morphology of extant and extinct Cebidae. Unpublished doctoral dissertation, Univ. of Washington.

86. Jones, T. C., Thorington, R. W., Jr., Hu, M. M., Adams, E. and Cooper, R. W. (1973). Amer. J. Phys. Anthrop., 38, 269-278

87. Baldwin, J. D. and Baldwin, J. I. (1981). The squirrel monkeys, genus Saimiri. In: A. F. Coimbra-Filho and R. A. Mittermeier (eds.) Ecology and Behavior of Neotropical Primates, Vol. I, pp. 277-330. (Rio de Janeiro: Brazilian Academy of Sciences)

88. Middleton, C. C. and Rosal, J. (1972). Weight and measurements of normal squirrel monkeys (Saimiri sciureus). Lab. Anim. Sci., 22, 583-586

89. Baldwin, J. D. and Baldwin, J. I. (1971). Squirrel monkeys (Saimiri) in natural habitats in Panama, Colombia, Brazil and Peru. Primates, 12, 45-61.

90. Coimbra-Filho, A. F. and Mittermeier, R. A. (1973). New data on the taxonomy of Brazilian marmosets of the genus Callithrix Erxleben, 1777. Folia primat., 20, 241-264

91. Vieira, C. C. (1955). Lista remissiva dos mamíferos do Brasil. Arq. Zool. Est. São Paulo, 13 (1), 341-474

92. Avila-Pires, F. D. de (1969). Taxonomía e zoogeografía do gênero "Callithrix" Erxleben, 1777 (Primates, Callithricidae). Rev. Brasil. Biol., 29 (1), 49-64

93. Coimbra-Filho, A. F. and Mittermeier, R. A. (1978). Tree-gouging, exudate-eating and the "short-tusked" condition in Callithrix and Cebuella. In: D. G. Kleiman (ed.) The Biology and Conservation of the Callitrichidae, pp. 105-115 (Washington, D. C.: Smithsonian Institution)

94. Sick, H. and Martins Texeira, D. (1979). Notas sobre aves brasileiras raras ou ameaçadas de extinção. Publ. Avul. Mus. Nac., Rio de Janeiro, 16

95. Soini, P. (1981). Informe de Pacaya no. 4: Ecologia y dinamica poblacional del pichico Saguinus fuscicollis (Primates, Callitrichidae). Unpublished report to the Peruvian Primate Project, Iquitos, Peru

96. Encarnación, F., Castro, N and De Rham, P. (1978). Observaciones de primates no humanos en el Río Yavineto (R. Putumayo), Loreto, Peru. Unpublished report to the Peruvian Primate Project

97. Soini, P. (1980). Informe sobre un estudio y cosecha experimental de Cebuella pygmaea (Primates: Callitrichidae). Bol. Comité Regional de Coordinación Proyecto Primates, 3 (1), 1-21

98. Soini, P. (1980). Hallazgo de una nueva subespécie de Saguinus fuscicollis (Callitrichidae) para el Peru. Bol. Comité Regional de Coordinación Proyecto Primates, 3 (1), 3 pp.

99. Soini, P. (1981). The pygmy marmoset, genus Cebuella. In: R. A. Mittermeier and A. F. Coimbra-Filho (eds.) Ecology and Behavior of Neotropical Primates, Vol. II, in press

Chapter 2

The Cebus Monkey *(Cebus apella)*

C. A. Nagle & J. H. Denari

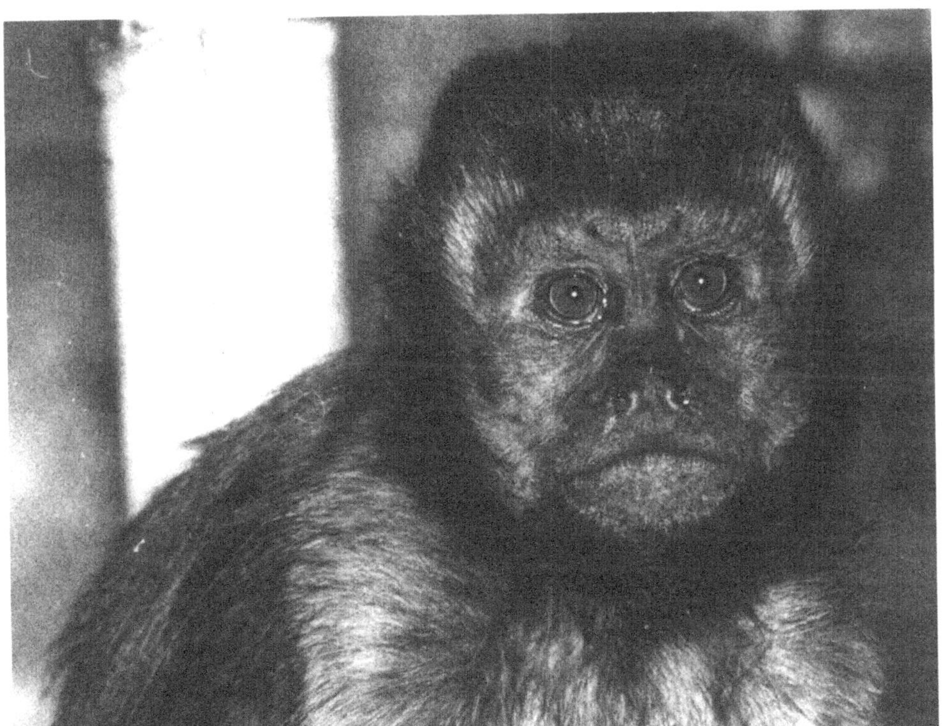

Cebus apella

THE CEBUS MONKEY (*Cebus apella*)

C.A. Nagle and J.H. Denari

Instituto Latinoamericano de Investigaciones Médicas
de la Universidad del Salvador (ILAIMUS ex ILAFIR)
Galván 4102 (1431), Buenos Aires, Argentina.

INTRODUCTION

The *Cebus* monkey, commonly called the Capuchin monkey, is widely distributed in Latin America. Its range extends from the southern part of Central America to the north east of Argentina.

On the basis of being either crested or uncrested, the main species of *Cebus* monkeys are grouped under Tufted (*C. apella*) and Untufted (*C. capucinus*, *C. albifrons*, *C. nigrivitatus*) capuchins[1,2].

The most common and widely distributed *Cebus* species in South America is *C. apella*. Although this species was considered distinct as a group[2], hybrids between it and *C. capucinus* or *C. albifrons* are reported[3]. All the capuchin species have the same chromosome number (2n = 54), with some similarity between their chromosome patterns and that of the Great apes and man[4].

Behavioral studies[5] have shown that there is little hierarchy in groups of capuchins and that the stability of the group depends on the relationship between all of the individuals in it.

The studies reported in this chapter were performed on *Cebus apella* cay. There is some uncertainty, however, as morphological indices suggest[2] that they may contain characteristics of *C. albifrons* and some animals may be *albifrons-apella* hybrids.

The *Cebus* monkeys included in this study had 54 chromosomes (52 autosomes and 2 sex chromosomes). The karyotype consisted of 32 acrocentrics, 20 submetacentrics and 2 metacentrics (Fig. 1).

The banded karyotype through the sequential staining for Q- band and C- band revealed striking similarities between the animals in spite of the differences in their external characteristics. Small variations between individuals were only observed after the sequential staining of chromosomes with Giemsa (G- band). In our controlled breeding program, hybrids could be obtained between phenotypically identified *C. albifrons* and *C. apella*.

MANAGEMENT OF LABORATORY COLONIES

A brief report of Hill[6] and other subsequent publications[7,8] concluded that the laboratory breeding and rearing of this intelligent and hardy primate species is

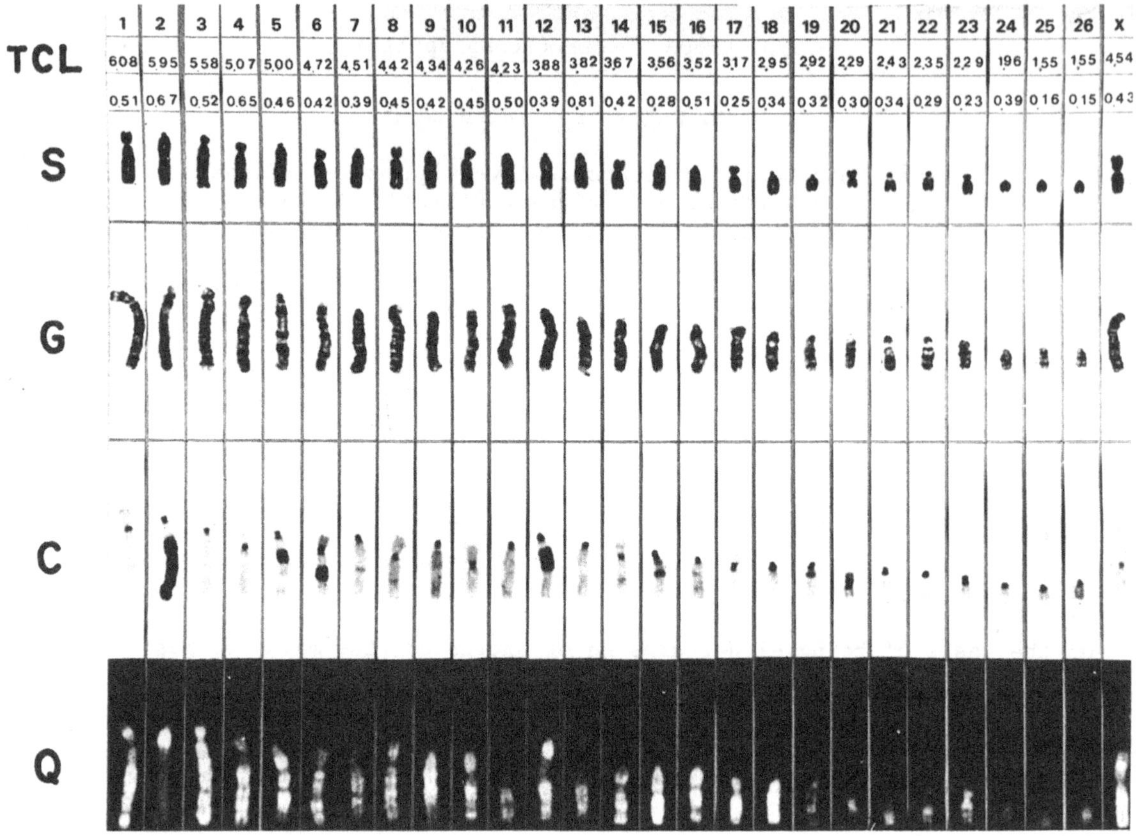

Figure 1. Standard (S) and banded (G, C, Q) karyotypes of the Cebus monkey. Chromosomes were displayed by size. Figures in the first row indicate chromosome order. Figures in the second and third rows indicate the size mean value and the standard error respectively. Size is expressed as the percentage of total complement length (TCL).

relatively simple. Our experience over the last four years largely confirms Hill's earlier experience.

In 1977 two hundred Cebus monkeys, trapped in Paraguay between the Parana and the Paraquay Rivers, were housed in a windowless, environmentally controlled animal house. The temperature is maintained between 22-24C^{o}, with a relative humidity of 50-70% and a lighting schedule of 14 h light and 10 h darkness.

There was a loss of 25% of the original imported stock, within 3 months of capture, due to the poor health of the animals when they arrived at the laboratory. Postmortem examinations of these animals showed a heavy parasitic load (Tapeworms sp, Filaria sp, Gongylonema sp, Trychostrongyle sp, Plasmodium sp, etc), which probably contributed to deaths when animals were in a debilitated state.

The Cebus monkeys were caged individually on arrival. A cage with dimensions 50 x 70 x 70 cm equipped with a restraining device, was found to be adequate for a single animal of this species. Animals were sedated with Ketamine hydrochloride (10-15 mg/kg) before handling. The animals were quarantined for a period of 90 days, during which period they were conditioned to captivity as follows:

a) General Clinical Care: monkeys were observed closely and given individual attention in any cases showing signs of illness. During the conditioning period

15% of the animals stopped eating and drinking and, if not observed frequently, could die of dehydration or starvation. Survival was helped by the administration of electrolytes with 5% dextrose solution and by hand feeding. Respiratory tract infections and gastrointestinal disorders (diarrhea) occurred frequently during the conditioning period but were overcome with the use of Penicillin 50,000 IU/kg/day, im, Chloramphenicol 30-50 mg/kg/day orally, and supportive treatment with electrolytes-5% dextrose, according to the degree of dehydration.

The food provided was a standard commercial diet with a protein content of 25% and supplemented with fresh fruit twice a week.

b) Tuberculosis control: 0.1 ml of Koch's old tuberculin was injected intradermally in the upper eyelid on arrival and again on being discharged from the quarantine room. Thereafter the animals were tested twice a year. Observations were made at 24, 48 and 72 hours after the test. The *Cebus* monkey is susceptible to tuberculosis but its incidence is extremely low[9]. No cases were found in the colony established here.

c) Antihelmintic treatment: was given immediately after arrival. Thiabendazole is effective against *Nematodes* when administered orally at doses of 70-100 mg/kg body weight. Niclosamide, 150 mg/kg body weight, or Praziquantel, 5 mg/kg body weight are effective against *Cestodes*. Two treatments with a 3-week interval were found to be sufficient.

d) A skin tattoo: was performed for permanent identification and maintenance of accurate records once quarantine was completed.

RESEARCH TECHNIQUES

Cebus monkeys have numerous advantages as laboratory primates. Their relatively large size, in comparison with other New World laboratory primates, make the repeated withdrawal of large quantities of blood feasible, facilitate experimental surgery and permit serial laparoscopy. Furthermore, the female *Cebus* monkey has a regular menstrual cycle.

Blood sampling. In the *Cebus* monkey the blood volume, determined through the Cr^{51} technique, is of 78.6 ± 10.4 ml/kg of body weight, whereas the packed cells volume is of 43.2 ± 4.0%. In an adult *Cebus* monkey up to 1.5 ml of blood can be withdrawn daily, with no effects on these parameters. The femoral veins and arteries, or alternatively the saphenous veins, are the best sites for bleeding. However, the *Cebus* monkey has a nervous and excitable disposition and this makes it difficult to train them to present limbs for bleeding.

Detection of menstruation. The detection of menses is performed by using vaginal swabs as with macaques. Menses are usualy detectable with swabs alone. However, the menstrual flow is not nearly as intense as it is in the rhesus and analysis of vaginal smears is recommended. The female *Cebus* can be trained to present her external genitalia to allow swabbing but the process is tedious and not all the animals will comply.

Endometrial biopsy. Transcervical endometrial biopsies that are used for serially sampling human endometrium, may also be performed on the Cebus monkey. As in the Great apes and parous baboons the female Cebus has a straight cervical canal offering an easy and direct access to the uterine cavity (Fig. 2). With

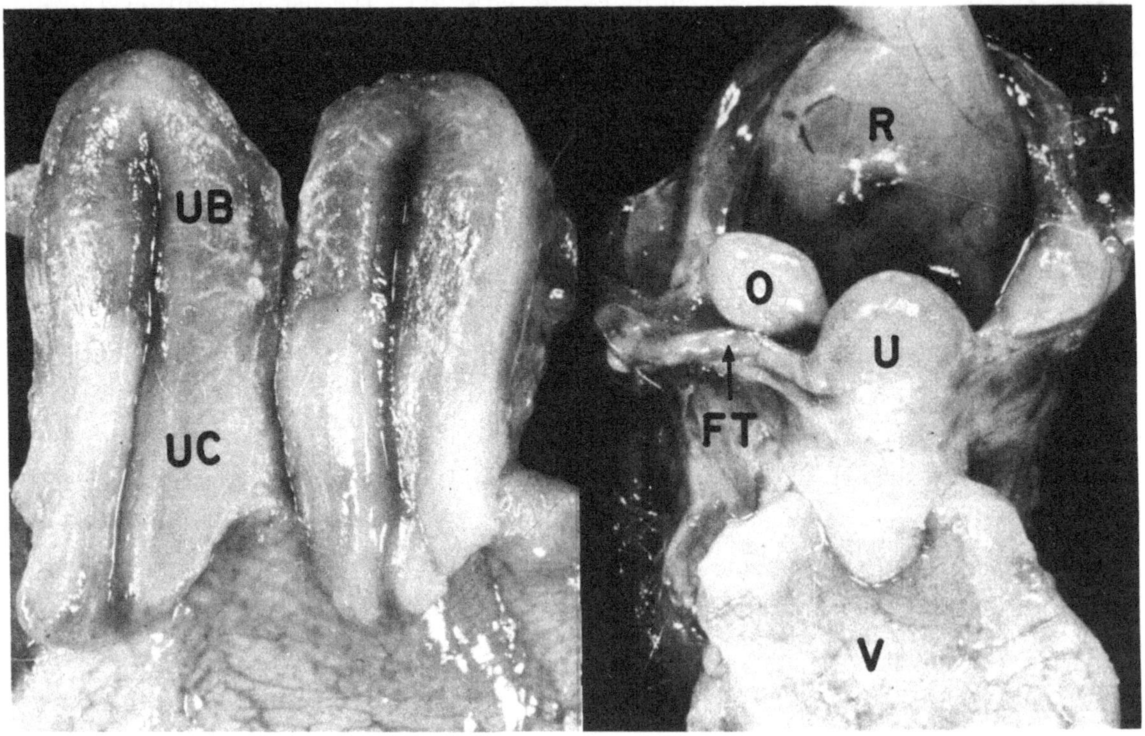

Figure 2. Morphological aspect of the genital tract of the female Cebus monkey. Right: the uterus (U) and its relationship with the vagina (V), ovaries (O), Fallopian tubes (FT) and rectum (R). Left: the uterus has been opened by means of a longitudinal section (antero-posterior plane) so as to show the cavity of the uterine body (UB) lined by the endometrium and the long and straight cervical canal (UC).

the aid of a vaginal speculum (nasal speculum for humans) and after cleansing the vaginal canal, a suction curette of 1 mm in diameter may be passed through the cervical canal into the uterine lumen. A gentle pressure is applied to the curette during passage so as to avoid penetration of the cervical or uterine wall. Suction is applied with a 5 ml syringe as the endometrium is gently scraped with the sharp edge of the curette.

Laparoscopy. The relatively large size of the Cebus monkey allows the repeated performance of laparoscopic examinations and manipulations of the internal genital organs without adverse side effects. As many as ten to fifteen laparscopic examinations performed in a 3-day period near the time of ovulation had no deleterious effects on ovulation[10] or on the animal's health. The procedure may be carried out under aseptic conditions and does not require absolute surgical sterility. A 5 mm-pediatric laparoscope is quite adequate for laparoscopic examination under Ketamine HCL anesthesia with an abdominal entry puncture in the median line, 1 cm below the umbilicus. The animal is placed in the

Trendelenburgh position, with abdominal pressure provided through an automatic insuflator of 12 mm Hg. The use of a Verres canula allows manipulation and examination of the uterus, fallopian tubes and ovaries with ease.

BREEDING TECHNIQUES

The most important factors to be considered in establishing a *Cebus* breeding group are: a) to identify animals of reproductive age, since most wild-caught animals are juvenile; and b) to ensure that the animals selected are fertile.

Sexual maturity in the *Cebus* monkey can be estimated from the stage of eruption of the canine teeth and by an approximate body weight of 2.5 kg for males and 1.8 kg for females. While these criteria will allow the recruitment of sexually mature animals they do not guarantee the animals to be successful breeders. Selection is more successful when regular menstrual cycles have been monitored in the female and when the quality of semen has been assessed in the male. The procedure used is to take daily vaginal smears for three consecutive cycles from the selected females and to obtain semen samples by electroejaculation from the males. The semen is collected into a 1 ml solution of 2% α-Quimotrypsine. After the enzymatic liquifaction, which occurs in about 5 minutes, the sperm concentration, total sperm count, motility and the ratio of live to dead spermatozoa is determined. Using this method of evaluation, it was found that *Cebus* males do not have any seasonal variation in their semen profiles.

Indoor breeding. The management of breeding in the laboratory colony is based on male-female pairs. The breeding male is housed permanently in a double cage (two compartments of 50 x 70 x 70 cm) with a removable separator. When menstruation starts the female is put in one of the compartments with the separator in place. The pair is observed over subsequent days to ensure that the male is not hostile. If they are compatible, the separator is removed on day 3 of the cycle and the pair are left together for 10 days. Under these laboratory conditions, copulation only occurs at night and is restricted to the period of maximum desquamation of the vaginal epithelial cells, a time that coincides with the mid-cycle rise in circulating estrogens in the plasma. The time that the female is left with the male may be shortened substantially if the optimal mating period is determined for each animal. In the *Cebus* female ovulation occurs between days 7 and 10 of the cycle and may be estimated through the vaginal smear or, more precisely, by measuring estrogens in blood[10]. This procedure can be specifically applied to studies of early embryonic development, where a precise knowledge of gestational age is essential.

Pregnancy in the *Cebus* monkey may be diagnosed routinely by rectal palpation of the uterus after about 30 days. The temperament of *Cebus* monkeys makes it unwise to handle pregnant females as abortions may ensue. If essential, pregnant females should first be sedated with Ketamine. Inadequate management of the pregnant females may result in an abortion rate approaching 100%. However, with proper management of the pregnant female the rate of fetal and neonatal loss need not exceed 20%.

Out-door breeding. *Cebus* monkeys can be bred and maintained in out-door enclosures and corrals without additional heat even at winter temperatures below freezing.

The out-door breeding programme at this Institute started in 1980 when 400 wild-caught *Cebus* monkeys were placed in out-door facilities located at a site 50 km from the indoor laboratory colony. The monkeys were lodged in compounds with two sections of 25 m^2 each, wire-net walls of 2.5 m high and a wire-net roof, half of which is covered with a metal sheet (Fig. 3). In addition, a

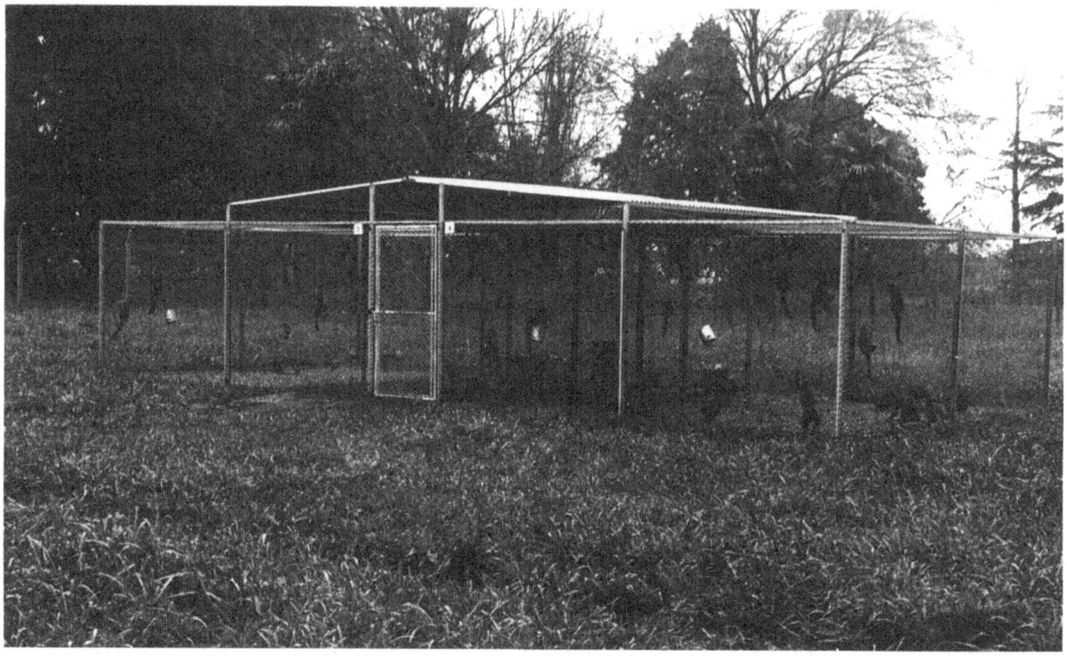

Figure 3. Out-door compound used for housing small breeding groups of *Cebus* monkeys. It has two compartments of 25 m^2 with a holding capacity of 20 monkeys in each.

large compound of 400 m^2 has walls as described above and a wire-net roof that covers it completely. Cement pipes are placed at random in the compound to provide a shelter from the cold wind in the winter and from aggressive behavior. Metal sheeting at the corners also protects the monkeys from the wind (Fig. 4).

The breeding groups are established in a harem breeding system. Ten females and two males constitute the breeding group in the small compounds and the same ratio is maintained in the larger compound, although the number of animals is larger. The breeding efficacy of both types of compound is currently being compared.

Our preliminary results show that initially there is a good deal of fighting, but this diminishes when balanced social relationships are established; once the group is settled it is difficult to introduce new animals.

In contrast to the observation of mainly nocturnal copulation in the indoor

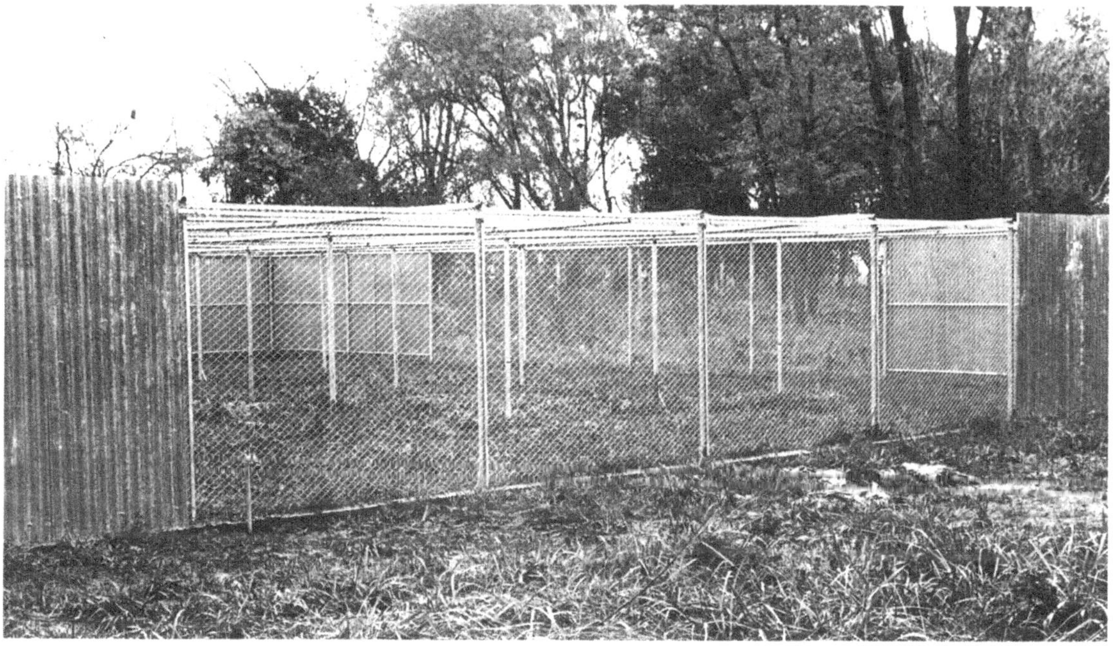

Figure 4. Out-door compound with a surface of 400 m^2 used for housing a large number of breeding groups.

breeding colony, in the out-door breeding facilities the animals copulate at any time of the day. In the first 6 months since the out-door colony was started with 30 females, 12 of these have become pregnant.

REPRODUCTIVE PHYSIOLOGY

Female

Menstrual cycle: The detection of uterine bleeding in the Cebus monkey was utilized as the parameter to determine the cycle length. The first day of vaginal bleeding was designated Day 1 of the menstrual cycle. Fig. 5 shows an analysis of the length of 108 menstrual cycles in the indoor colony. In 69.4% o the cycles, the length ranged from 18 to 23 days, with a mean value of 20.8 ± 1. days, while the period of menstruation was of 2.8 ± 0.4 days with a range from 1 to 5 days. It is noteworthy that most individuals have regular cycles of predictable duration. The results of studies on six regularly cycling females (Fig. 6) showed a follicular phase of 8.3 ± 1.2 days and a luteal phase of 11.7 ± 0.7 days.

a) Profile of reproductive hormones. Plasma levels of 17-β estradiol and progesterone during the menstrual cycle were measured by radioimmunoassays as described elsewhere[11]. In addition, LH was measured according to the method of Niswender[12] utilizing ovine LH antiserum, ovine LH standard LER-1056-C_2 and ovine $LH^{125}I$.

17-β estradiol: Plasma concentrations of estradiol increased gradually during the first five days of the cycle, from 50 to about 150 pg/ml (Fig. 6). This was followed by a rapid increase to a peak of 540 pg/ml on days 7-10, falling

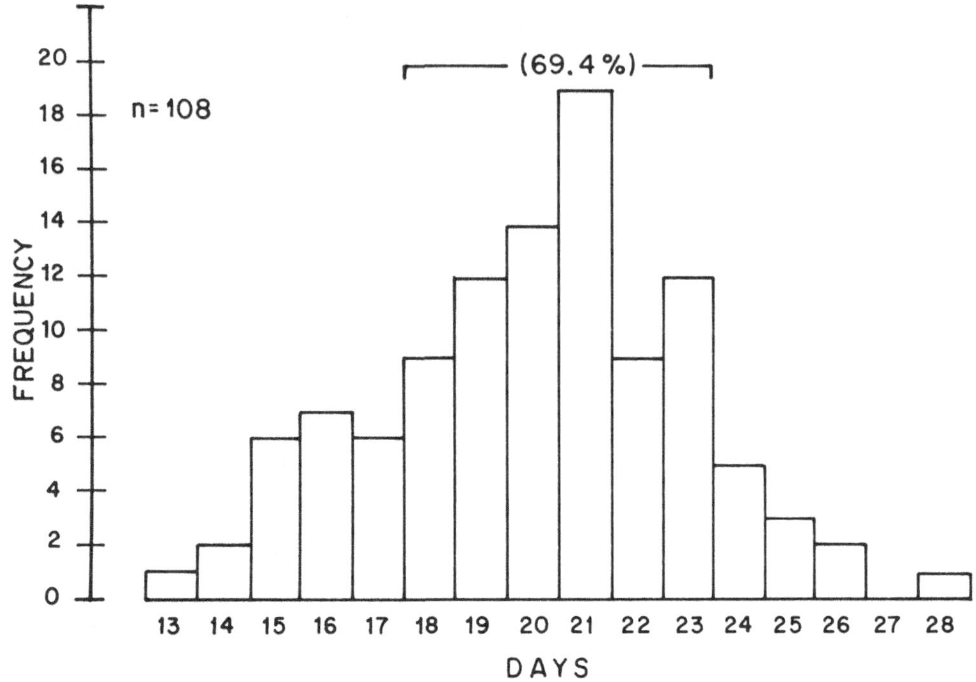

Figure 5. Histogram showing the variation in length of the menstrual cycle in *Cebus* monkeys.

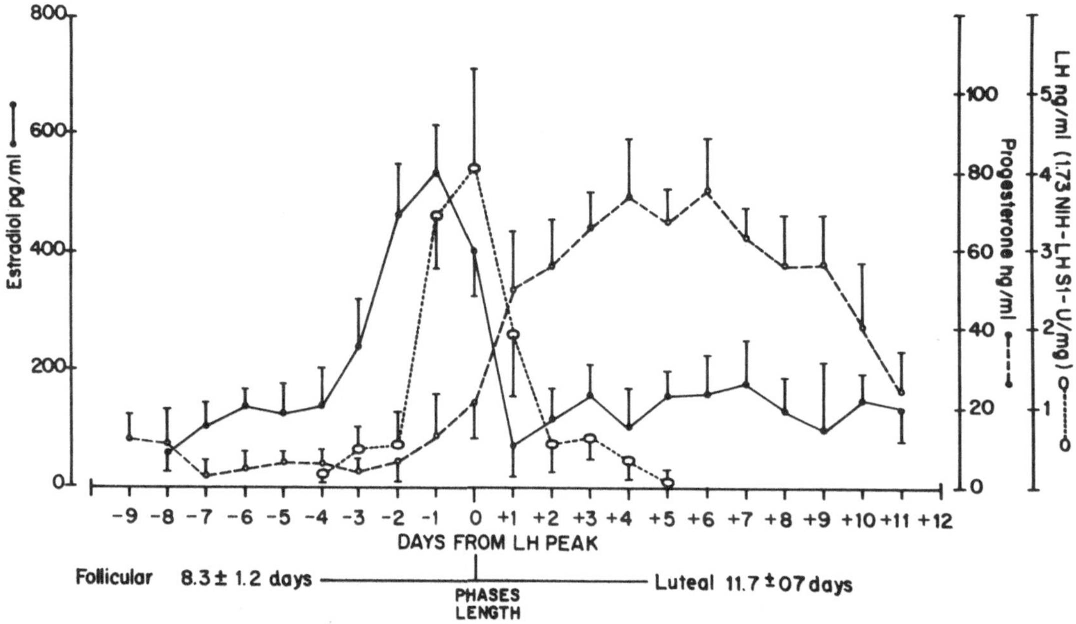

Figure 6. Mean (±SE) concentrations of estradiol, progesterone and LH like activity in plasma samples taken daily from 6 *Cebus* monkeys during an entire menstrual cycle. The data were centered around the sample with the highest LH concentrations in each cycle.

with the start of the luteal phase to the same amounts (about 150 pg/ml) observed during the early follicular phase. These concentrations then remain stable until the onset of menstruation. Thus, the plasma levels of estradiol in the Cebus monkey are similar to those observed in women[13], with peak values (420 to 600 pg/ml) rather higher in the monkey, but the estradiol rise observed in women during the mid-luteal phase is not usually seen in the monkey. The levels of circulating estradiol were shown to originate from the ovary as levels were virtually undetectable after ovariectomy (Fig. 7).

Progesterone: Plasma concentrations of progesterone were low during the follicular phase (5 ng/ml) but increased gradually from one day before the LH peak. On the day after the LH peak progesterone levels rose significantly above those observed during the beginning of the cycle (50 ng/ml). Maximal levels, 60-100 ng/ml, were detected during the mid-luteal phase. Approximately 2-3 days before the onset of menstruation progesterone concentrations declined to 10-20 ng/ml.

Progesterone levels during both follicular and luteal phases of the menstrual cycle in Cebus monkeys are 6 to 10 times higher than those in humans and 8 to 12 times higher than those in Old World monkeys.

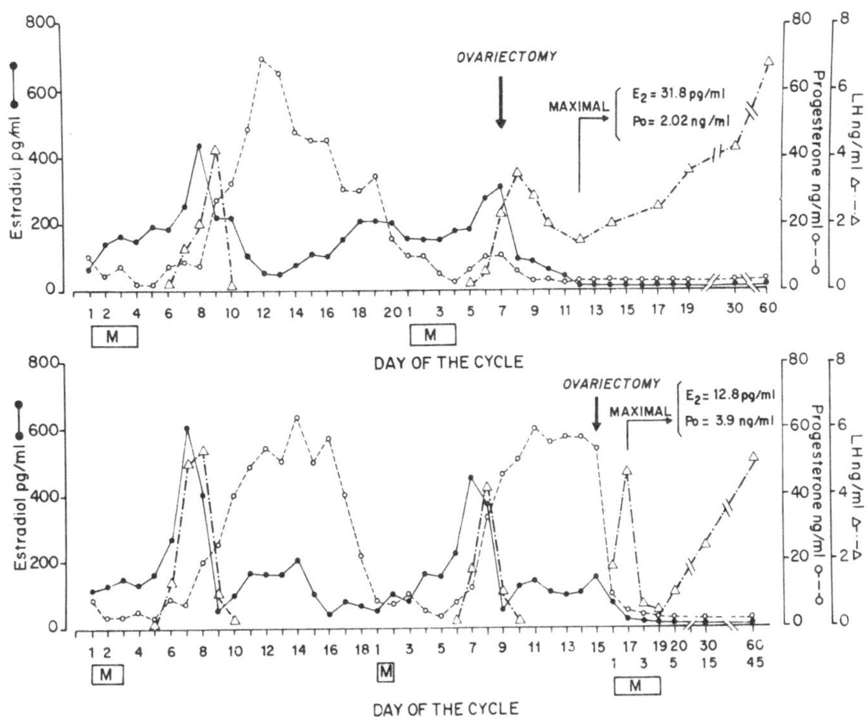

Figure 7. Plasma levels of estradiol, progesterone and LH-like activity in two monkeys that were followed during two consecutive cycles. Bilateral ovariectomy was performed in the second cycle (arrow). The maximal levels of estradiol and progesterone are given for the day after ovariectomy. (M = menstruation).

The high concentrations of plasma progesterone described here for the Cebus

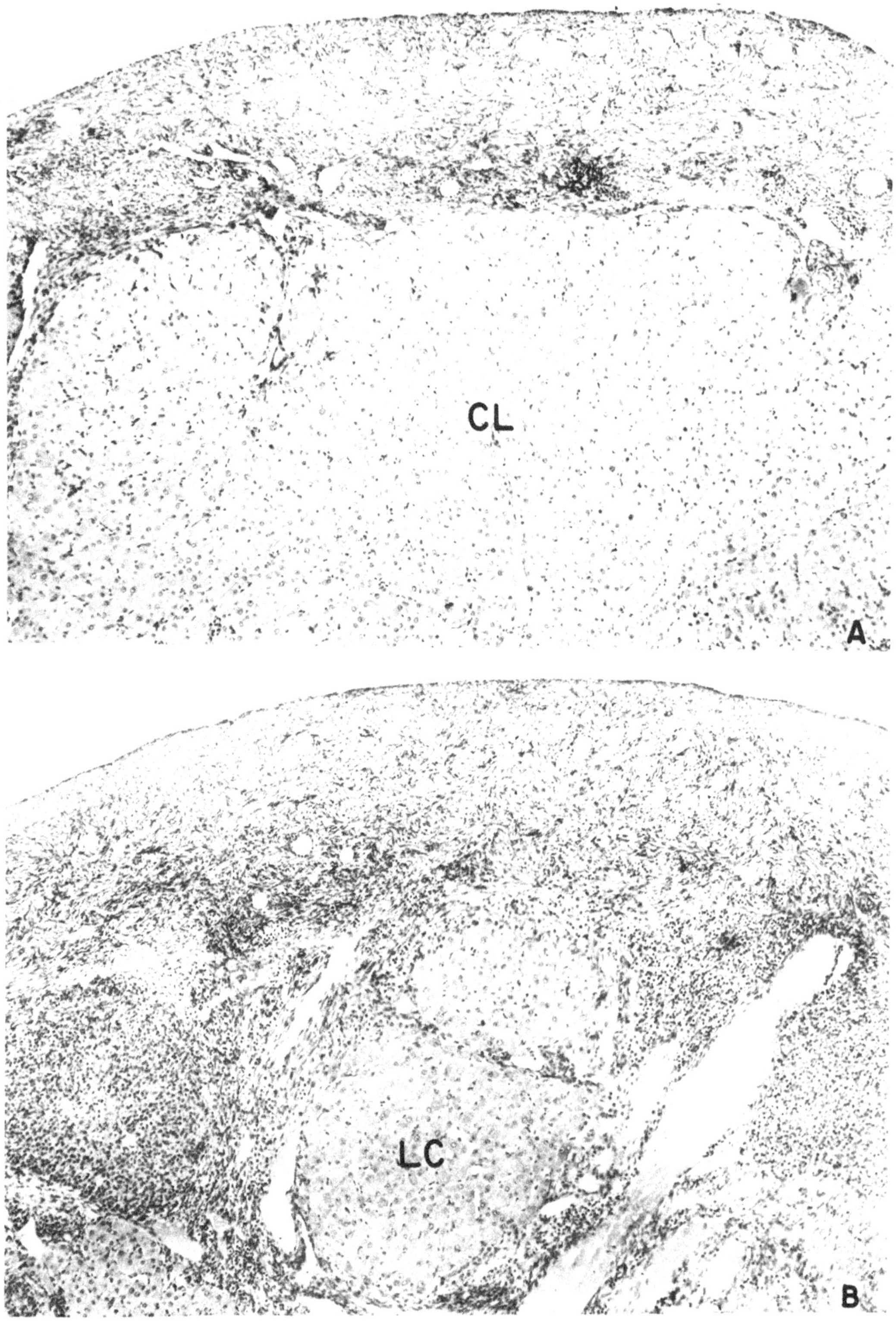

Figure 8. Photomicrographs of sections of both ovaries from biopsies performed in a Cebus monkey on day 15 of the cycle. The right ovary (A) developed a well defined corpus luteum (CL) whereas the left one (B) shows lobular formation of luteal cells (LC) in the stroma (H & E 45 x)

monkey seem to be a common feature of New World monkeys, as similar levels were described for Aotus trivirgatus[14], Saimiri sp[15] and Saguinus sp[16]. Though the ovary is the principal source of progesterone secretion other structures may be functional in the female Cebus monkey as plasma progesterone levels range from 0.9 to 3.9 ng/ml even in ovariectomised animals (Fig. 7). Further development and validation of the assays in use should clarify this anomaly.

Histological studies show the presence of abundant luteal tissue in both ovaries irrespective of the ovulation site and corpus luteum, with lobular areas of luteinized cells present in the stroma (Fig. 8). The contribution of each ovary to the levels of circulating steroids was assessed in a series of studies in which blood was drawn from the ovarian veins of both ovaries and the levels of estradiol and progesterone analysed on days 7, 9, 11, 13, 15 and 17 after the spontaneous onset of menses. The results were correlated with the presence or absence of follicles and corpora lutea, as well as the concentrations of these steroids in the peripheral circulation. Table 1 indicates that high steroid levels are detected in the ovarian veins from both ovaries.

Table 1. Estradiol (E_2) and progesterone (P=0) concentrations in the femoral and ovarian veins of six female Cebus monkeys

MONKEY Nº	Day of the Cycle	FEMORAL VEIN		OVARIAN VEIN			
				OVULATORY SIDE		NON-OVULATORY SIDE	
		E_2	P=0	E2	P=0	E_2	P=0
35*	7	333.2	3.6	2800.6	170.8	2140.8	166.4
163 *	9	520.8	18.6	4316.8	1016.6	4122.6	919.1
37*	11	118.7	9.8	1580.1	290.2	1561.4	270.6
20	13	174.6	63.1	1411.5	3090.6	1671.4	4810.0
69	15	96.5	62.3	1540.5	5350.3	1140.8	2010.3
60	17	99.6	89.8	1130.9	5380.1	1170.1	6220.0

Estradiol pg/ml -Progesterone ng/ml

*** Preovulatory follicle**

Nevertheless, monkeys subjected either to surgical lutectomy (Fig. 9) or to removal of the ovulating ovary showed a drastic and immediate diminution of peripheral plasma progesterone.

In this latter experiment, although progesterone concentrations were very similar in both ovarian veins 30 minutes after removal of the ovary with a fresh corpus luteum, the vein from the remaining ovary contained only 28% of the basal value (Table 2). These data suggest strongly that these steroids in the peripheral blood originate mainly from the ovulating ovary. The similar hormonal

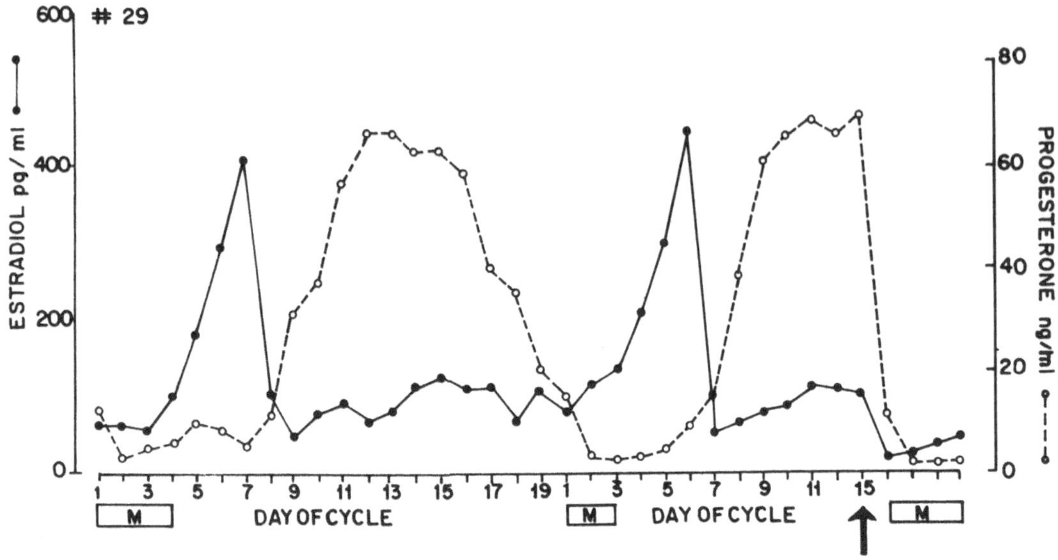

Figure 9. Plasma levels of estradiol and progesterone in a <u>Cebus</u> female subjected to surgical removal of the corpus luteum (arrow). The animal was followed during two consecutive cycles. Surgery was performed on day 15 of the second cycle (M = menstruation).

levels found in both ovarian veins may be explained by venous anastomoses between the two sides, as described in the rhesus monkey[17].

Table 2. The concentration of plasma progesterone before and after unilateral ovariectomy.

	Before	30 minutes after
Femoral vein	48.9 ng/ml	48.4 ng/ml
Right ovarian vein*	5.9 μg/ml	-
Left ovarian vein	4.2 μg/ml	1.5 μg/ml

* Ovary containing a recently formed corpus luteum

Measurements of progesterone in urine samples collected throughout the menstrual cycle suggest that large amounts of progesterone are excreted unmetabolised. Progesterone measured in urine reflects the plasma steroid pattern as shown in Fig. 10. Surprisingly, the levels of pregnanediol measurable in urine during the menstrual cycle is practically undetectable.

Gonadotropin hormones: Plasma LH levels during the mesntrual cycle, as measured by a previously described heterologous radioimmunoassay method, closely resemble the time course of this gonadotropin during the human cycle[13] (Fig. 6). The LH concentration in plasma during the mid-cycle surge is about 8-10 times higher than during the rest of the cycle. These relative changes are also similar to those occuring in women[13] and in rhesus monkeys[18]. Unfortunately, no <u>Cebus</u> LH standard is available in order to compare LH absolute values during the

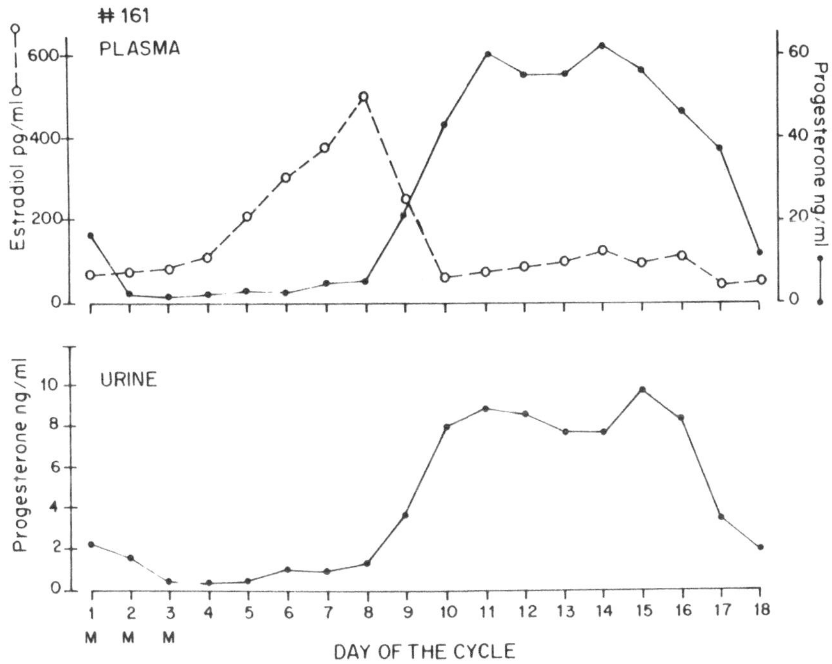

Figure 10. Estradiol and progesterone concentrations in plasma and urinary progesterone levels in an individual Cebus monkey (M = menstruation)

Cebus menstrual cycle with those in other species.

In samples collected daily, the day of the LH peak usually occurs one day after the estradiol surge. The LH peak value in all these cases is associated with the initial increase of plasma progesterone. The elevation in peripheral estrogen concentrations prior to the detected LH surge is clear evidence of the usual positive feedback control of gonadotropin secretion seen in mammals. Direct observation of the ovaries during the periovulatory period confirms the relationship between the LH surge and ovulation (see Ovulation below).

The negative feedback of ovarian steroids on circulating levels of LH was seen in two animals after bilateral ovariectomy (Fig. 7), with normal low levels of LH before ovariectomy and the initial and chronic changes in plasma LH, estradiol and progesterone following surgery. These data showed a rapid rise in LH levels after the removal of ovarian steroids from the circulation.

A suitable method of measuring FSH in Cebus plasma is not yet available so that the profile of this gonadotropin is unknown.

b) Vaginal cytology. Other authors[7,19-21] have studied the vaginal cytology pattern during the menstrual cycle of the Cebus monkey. In our studies the sequential cytological changes of the Cebus vaginal epithelium were correlated with the plasma profile of 17β-estradiol and progesterone during the menstrual cycle.

Five phases could be differentiated during the menstrual cycle according to the state of exfoliated vaginal cells and the presence or absence of erythrocytes

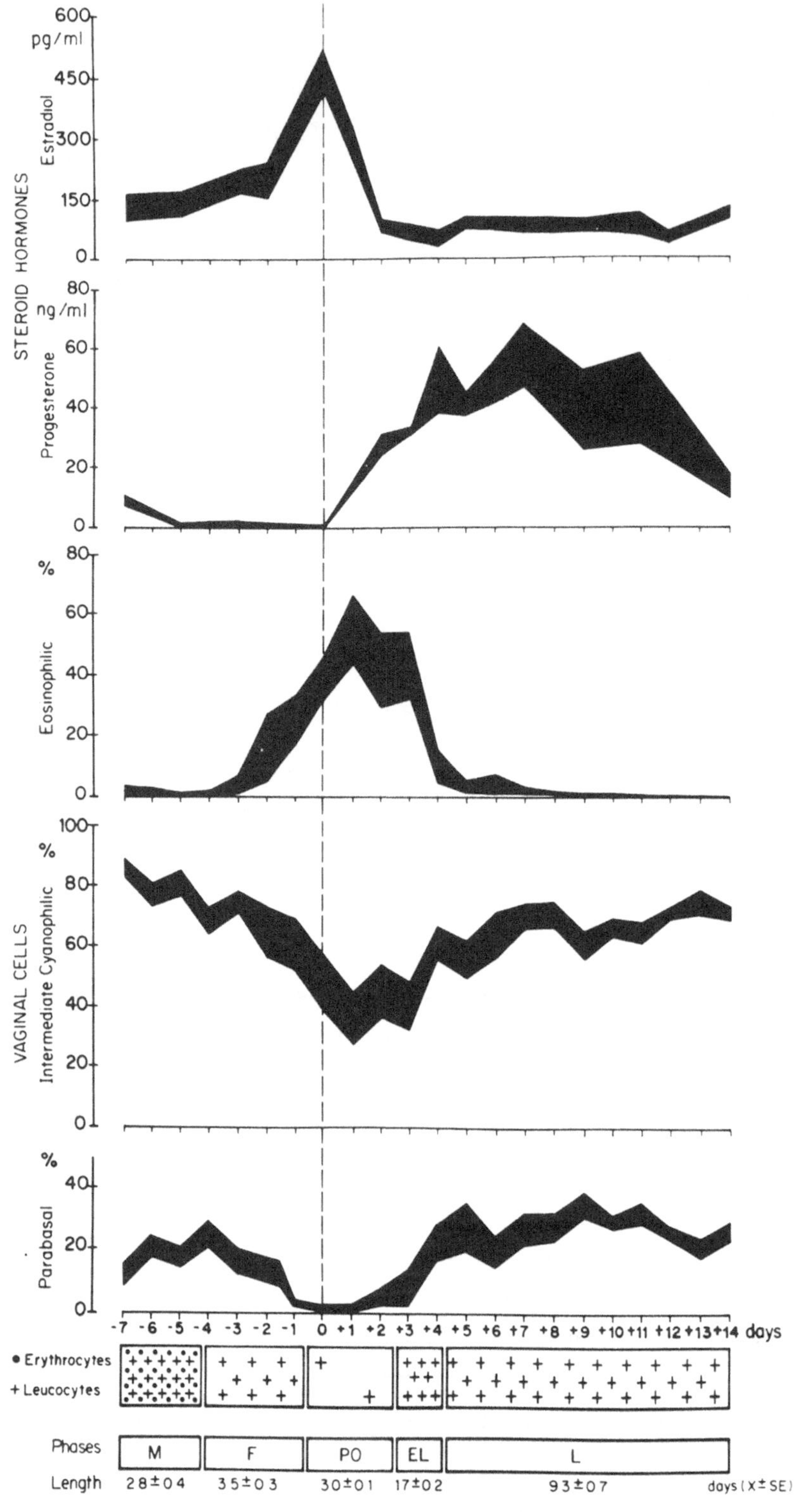

Figure 11. Composite figure showing the plasma profiles of ovarian steroids and their correlation with the cytological pattern found in vaginal smears of Cebus females. M = menstruation; F = follicular; P.O = periovulatory; EL = early luteal; L = luteal. (X ± SE, n=8)

and leucocytes (Papanicolau's staining technique). Figure 11 shows the cytological pattern of these five phases (menstrual, follicular, periovulatory, early luteal and luteal) and the steroid hormone profile. In contrast to the rhesus monkey and baboon[22,23], eosinophilia in the Cebus monkey was present not only in superficial but also in intermediate cells. Thus, the percentage of superficial cells, which is the normal index for the evaluation of follicular maturation and a marker for ovulation in women, rhesus and baboons, does not denote clear changes during the Cebus menstrual cycle. In this monkey the percentage of both types of eosinophilic cells, which increase sharply during the periovulatory period, is a useful parameter for detecting the start and finish of this phase. As each phase of the menstrual cycle has a distinctive cytology the evaluation of vaginal smears gives a reliable and simple technique for monitoring ovarian function in the Cebus monkey.

c) Endometrial changes. The endometrium presents a well-defined cyclicity through the menstrual cycle and during the period of bleeding shows this monkey to be a regularly menstruating animal. However, in between menses the endometrial changes show striking peculiarities that may be correlated with the levels of circulating estradiol and progesterone.

During the menstrual period the superficial layer of the functional endometrium showed a partial desquamation and necrosis of glands and stroma, with some vessels containing fibrin's thrombi. During this period the plasma values of the ovarian hormones are the lowest of the cycle. At the end of menses, while the plasma progesterone level was low and estradiol values started to increase, the endometrium was completely regenerated. The functional layer was thin and no mitosis was detected either in the glands or in the stroma, which is in contrast to other primate species.

Around the periovulatory period, characterized by the highest estradiol values in plasma and by an increasing progesterone concentration, the functional endometrium was well-developed. The most conspicuous features of this period was the presence of mitoses in both glands and stroma with glandular intraluminal secretion (Fig. 12-1). During the luteal phase the plasma hormonal pattern showed low levels of estradiol while those of progesterone reached the highest values. The endometrium during this period was characterized by the persistence of epithelial cell mitoses, abundant glandular secretion, and the absence of coiled arterioles (Fig. 12-2). Predecidual cells were present around vessels and distributed in patches (Fig. 12-3).

d) Ovulation. The analysis of hormonal events at mid cycle and their temporal relationship to ovulation were studied carefully in this New World monkey[10]. Serial laparoscopy allowed identification of the developing (preovulatory) follicle 4 days before ovulation; it was recognized by the swelling and darkening of an ovarian area which appeared translucent. At this time estradiol and progesterone concentrations in the femoral vein were relatively low.

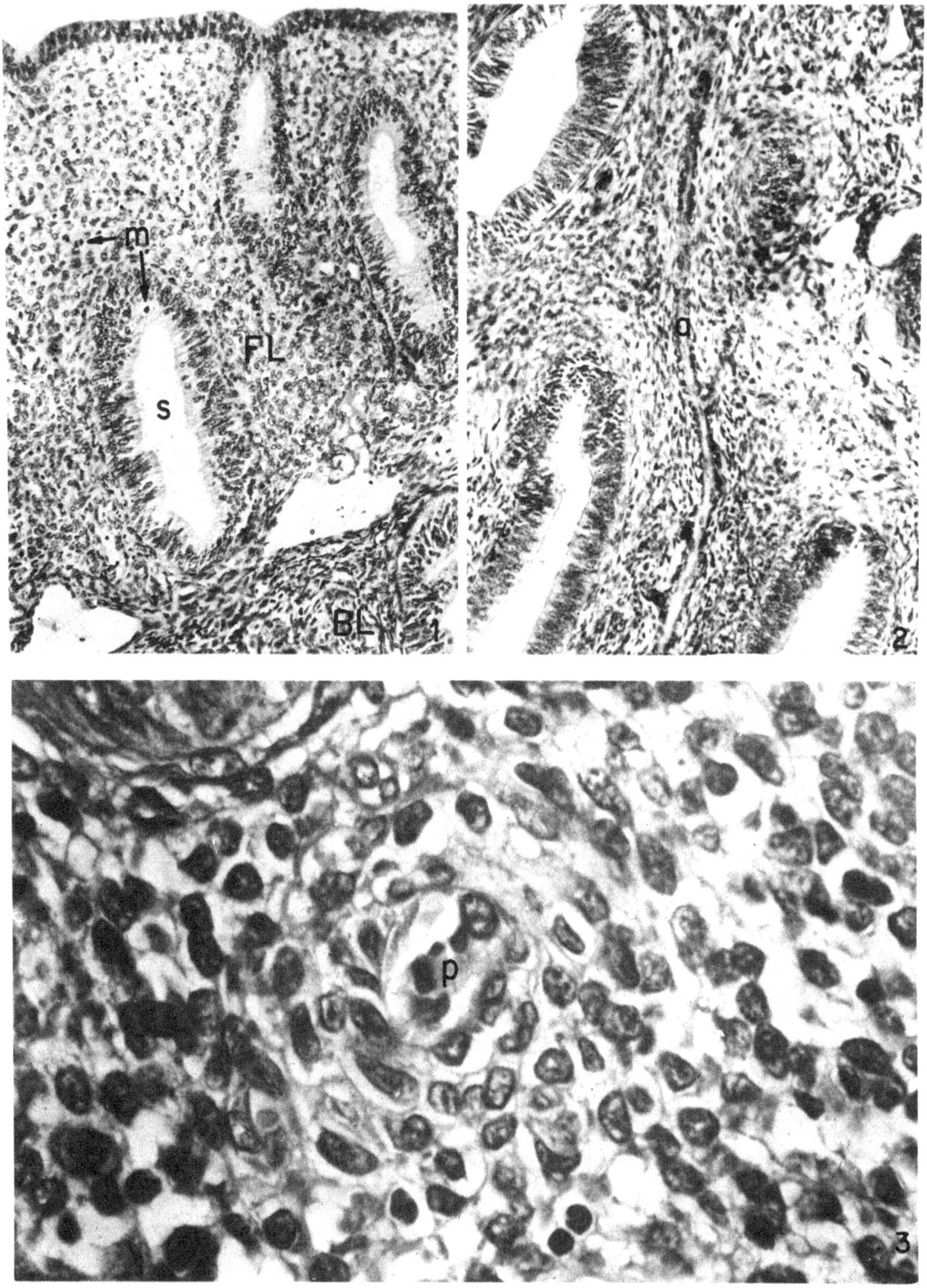

Figure 12. Microphotographs of the endometrium of Cebus monkeys. 1. Functional (FL) and basal (BL) layers around the perivoulatory period. Epithelial and stromal mitosis (m) and glandular secretion were typical features of this period (H & E-84x). 2. During the luteal phase the well developed functional layer showed arterioles (a) running straight (PAS-133x). 3. The second half of the luteal phase is characterized by the appearance of perivascular predecidual reactions (p) (H & E-840x).

Two days later and concomitant with the ascending slope of the estradiol peak in plasma, the preovulatory follicle enlarged dramatically. About 30 hours before ovulation blood vessels were clearly seen in the follicle wall. This vascularization increased as did the rising level of LH in plasma. Subsequently the follicle became conical in shape, with small hemorrhages on its walls. The fimbria completely covered the follicle and it was difficult to separate the two structures. Although not yet proven, the adherence of the fimbria to the follicular wall could be associated with ovum pick-up since by about 4 hours later the follicle appeared deflated and the stigma caused by follicular rupture was evident.

The relationships between hormonal events and ovulation are shown in Table 3. The events occurred over a shorter time span than that described for rhesus[18], bonnet monkeys[24] and women[25]; perhaps a consequence of the shorter follicular phase of this monkey.

On the basis of these data, plasma estradiol and progesterone levels are useful indicators of ovulation, to within a few hours, enabling experiments to be carried out that require the prediction and detection of ovulation.

Ageing the corpus luteum of the *Cebus* monkey presents problems as it regresses in different ways. The ovulation-stigma may subside and the CL remain very similar when viewed through a laparoscope for the remainder of the cycle or even during subsequent cycles. Consequently it is difficult to diagnose ovulation and estimate the age of the corpus luteum with a single laparoscopic observation.

Table 3. Time intervals between hormonal events and ovulation in the *Cebus* monkey.

Monkey Nº	Estradiol Peak		LH Peak		Ovulation* Diagnosis		Time intervals (hours)		
	day	hour	day	hour	day	hour	Estradiol LH	Estradiol Ovulation	LH Ovulation
123	10	12	10	20	10-11	(1) (2) 22-4	8	10-16	2-6
96	8	17	9	9	9	10-15	17	17-22	1-6
120	7	20	8	9	8	10-12	13	14-16	1-3
165	8	14	8	24	9	10-14	10	10-14	10-14
107	10	12	10	23	11	24-9	11	12-21	1-9
137	10	17	11	8	11	10-14	15	17-21	2-6

*Ovulation was assumed to occur in the period elapsed between two consecutive laparoscopic examinations; the former (1) showing a follicle or the fimbria covering it, and the latter (2) showing a newly formed corpus luteum.

The ovulatory process in the Cebus monkey is similar but more rapid than that described for women. This New World monkey has potential for studies of the mechanisms controlling follicular growth, rupture and the pick-up and transport of the ovum.

Male

There is little information available on the reproductive physiology of the male Cebus monkey. The data presented here were obtained from adult males selected as breeders in our indoor colony.

Endocrinology: Plasma testosterone levels in Cebus males ranged between 5-110 ng/ml (Fig. 13); peak values being approximately 7-fold higher than plasma testosterone values reported for Old World primates[26].

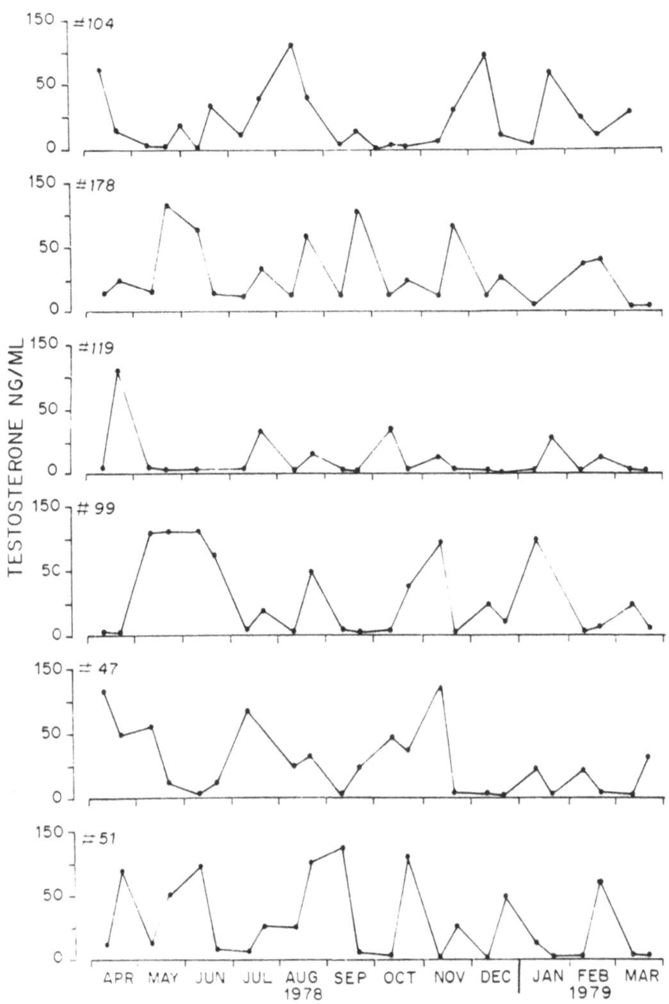

Figure 13. Plasma testosterone profiles in six individual male Cebus monkeys followed during a period of one year. Blood was drawn twice or three times a week at a fixed time (14.00 - 16.00 hours).

Generally, there was no consistent pattern in plasma androgen levels with striking variations within or between animals evident through the year. The significance of these individual variations remains to be elucidated.

Dorfman et al[27] studied the in vitro synthesis of testosterone by Cebus testis homogenates, investigating testosterone production from different precursors such as progesterone, DHEA, 17α-hydroxyprogesterone and androstenedione and finding the well-known pathway of progesterone → 17α-hydroxyprogesterone → testosterone in the human present also in the Cebus.

Semen properties: All monkey species[28], Cebus included, have semen with a fast coagulation time and no spontaneous autolysis of the coagulum for several hours after ejaculation.

The solubilization effects of different treatments on specimens of coagulated semen obtained by electroejaculation are shown in Table 4. The best results

Table 4. Solubilization of coagulated semen and recovery of motile spermatozoa from Cebus monkey

TREATMENT	CONCENTRATION (%)	TEMPERATURE	SOLUBILIZATION TIME (min)	POSITIVE RESULTS (%)	* MOTILITY	** MOTILITY RATING
SALINE	--	20-35	NS	0	0	0
SALINE + CUT	--	20	Instant.	40	9	9/4
HEPARINE	1-2	20	NS	0	0	0
TRYPSIN	1-2	20-35	> 15	100	7	7/3
& CHYMOTRYPSIN	1	20-35	>15	100	7	7/3
& CHYMOTRYPSIN	2	20-35	< 5	100	8	8/4
& CHYMOTRYPSIN	3	20-35	< 3	100	7	7/3

* PERCENT/10 OF THE SPERMATOZOA SHOWING ANY MOTILITY.

** UPPER NUMBER REFERS TO THE PERCENT/10 OF MOTILE SPERMATOZOA AND THE LOWER REFERS TO THE PERCENTAGE SHOWING PROGRESSIVE MOTILITY

yielding motile spermatozoa were obtained when the ejaculate was immersed in saline solution and an area showing a dense population of spermatozoa excised (saline + cut). However, this procedure was effective in only 40% of the samples. Treatment with α-chymotrypsin (2%) is effective in 100% of the attempts, without any serious modification of sperm motility, but the effects of this enzymatic treatment on the fertilizing capacity of the spermatozoa is unknown.

Table 5 summarizes the characteristics of the seminal fluid in six male Cebus subjected to electroejaculation and subsequent treatment of the ejaculated semen with α-chymotrypsin. Under these conditions the concentration of spermatozoa varied between 38 x 10^6 and 30 x 10^7/ml with a high percentage of motility and an acceptable live/dead ratio in all samples.

Pregnancy

Observations of female monkeys with regular menstrual cycles caged with fertile males indicate that mating occurs only once or twice during the menstrual cycle and this during the periovulatory period, when peak or declining levels of

Table 5. Motility and viability of α-chymotrypsin-treated Cebus monkey spermatozoa

ANIMAL No.	VOLUME EJACULATED (ml)	α CHYMOTRYPSIN - 2%			
		SOLUBILIZATION TIME (min)	CONCENTRATION $\times 10^6$	MOTILITY *	LIVE ** %
104	2.2	2	308.0	8.0	80
178	1.9	5	120.0	7.0	72
119	2.6	2	38.7	8.5	81
99	1.6	2	400.0	9.5	95
47	2.0	3	160.0	7.5	77
51	1.2	4	220.0	7.0	68

* PERCENT /10 OF SPERMATOZOA SHOWING ANY MOTILITY.

** COUNTING OF 200 TO 300 SPERMATOZOA

prevoulatory estrogen are present. Calculating the first day of pregnancy as the day of mating, the length of gestation was estimated to be 155 ± 7 days and one fetus is usually produced. There was no evident seasonality in breeding patterns as births occurred throughout the year. Table 6 shows the conception rate for Cebus monkeys maintained in the indoor colony.

Table 6. Conception data of female Cebus monkeys from the indoor colony.

Period	Total number Females	Matings	Conceptions	Matings per conception	Conception rate %
March-August 1979	14	16	10	1.6	62.5
September 1979-February 1980	6	9	5	1.8	55.5
March-August 1980	7	11	6	1.8	54.5

Three methods were used for the diagnosis of pregnancy, 1) rectal palpation of the uterus, 2) chorionic gonadotropin in urine, and 3) progesterone levels in urine. Rectal palpation of the uterus yielded satisfactory diagnosis 5 to 6 weeks after mating. Chorionic gonadotropin determinations in urine, using the Hemagglutination Inhibition test (NICHD), detected pregnancy during the third week after mating, but only showed positive until the sixth week of pregnancy. Detection of elevated levels of progesterone in urine from the second week after mating onwards was a reliable method for diagnosis of pregnancy in the Cebus monkey.

'Placental sign' was not seen frequently in this monkey, but was observed occasionally in the second week of pregnancy.

The progesterone concentrations in plasma and urine during pregnancy and the percentage of pregnant monkeys giving positive MCG tests are summarized in Table 7.

Table 7. Plasma and urinary levels of progesterone and the percentage of positive hemagglutination-inhibition tests for monkey chorionic gonadotropin (MCG) during pregnancy in the Cebus monkey.

			DAYS FROM THE ONSET OF MENSES															
			11-20	21-30	31-40	41-50	51-60	61-70	71-80	81-90	91-100	101-110	111-120	121-130	131-140	141-150	151-160	161-170
PROGESTERONE ng/ml	PLASMA	mean	67.1*	72.4	126.3	142.9	101.8	119.3	118.6	99.9	101.1	121.5	113.0	119.9	121.1	125.8	103.3	103.7
		s.e.	6.6	10.2	12.4	21.0	6.9	7.8	9.1	9.0	7.1	8.8	5.9	7.5	6.9	7.3	4.8	6.9
		n	5	8	9	9	11	9	8	9	8	7	10	10	9	5	11	7
	URINE	mean	28.6	33.5	51.9	58.9	48.0	54.4	52.5	47.1	44.8	62.6	52.1	55.4	56.9	61.7	62.7	51.1
		s.e.	2.1	8.9	10.7	4.4	5.5	3.8	4.7	3.9	5.0	5.8	5.5	6.6	3.3	2.5	5.7	4.5
		n	12	18	12	25	26	24	13	18	12	10	13	18	11	14	13	9
Positive MCG Test %			-	-	57.1	85.7	42.8	-	-	-	-	-	-	-	-	-	-	-

* Mean values for samples obtained in a period of 10 days.

In a group of mated females the mean value of plasma progesterone during the luteal phase of the fertile cycle was 67.1 ± 6.6 ng/ml. Subsequently plasma progesterone values increased to reach 142.9 ± 21.0 ng/ml on days 30-40 of gestation and then decreased slightly to values of 101.8 ± 6.9 ng/ml which were maintained until the end of pregnancy. Urinary progesterone values measured were approximately one half of those of the steroid in plasma but the profile in urine was similar to that in plasma.

These data indicate that urinary progesterone, measured by a direct radioimmunoassay, provides a reliable monitor of gestation in the Cebus monkey. It was noted with interest that positive MCG tests were associated with the highest progesterone levels found during pregnancy. A peculiar feature of Cebus monkey pregnancy was the high levels of progesterone recorded throughout gestation, with no secondary rise in late gestation as seen in women.

Figure 14 summarizes the mean values (± SE) of urinary progesterone around parturition in seven pregnant monkeys. The values given are centered on the time of delivery.

From parturition onwards the progesterone concentrations in urine show a continuous decrease reaching values of about 10 ng/ml 10 days after delivery. Progesterone levels remain low during lactation and weaning commences between 16 and 20 weeks after parturition.

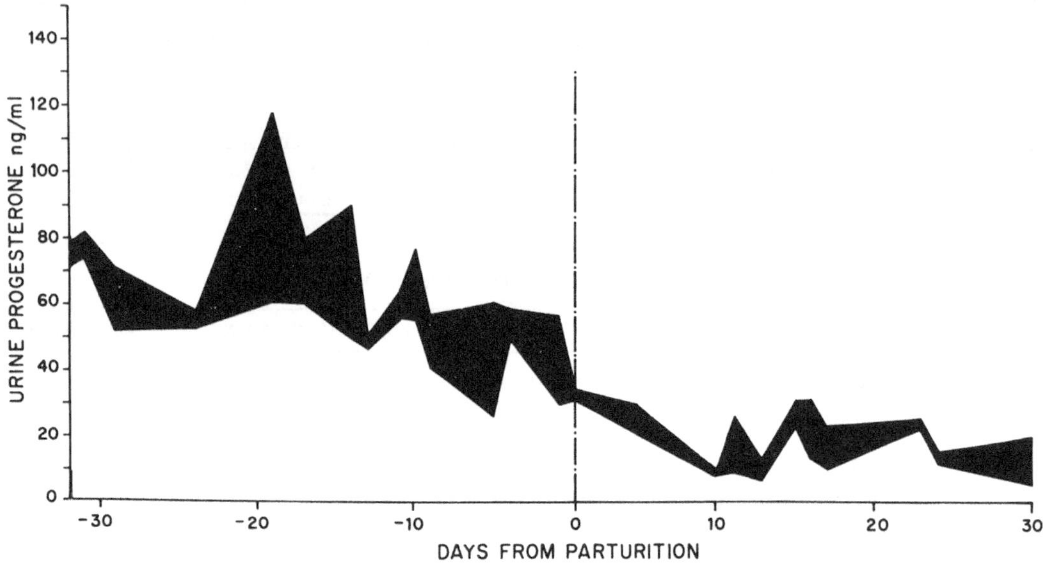

Figure 14. Mean ± SE values of urinary progesterone around parturition. The data were normalized to the day of parturition (day 0).

APPLIED STUDIES

Cebus monkeys are the subject of increasing interest and research in biomedical science. This interest is focussed at present mainly on applied research in the field of infectious diseases, since these monkeys have proven particularly susceptible to some human pathogens[29-31]. To date no applied studies in reproductive physiology have been reported using this animal as an experimental model. However, the data reported in the present chapter on the reproductive characteristics of this animal make feasible the future development of this primate to applied studies on reproduction.

Reproductive physiology

The data presented in this chapter suggest some areas in which the Cebus monkey may be useful for applied studies on human reproduction:

1) The endocrinology of the menstrual cycle
2) The mechanisms of ovulation
3) Endometrial physiology and pathology
4) The developing and testing of contraceptive devices such as IUDs or ICDs
5) The developing and testing of hormonal contraceptives
6) Embryology and teratology.

Other nonhuman primates, especially Old World monkeys, are being used successfully in research in these areas, but the current and potential demands for Old World primates exceed supply and the Cebus monkey should be considered as an alternative.

Infectious diseases

There are many species within the families of Cebidae of unquestionable value as experimental models in this extended biomedical area; almost every species may be useful for research in various types of disease. For example, the Cebus species have proved valuable as models for studies on Herpes virus Saimiri[32]; schistosoma haematobium-induced urinary bladder neoplasm[33]; induced malaria of Plasmodium vivax[34] and Plasmodium falciparum type[30]; Argentina Haemorrhagic fever[35]; South American Trypanosomiasis (Chagas-Mazza disease)[36]; and others. However, we will consider here just those areas of research for which the Cebus monkey is essential and where no other alternative model has been found.

Herpes virus and cervical cancer. The Cebus monkey is susceptible to herpes virus infection and constitutes a unique nonhuman primate model in research on herpes virus hominis type II-genital infection in man. The model is relevant to understanding the role of this virus in the etiology of cervical cancer in women[37]. The Cebus female develops a localized herpetic cervical infection following intravaginal inoculation[29]. The evolution of these lesions to cervical cancer may be studied with colposcopic and cytological examinations[38]. The incidence of anaplasia-type lesions among the inoculated monkeys is about 20%, but progression of these lesions to carcinoma has not yet been reported, indicating a long latent period in humans.

Chagas-Mazza disease. Cebus monkeys are susceptible to and may become naturally[39] or experimentally[36] infected with Trypanosoma cruzi. In our experience about 10% of wild-caught Cebus monkeys present signs of T. cruzi infection as determined by xenodiagnosis or indirect immunofluorescence techniques against T. cruzi. Although naturally infected animals generally manifest no sign of illness the association of myocarditis with natural T. cruzi infection has also been reported[40].

After experimental inoculation of metacyclic forms of T. cruzi by the conjunctival route, Cebus monkeys develop a persistent infection without any major acute manifestation of the disease. However, after 9-10 months of infection the Cebus monkey develops chronic lesions of the heart and colon similar to those found in human Chagas disease[36].

Both the electrocardiographic and the pathological characteristics of the cardiac disease, observed in the Cebus monkey, resemble the human disease, especially those concerning conduction disturbances and fibrotic myocardial lesions.

It seems reasonable to suppose that a primate model in which the full development of Chagas disease takes 10-12 months may be a useful tool for advancing our knowledge of the pathological mechanisms operating in human Chagas disease.

ACKNOWLEDGEMENTS

The authors are especially grateful to Drs S. Quiroga, A. Riarte and A. Merlo of the Biochemistry, Morphology and Pharmacology Departments respectively; to Drs A. Mendizábal and M. Carril of the CEMIC, Gynecology Department, to Dr E. Gadow and T. Matayoshi for their contributions in the genetic studies; to WHO Fellows R. Zárate and F. Gómez Argaña; to Drs M. Scarci and D. Grana and to Mr C. Malateste, H. Arance, J. Riva and Miss E. Gómez for their expert technical assistance.

Appreciation is extended to the World Health Organization Special Programme in Human Reproduction, and to the UNDP/World Bank/WHO Special Programme for Research and Training in Tropical Diseases, for their support which made possible the studies reported here.

The authors are members of the National Research Council of Argentina (CONICET).

The authors are indebted to Dr G. Niswender and Dr L. Reichert Jr for providing the LH antiserum and the LH standard respectively, and to NICHD for the provision of the Sub-Human Primate Test for Pregnancy Detection.

REFERENCES

1. Hill, W.C.O. (1960) Primates, Comparative Anatomy and Taxonomy. IV Cebidae Part A. pp.523. (University Press : Edinburgh).
2. Hershkovitz, P. (1949) Mammals of northern Colombia. Preliminary report No. 4: Monkeys (primates) with taxonomic revisions of some forms. Proc. US natn. Mus., 98: 323-427.
3. Thorington, R.W. Jr (1976) The systematics of New World monkeys. In: PAHO Scientific Publication No. 317. First Inter-American Conference on Conservation and Utilization of American Nonhuman Primates in Biomedical Research, pp.8-17. (PAHO/WHO : Washington).
4. Dutrillaux, B. (1979) Very large analogy of chromosome banding between Cebus capucinus (Platyrrhini) and man. Citogenet. Cell. Genet., 24: 84-94.
5. Welker, C. (1979) Zum sozialverhalten des kapuzineraffen Cebus apella cay ILLIGER, 1815, in Gefangenschaft I. Philippia, 4: 154-168.
6. Hill, W.C.O. (1941) Reproduction in Capuchin monkeys. Nature, 148: 408.
7. Castellanos, H. and McCombs, H.L. (1968) The reproductive cycle of the New World monkey. Gynecologic problems in a breeding colony. Fertil. Steril., 19: 213-227.
8. Hayes, K.C., Fay, G., Roach, A. and Stare, F.J. (1972) Breeding New World monkeys in a laboratory environment. In: Beveridge W.I.B. (ed.) Breeding Primates, pp.122-129. (Karger : Basel).
9. Moreland, A.F. (1970) Tuberculosis in New World primates. Lab. Anim. Care, 20: 262-264.
10. Nagle, C.A., Riarte, A., Quiroga, S., Moreno Azorero, R., Carril, M., Denari, J.H. and Rosner, J.M. (1980) Temporal relationship between follicular development, ovulation and ovarian hormonal profile in the Capuchin monkey (Cebus apella). Biol. Reprod., 23: 629-635.
11. Nagle, C.A., Denari, J.H., Quiroga, S., Riarte, A., Merlo, A., Germino, I,

Gómez Argaña, F. and Rosner, J.M. (1979) The plasma pattern of ovarian steroids during the menstrual cycle in the capuchin monkey (Cebus apella). Biol.Reprod., 21: 979-983.

12. Niswender, G.C., Monroe, S.E., Peckham, W.D., Midgley, A.R., Jr, Knobil, E. and Reichert, L.E., Jr (1971) Radioimmunoassay for rhesus monkey luteinizing hormone (LH) with anti-ovine LH serum and ovine LH^{131}I. Endocrinology, 88: 1327-1331.
13. Ross, G.T., Cargille, C.M., Lipsett, M.F., Rayford, P.L., Marshall, J.R., Strott, C.A. and Rodbard, D. (1970) Pituitary and gonadal hormones in women during spontaneous and induced ovulation cycles. Recent Prog.Hormone Res., 26: 1-48.
14. Bonney, R.C., Dixson, A.F. and Fleming, D. (1979) Cycle changes in the circulating and urinary levels of ovarian steroids in the adult female owl monkey (Aotus trivirgatus). J.Reprod.Fert., 56: 271-280.
15. Wolf, R.C., O'Connor, R.F. and Robinson, J.A. (1977) Cyclic changes in plasma progestines and estrogens in squirrel monkeys. Biol.Reprod., 17: 228-231.
16. Preslock, J.P., Hampton, S.H. and Hampton, J.A. (1973) Cyclic variations of serum progestines and immunoreactive estrogens in marmosets. Endocrinology, 92: 1096-1101.
17. Gunther, O.J., Dierschke, D.J., Walsh, S.W. and Del Campo, C.H. (1974) Anatomy of arteries and veins of uterus and ovaries in rhesus monkeys. Biol. Reprod., 11: 205-219.
18. Weick, R.F., Dierschke, D.J., Karsh, F.J., Butler, W.R., Hotchkiss, J. and Knobil, E. (1973) Periovulatory time courses of circulating gonadotropic and ovarian hormones in the rhesus monkey. Endocrinology, 93: 1140-1147.
19. Dempsey, E.W. (1939) The reproductive cycle of the New World monkeys. Amer.J.Anat., 64: 381-405.
20. Hamlett, G.W.D. (1939) Reproduction in American monkeys. Anat.Rec., 73: 171-187.
21. Wright, E.M. and Bush, D. (1977) The reproductive cycle of the capuchin (Cebus apella). Lab.Anim.Sci., 27: 651-654.
22. Allende, I., Shorr, E. and Hartman, C. (1945) A comparative study of the vaginal smear cycle of the rhesus monkey and the human. Contrib.Embryol., 198: 3-26.
23. Hendrickx, A.G. (1967) The menstrual cycle of the baboon as determined by vaginal smear, vaginal biopsy and perineal swelling. In: Vagtborg, H. (ed.) The Baboon in Medical Research, Vol. II, pp.437-459. (Texas University Press : Houston).
24. Lasley, B., Hendrickx, A.G. and Stabenfeldt, G.H. (1974) Estradiol levels near the time of ovulation in the bonnet monkey (Macaca radiata). Biol. Reprod., 11: 237-244.

25. Croxatto, H.B., Ortiz, M.E., Díaz, S., Hess, R., Balmaceda, J. and Croxatto, H.D. (1978) Studies on the duration of egg transport by the human oviduct. II. Ovum location at various intervals following luteinizing hormone peak. Am.J.Obstet.Gyn., 132: 629-634.

26. Snipes, C.A., Forest, M.G. and Migeon, C.J. (1969) Plasma androgen concentrations in several species of Old and New World monkeys. Endocrinology, 85: 941-945.

27. Dorfman, R.I., Menon, K.M.J., Sharma, D.C., Joshi, S. and Forchielli, E. (1967) Steroid hormone biosyntehsis in rat, rabbit and capuchin testes. Ciba Fdn.Collq.Endocr., 16: 91-104.

28. Dukelow, W.R. (1971) Semen and artificial insemination. In: Hafez, E.S.E. (ed.) Comparative Reproduction of Nonhuman Primates, pp.115-130. (Charles C. Thomas : Springfield, USA).

29. Nahmias, A.J., London, W.T., Catalano, L.W., Fuccillo, D.A., Sever, J.L. and Graham, C. (1971) Genital Herpes virus hominis type 2 infection: an experimental model in Cebus monkeys. Science, 171: 297-298.

30. Young, M.D. and Barerg, D.C. (1969) Experimental infection of Plasmodium falciparum in Cebus capucinus (White-faced capuchin) Monkey. Milit.Med., 184: 767-771.

31. Kalter, S.S., Kuntz, R.E., Heberling, R.L., Smith, G.C., Moore, J.A. and McCullough, B. (1977) Type C-oncorna viruses in a capuchin monkey (Cebus apella) previously infected with Schistosoma haematobium. Lab.Anim.Sci., 23: 533-539.

32. Melendez, L.V., Hunt, R.D., Daniel, M.D., Fraser, C.E.O., García, F.G. and Williamson, M.E. (1970) Lethal reticulopreoliferative disease induced in Cebus albifrons monkeys by Herpes virus saimiri. Int.J.Cancer, 6: 431-435.

33. Kalter, S.S., Kuntz, R.E., Heberling, R.L., Helmke, R.J. and Smith, G.C. (1974) C-type viral particles in a urinary bladder neoplasm induced by Schistosoma haematobium. Nature, 251: 440.

34. Young, M.D. and Porter, J.A. (1969) Susceptibility of Ateles fusciceps, Ateles geoffroyi and Cebus capucinus to Plasmodium vivax. Trans.R.Soc.Trop. Med.Hyg., 63: 203-205.

35. Carballal, G., Cossio, P.M., Arana, R.M., Nagle, C. and Casanova, M.B. (1980) El Cebus sp como modelo experimental para la Fiebre hemorrágica Argentina. Medicina (Buenos Aires), 40 ($^{6}/1$): 734.

36. Bolomo, N., Milei, J., Cossio, P.M., Segura, E., Laguens, R.P., Fernandez, L.M. and Arana, R.M. (1980) Experimental Chagas disease in a South American primate (Cebus sp). Medicina (Buenos Aires), 40: 667-672.

37. London, W., Nahmias, A., Naid, Z., Fuccillo, D., Ellenberg, J. and Sever, J. (1974) A non-human primate model for the study of the cervical oncogenic potential of Herpes Simplex virus Type 2. Cancer Res., 34: 1118-1121.

38. Tunca, J., Palmer, A., Nahmias, A., Mihalik, K., Naib, Z., London, W. and Sever, J. (1978) Colposcopic examination of the cervix of _Cebus_ monkeys. _Obstet.Gynecol._, _52_, 634-639.

39. Baker, J.R. (1972) Protozoa of tissues and blood (other than the Haemosporina). In: Fieness, R.N.T.W. (ed.) _Pathology of Simian Primates. Part II. Infectious and Parasitic Diseases_, pp.29-56. (Karger : Basel).

40. Bullock, B.C., Wolf, R.H. and Clarkson, T.B. (1967) Myocarditis associated with trypanosomiasis in a Cebus monkey (_Cebus albifrons_). _J.Am.Vet.Med. Assoc._, _151_: 919-922.

Chapter 3

The Owl Monkey *(Aotus trivirgatus)*

A. F. Dixson

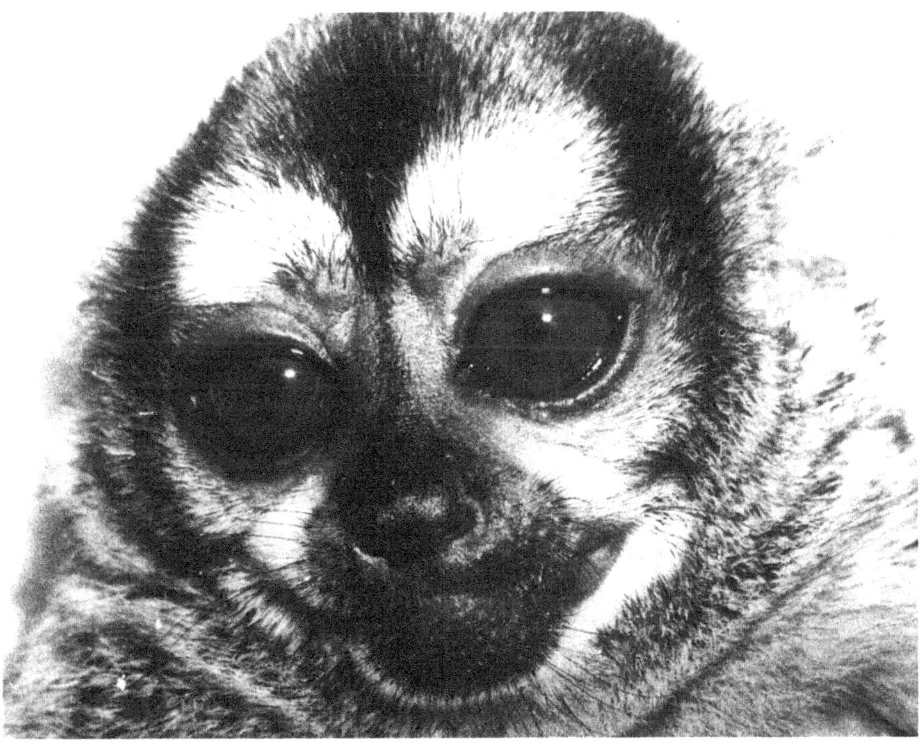

Aotus trivirgatus griseimembra

THE OWL MONKEY (*Aotus trivirgatus*)

Alan F. Dixson
The Institute of Zoology
The Zoological Society of London
Regent's Park
London NW1 4RY, U.K.

INTRODUCTION

The owl monkey is the only anthropoid primate which has exploited a nocturnal niche and in this respect it has proven extremely successful. It occurs in Northern Argentina, Bolivia, Brazil, Colombia, Ecuador, Panama, Paraguay, Peru and Venezuela, which represents the widest distribution range of any South American monkey. Throughout this range, various populations of owl monkeys exhibit considerable genetic diversity. Reumer and De Boer[1] have defined seven karyomorphs for the owl monkey, with diploid numbers ranging from 46 to 56. Ma *et al*[2] describe four phenotypes for the genus based on differences in the pelage of animals captured in various parts of South America. The taxonomic significance of these variations remains a matter of dispute and is beyond the scope of this review. All the observations on captive owl monkeys reported here refer to the Colombian subspecies (Plate I: *Aotus trivirgatus griseimembra*)[3,4] which belongs to phenotype B in Ma *et al*'s scheme. These monkeys have diploid chromosome numbers of 52, 53 or 54 and one specimen with a diploid number of 46 has been described. Naturally occurring "hybrids" between such animals have been studied by Yunis *et al*[5]. The sexes are of equal size and general appearance (Plate I) and adults weight about 1 kilogramme (males N = 20, mean weight ± standard deviation = 1009 ± 200g; females N = 16, mean weight = 923 ± 63g). The pelage is greyish brown dorsally and the ventrum is pale yellow. In the author's experience these animals are readily distinguishable from other owl monkey phenotypes. The Bolivian form (phenotype D of Ma *et al*) is larger and a little heavier than the Colombian subspecies (males N = 7, mean body weight = 1091g; females N = 7, mean weight = 1141g) and the hair on the ventrum is brighter yellow or orange in colour. The Brazilian owl monkey (phenotype A) is also a large animal with a bright orange ventrum. The orange hairs extend to the point of the chin and as far as the elbows and knees. In phenotype C, which occurs in Peru and which I have not observed, orange hair extends as far as the wrists and ankles whilst there is a broad mantle of white hair around the face.

The limited information available from field studies indicates that owl monkeys live in family groups, numbering 2-4, and that larger groups of up to

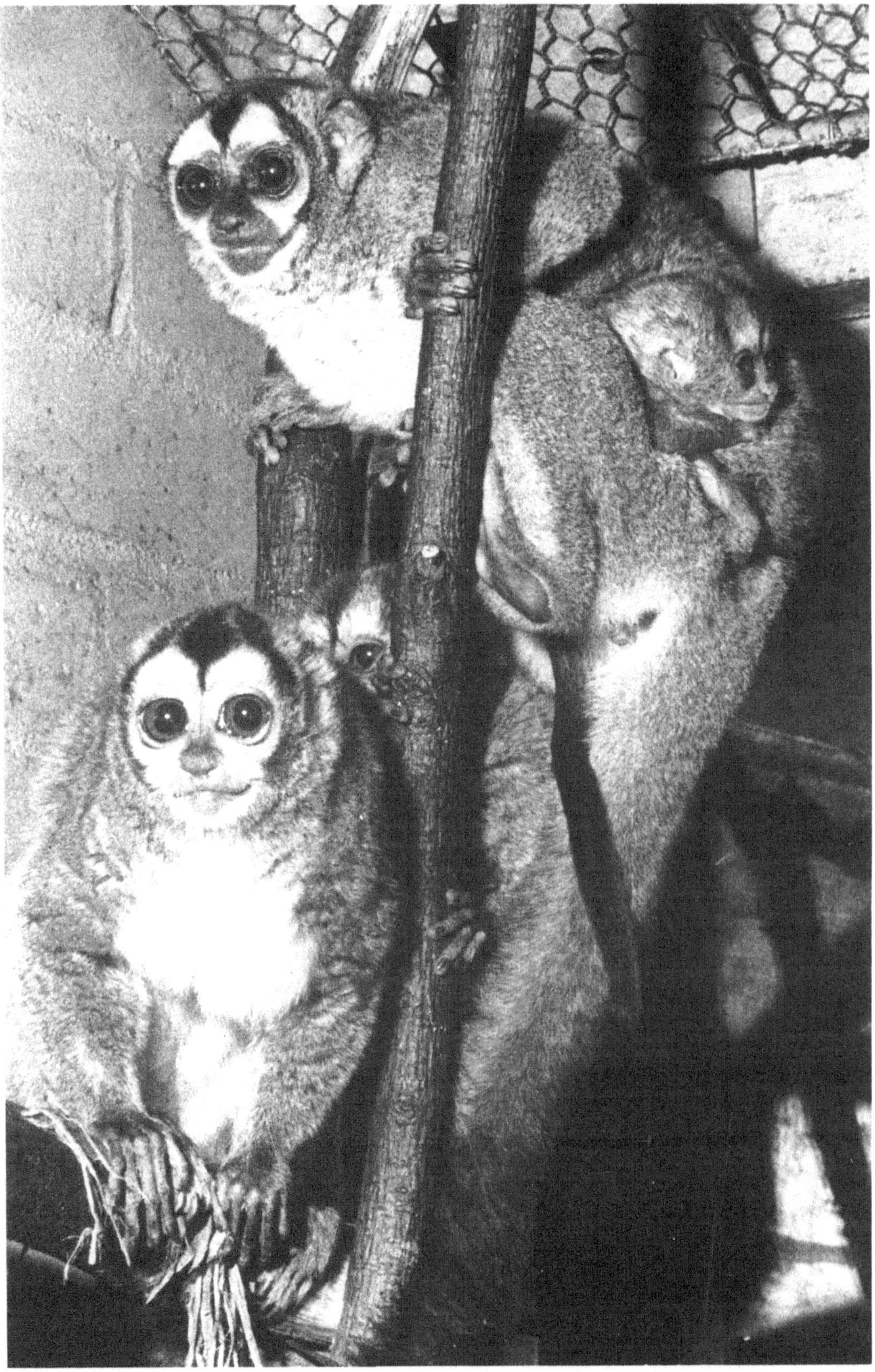

PLATE I. A family group of owl monkeys (Aotus trivirgatus griseimembra). The adult female is in the foreground and the adult male is carrying the infant.

6 monkeys occasionally occur[6-10]. Estimates of population density are extremely variable, ranging from 1.5/km^2 to 150/km^2[9,10]. The task of studying a small nocturnal, arboreal monkey in its natural habitat is a difficult one, so that some of these population estimates are doubtless inaccurate. The scarcity of data on the reproductive biology, behaviour and ecology of wild owl monkeys is attributable to similar problems. Family groups are apparently territorial and are primarily frugivorous, although they also include small mammals, birds and insects in their diet[6,7]. At the present time it is not known whether seasonal factors influence reproduction or behaviour in owl monkeys.

Large numbers of owl monkeys have been removed from the wild because of their unique interest as subjects for malarial and cancer research[11-14]. Only the Colombian form has proven suitable for research on falciparum malaria and its numbers in the wild have been drastically reduced due to collecting and deforestation. Several centres have established captive breeding programmes and a number of publications dealing with husbandry of the owl monkey are available[15-18]. This chapter will review information on various aspects of reproductive physiology and behaviour in captive owl monkeys. Previously unpublished data will be presented as well as information from published accounts[19-25].

CAGING, DIET AND GENERAL HUSBANDRY

The owl monkey has the undeserved reputation of being "difficult" to breed in captivity. However, most laboratories which maintain owl monkeys use them for malarial or cancer research and little attention is paid to their husbandry or reproductive biology. Most of the animals we have paired for breeding purposes have produced offspring. Monkeys newly imported from the wild sometimes fail to breed for the first 12-18 months in captivity but thereafter births occur every 8 months on average and at all times of year. Of 47 infants born at the Institute of Zoology, 43 have survived and have been reared by their parents. Meritt and Meritt[26] have provided useful guidelines for hand-rearing owl monkeys but this should not be necessary except in rare instances.

A cage measuring 102 x 55 x 66 cms is adequate for a family group of 4 or 5 owl monkeys provided that it contains branches or other types of perches so that the monkeys can make maximum use of the available space. A "nest box" should be attached to the cage since this provides sleeping quarters for the animals and a simple means of trapping them. We use nest boxes which have a detachable front and which can be fitted internally with a draw bar and vertical plate. This allows the animals to be restrained without handling them or using a net.

The monkeys are fed daily with pelleted diet (Mazuri), cereal (Farex), vegetables (carrot, lettuce), fruit (apple, orange, banana, tomato, dates, grapes) and seeds (sunflower, groundnut). Locusts and mealworms are provided regularly and water is always available. Temperatures in the animal room are maintained between 20°-25°C and no attempt is made to control humidity levels. A reversed lighting regime is employed (artificial light 02:00-14:00h, dim red light 14:00-02:00h) so that it is possible to carry out routine procedures in the morning (cleaning, feeding, collections of blood samples, etc.) and to make behavioural observations in the afternoon.

THE OVARIAN CYCLE

In common with other New World primates, the owl monkey exhibits no changes in the external genitalia during the ovarian cycle. Minor changes have been observed in some female squirrel monkeys but careful daily observations of female owl monkeys failed to reveal any alterations in swelling or colouration of the vulva. Changes in vaginal cornification may be used to monitor ovarian cycles in certain species (eg. *Saimiri sciureus*[27]; *Cebus apella*[28]), but this is not the case in the owl monkey. Cicmanec and Campbell[17] reported that in 3 out of 6 females they studied squamous cell counts in vaginal smears increased every 10-15 days. No quantitative data were presented, however, and we have been

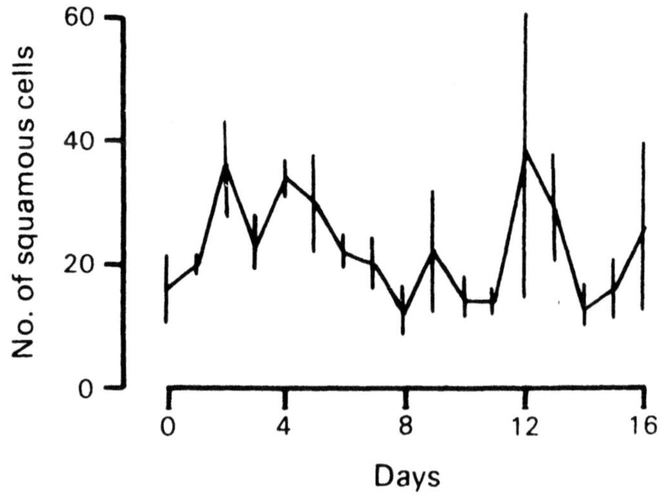

Fig. 1. Mean (±s.e.m.) number of squamous cells counted in vaginal smears from 4 owl monkeys throughout a single ovarian cycle, related to the oestradiol peak (day 0).

unable to confirm these observations. Vaginal smears were collected daily from 4 adult females in which ovarian cycles were normal (as revealed by concurrent hormonal measurements). Squamous cells were counted in 100 regularly spaced fields on each slide, giving a total area of 3528 $\mu m^2 \times 10^3$ and using an automatic stepping stage to eliminate possible bias in the selection of fields. There were no significant changes in numbers of squamous cells during the cycle and in all smears the total cell population was sparse (Fig. 1).

Menstruation does not occur in the owl monkey and erythrocytes are never present in appreciable numbers in vaginal smears. Menstruation is absent in other New World monkeys such as *Callithrix jacchus*[29], and *Saimiri sciureus*[27] except in *Cebus* in which its occurrence has been documented by Nagle *et al*[28]. Vaginal smears taken from owl monkeys are occasionally tinged with an orange-brown material referred to as "smegma" by Hill[30]. In fact this substance is not produced by the genital tract and serial secretions through the tract of one female failed to reveal any glands containing the material. Orange-brown secretions are produced by the subcaudal cutaneous glands in the owl monkey and sometimes these secretions are introduced into the vagina if the animal sits with the gland pressed against its genital region. Measurements of circulating oestrogens and progesterone provide the most reliable means of studying the ovarian cycle of the owl monkey. Fig. 2 shows the cyclic changes in oestrone

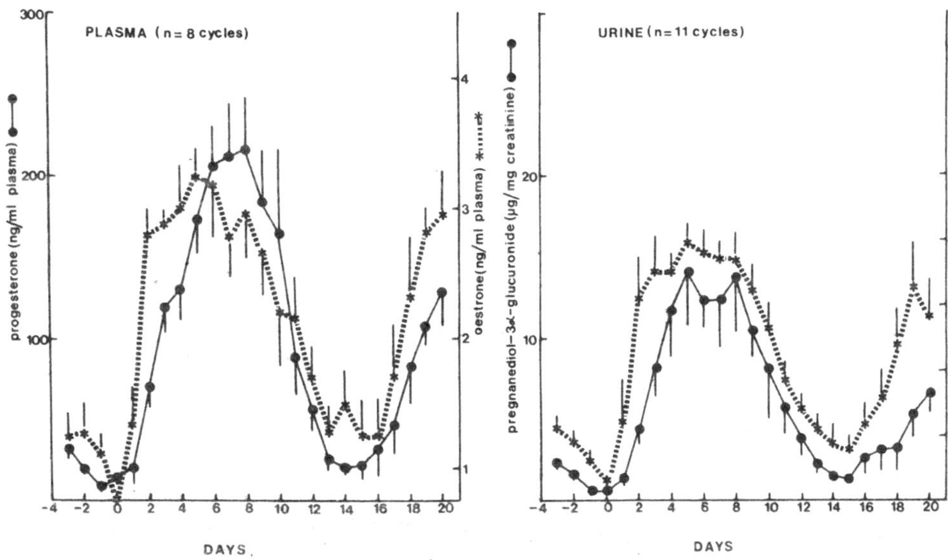

Fig. 2. Cyclic changes in plasma and urinary levels of ovarian steroids in owl monkeys. Data are means ± s.e.m. for plasma oestrone and progesterone and urinary oestrone and pregnanediol-3α-glucuronide.

and progesterone levels in 8 cycles from three females. The average duration of the cycle, based upon nadir to nadir intervals of oestrone or progesterone, was estimated to be 15.75 ± 0.09 and 15.38 ± 0.22 days respectively. Typically, oestrone concentrations rose sharply from day 0, peaked on day 5 of the cycle, and then declined to basal concentrations by day 13 remaining low until day 16. Plasma progesterone levels began to increase about 24 hours after the oestrone rise and peaked on day 8. Progesterone then declined to basal levels by day 11. The peak levels of these steroids during the cycle were extremely high; oestrone: 3.59 ± 0.066 ng/ml and progesterone: 250.48 ± 11.37 ng/ml. This finding applies to a number of New World monkeys such as the squirrel monkey and various marmoset and tamarin species and is clearly different from catarrhine primates. The ovaries of New World monkeys are larger than those of Old World species relative to body size and this is mainly due to the large amounts of interstitial gland tissue[31]. The extensive luteinization of the ovaries in New World monkeys may be responsible for the high levels of steroids measurable in their plasma. Hertig, Barton and Mackey[32] were unable to identify a distinct corpus luteum in ovaries obtained at post mortem from owl monkeys. However, laparotomies on females which show ovarian cyclicity confirm that a corpus luteum does occur (Bonney and Hearn, personal communication).

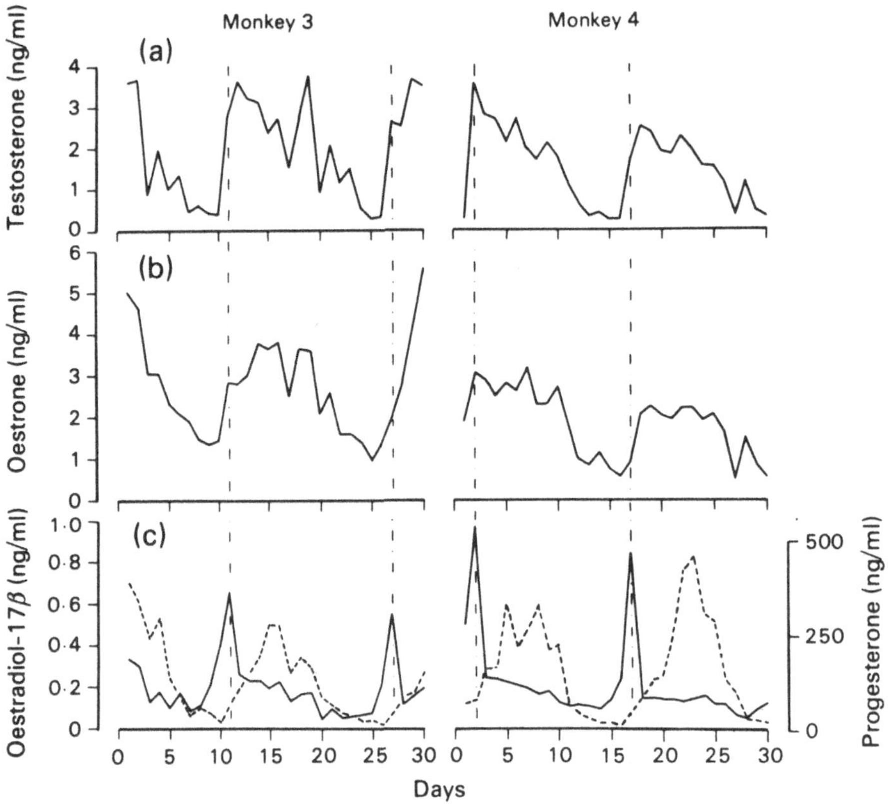

Fig. 3. Concentrations of ovarian steroids in peripheral plasma during two consecutive cycles in two female owl monkeys. (a) testosterone, (b) oestrone and (c) oestradiol-17β (solid line) and progesterone (broken line). Vertical lines are placed at the oestradiol peaks.

The oestrone and progesterone profiles for the owl monkey are almost superimposed and the follicular and luteal phases of the cycle are not clearly differentiated. However, measurements of circulating oestradiol-17β shown in Fig. 3 indicate that the follicular phase lasts approximately 6 days and the luteal phase 10 days, as is also the case in the common marmoset[33]. Basal levels of oestradiol average 0.1-0.2 ng/ml and peak levels (0.68 ± 0.05 ng/ml) occur at intervals of 15.5 days. These levels of oestradiol are similar to those recorded for the common marmoset although plasma progesterone levels are much higher in the owl monkey than the values of 20-140 ng/ml reported for marmosets.

Measurements of steroids excreted in the urine confirm these findings on the duration of the cycle in owl monkeys (Fig. 2). Sedation, using ketamine hydrochloride in order to collect blood samples, has no effect on the characteristics of the cycle in these animals, as is also the case in some other species (rhesus monkey[34]; baboon[35]). Oestrone is the major oestrogen excreted in the urine of owl monkeys as in some other New World primates (Saguinus fuscicollis, Saimiri *sciureus*, *Cebus albifrons*, *Ateles fusciceps*[36]). The owl monkey excretes progesterone mainly as 6β-hydroxypregnanolone[37] and this is also the case in the marmoset[38,39]. Pregnanediol and 16α-hydroxypregnanolone are also major urinary metabolites in the owl monkey and radioimmunoassay of pregnanediol-3α-glucuronide proves a reliable means of monitoring progesterone excretion during the cycle.

EFFECTS OF THE OVARIAN CYCLE UPON BEHAVIOUR

Owl monkeys do not exhibit consistent changes in the frequencies of copulatory behaviour, scent-marking or grooming when paired together daily throughout the ovarian cycle. Five pairs of monkeys were studied and each female was placed in the male's home cage for 15 minutes daily. The experiment lasted for 30 days and urine samples were collected from females in order to monitor levels of oestrone and pregnanediol-3α-glucuronide.

Three females exhibited regular ovarian cycles and one example is shown in Fig. 4 of a female which showed two complete cycles during the study. Frequencies of anogenital inspections by the male, mounting attempts and mounts with pelvic thrusting did not vary in a predictable fashion during these cycles, nor were there any changes in the latencies to the male's first attempted mount or the duration of the mounts. Male owl monkeys do not exhibit a noticeable body tremor or pause in thrusting behaviour such as occurs in males of many other primate species during ejaculations. It is not known if ejaculations occurred during every test, although mounts with pelvic thrusting did occur throughout the ovarian cycle.

Similar results to those shown in Fig. 4 were also obtained from two other pairs of owl monkeys in which females showed regular ovarian cycles. Thus, under these testing conditions, female owl monkeys remain sexually attractive and receptive to males throughout the cycle. Females rarely refused the males' mounting attempts in these experiments. Sexual presentations and other proceptive behaviours were never observed and, as far as could be ascertained, all copulations were initiated by the males. Although both sexes employed scent marking behaviours (rubbing with the subcaudal gland and "urine washing") the frequencies of these behaviours bore no relationship to the stages of the ovarian cycle.

In the fourth pair of monkeys studied, changes in urinary oestrone and pregnanediol-3α-glucuronide were erratic. Nonetheless, copulatory activity was high (Fig. 5) and the behaviour of this pair was indistinguishable from that of pairs in which females exhibited regular cycles. Comparable results were obtained from a fifth pair in which the female conceived during the first few days of the study and continued to mate regularly during early pregnancy.

The only other New World primate which has been studied thoroughly in order to establish the effects of ovarian cyclicity upon sexual behaviour is the

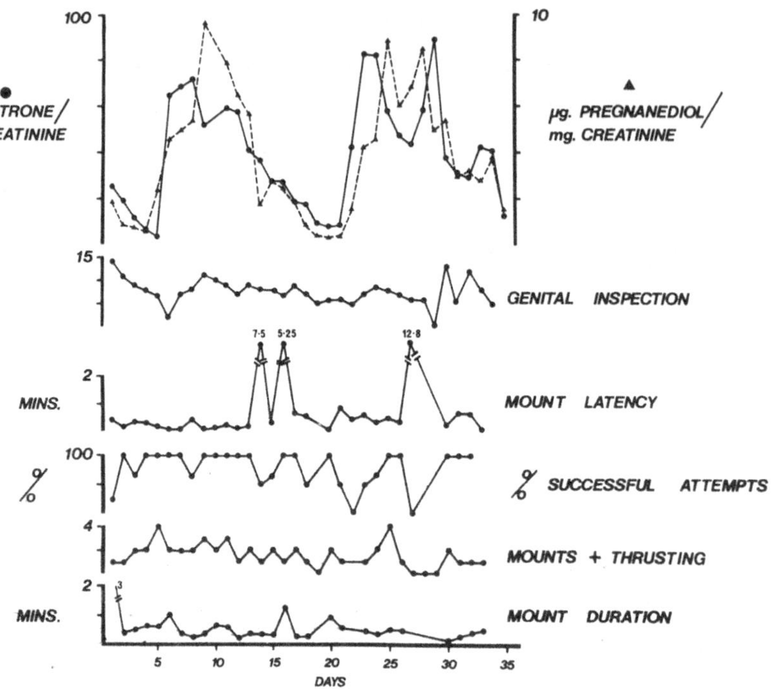

Fig. 4. Sexual interactions during two consecutive ovarian cycles of a female owl monkey paired daily with the same male. The upper graph shows the urinary level of oestrone (●——●) and pregnanediol-3α-glucuronide (▲——▲). Other graphs show measurements of the male partner's sexual activity: genital inspections, latency to onset of mounting, % of the male's attempts to mount which were successful, number of mounts with pelvic thrusting and the duration of mounts with thrusting.

squirrel monkey. In that species, copulations are limited to the day of ovulation during the 7-9 day cycle when females are maximally receptive (and probably maximally attractive) to males[40]. Clearly, the effects of ovarian hormones upon sexual behaviour must vary among New World primates and this is certainly true of the Old World monkeys and apes. In some Old World monkeys (eg. mangabeys, talapoins), pronounced peaks in copulatory activity occur at mid-cycle and this is also true of the gorilla. In others (such as the pigtail or rhesus monkey) copulations are frequent throughout the follicular phase and mid-cycle peaks are less obvious (Table 1). There is a tendency for many species to show less copulatory activity during the luteal phase of the ovarian cycle, although it was not possible to measure such a decrease in the owl monkey. The information in Table 1 indicates that there is no simple relationship between phylogenetic position and control by ovarian hormones of sexual behaviour in primates. One fair generalization is that among prosimian species, females exhibit clearly defined periods of sexual receptivity. In monkeys and apes, however, females of certain species remain sexually receptive throughout the ovarian cycle and changes in their sexual attractiveness (or proceptivity) are

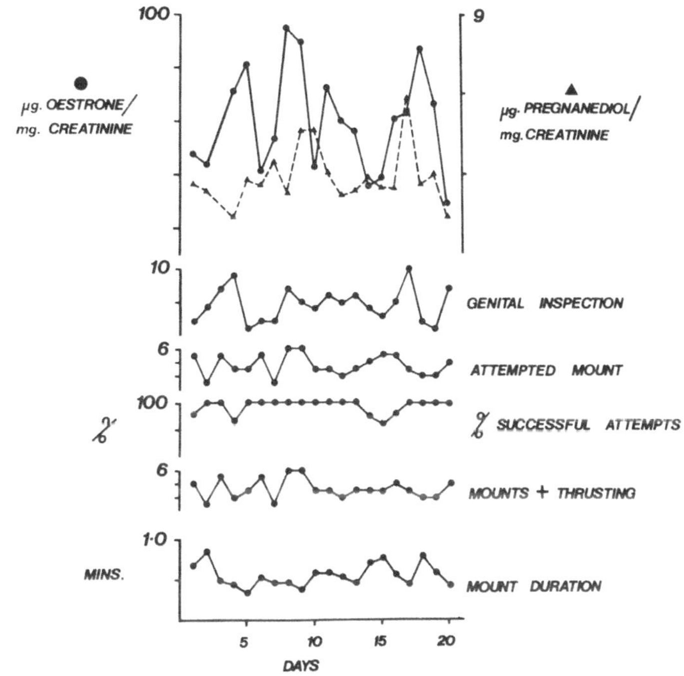

Fig. 5. Sexual interactions in a pair of owl monkeys correlated with daily measurements of urinary oestrone and pregnanediol-3α-glucuronide in the female. Frequent mounts occur although the female does not exhibit ovarian cyclicity. For further explanation see text and caption to Fig. 4.

more important in the regulation of mating behaviour. It is also the case that individual differences in behaviour, sexual preferences for particular partners, or social factors may override hormones as the major determinants of copulatory activity[51,52].

Table 1. Maximum frequencies of copulation during the ovarian cycle in various primate species.

Species	Highest frequency of ejaculatory mounts during ovarian cycle	Reference source
PROSIMIANS		
Galago crassicaudatus	Peri-ovulatory phase	41
Lemur catta	Peri-ovulatory phase	42
NEW WORLD MONKEYS		
Aotus trivirgatus	Throughout cycle	Present study
Saimiri sciureus	Peri-ovulatory phase	40
OLD WORLD MONKEYS		
Miopithecus talapoin	Peri-ovulatory phase	43
Macaca mulatta	Follicular and peri-ovulatory phase	44
Macaca nemestrina	Follicular and peri-ovulatory phase	45
Cercebus albigena	Peri-ovulatory phase	46
Papio ursinus	Follicular and peri-ovulatory phase	47
APES		
Pan troglodytes	Follicular and peri-ovulatory phase	48
Gorilla gorilla	Peri-ovulatory phase	49
Pongo pygmaeus	Throughout cycle	50

Under normal social conditions mating occurs very infrequently in the owl monkey. During 278 hours of observation on 5 captive groups only 19 attempts at copulation occurred (Table 2). As in the pair tests, females exhibited no obvious proceptive behaviours and did not refuse the males' mounting attempts. One explanation of these findings is that subtle changes in female attractiveness control sexual interactions in family groups of owl monkeys, so that matings occur at the appropriate time to ensure conception. In the highly artificial conditions of a pair test, such cues are less important and males initiate sexual activity irrespective of the females' endocrine status.

Sexual interactions are usually infrequent in primates which live in monogamous family groups[53]. In certain callitrichid species, matings may occur frequently (as in the owl monkey) if the animals are caged singly and pair-tested throughout the ovarian cycle (Saguinus oedipus: Brand, personal communication; Saguinus fuscicollis[54]). In owl monkeys some other behaviours also occur more frequently during pair tests. Thus "arching" (Fig.22) which is believed by Moynihan[55] to act as a "hostile" display, occurs quite frequently in pair tests but rarely in family groups. Female owl monkeys also "tail rub" more often when introduced into the home cages of male animals (Table 2). Arching and tail rubbing (ie. marking with the subcaudal gland) have been observed during intergroup agonistic interactions in wild owl monkeys[6]. It is possible that heightened levels of these behaviours occur in captivity when animals are not thoroughly familiar with one another or with the cage in which they are tested.

Table 2. Hourly frequencies of selected behaviours in family groups of owl monkeys or during daily pair tests.

	Five family groups*		Five pairs**	
	♂ + ♀		♂ + ♀	
Arching displays	0		2.44	
Copulations	0.07		3.87	
	♂	♀	♂	♀
Urine mark	8.3	5.5	3.93	3.93
Tail mark	7.4	0.56	3.13	7.25

* 278 hours of observations
** 150 tests of 15 minutes duration

TESTICULAR FUNCTION IN THE ADULT MALE

Captive adult male owl monkeys exhibit a condition which has been described by some workers as partially arrested spermatogensis[56,57]. This phenomenon occurs at all times of the year in captivity. We have examined sections of whole testes or testicular biopsies from 19 males and have found a similar histological picture to that described by Hunt et al[56]. Few spermatozoa are present, many of the spermatocytes may appear degenerate and deposits of an orange-brown pigment are present in the inter-tubular tissues. These observations have been attributed to a vitamin E deficiency which is irreversible[56,57]. However, three captive-born males in our colony exhibited the same condition as animals originating from the wild, although their diet should have provided adequate vitamin E. A fourth captive-born male was treated with vitamin E once weekly between the ages of 72 and 577 days. A total of 1940 mg of the vitamin was administered to this male by intramuscular injection (an average dose of 26 mg/week). A testicular biopsy was taken at close of treatment which was histologically similar to those taken from other adult males. The pilot study did not confirm the hypothesis that owl monkeys are prone to an irreversible vitamin E deficiency which affects testicular function.

Serial sections were prepared of testes from four adult males and it transpired that a few spermatozoa were present in some seminiferous tubules. Very few spermatozoa were found in the epididymis. When electroejaculation was attempted (using a rectal probe) a few spermatozoa were present in emissions from several males but it was not possible to produce a full ejaculation. Whatever the causes of the unusual testicular structure of male owl monkeys might be, it is apparent that these animals are fertile and it would be premature to assume that the condition is pathological. Five males in our colony which have a successful breeding history also exhibit the same histological features of their testes. As described previously, copulatory activity is extremely infrequent in family groups of owl monkeys yet conceptions occur regularly and there is no indication of male infertility. Levels of plasma testosterone in male owl monkeys are apparently normal and are subject to a diurnal rhythm (Fig. 6). The highest levels of testosterone (mean ± s.e.m., 24.8 ± 5.3 ng/ml) occur during the illuminated phase of the lighting cycle and the lowest levels (4.7 ± 1.2 ng/ml) occur during the periods of darkness. These daily changes in circulating testosterone are the reverse of those reported in some diurnal primates (eg. rhesus monkey[58], bonnet monkey[59], ring-tailed lemur[60]). However, all these species agree in having high levels of testosterone during periods of rest or sleep and lowest levels during periods of activity.

There has been no study of testicular function in wild owl monkeys and this would be useful. We have examined one adult specimen which was collected by Osman-Hill in the Canal Zone and its testicular structure was indistinguishable from that of captive males. It is not known whether this specimen was obtained directly from the forest or had been held in captivity for some time. Testes from a range of New World monkeys which died in captivity all exhibited a normal testicular structure (*Cebus apella*, *Lagothrix lagotricha*, *Ateles geoffroyi*, *Pithecia pithecia*, *Saguinus oedipus*, *Saguinus fuscicollis*, *Leontopithecus rosalia* and *Callithrix jacchus*). A scanning image analyser was used to measure cross-sectional areas of seminiferous tubules and intertubular tissue in testes from *Aotus* and other New World primates (Fig. 7). Although owl monkeys had a large

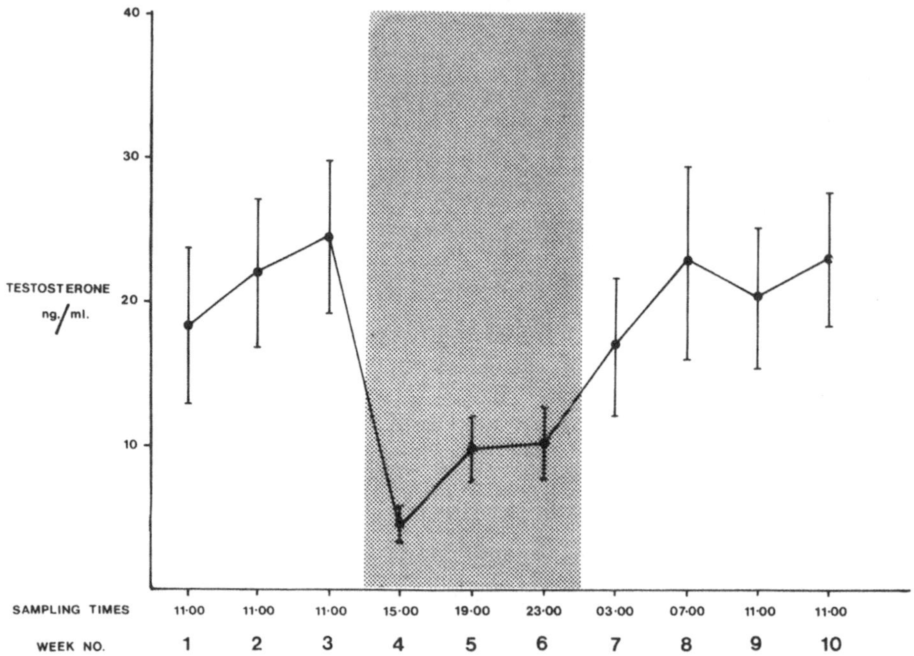

Fig. 6. Concentrations of plasma testosterone (mean ± s.e.m.) in adult male owl monkeys sampled once weekly at different times of day during 10 consecutive weeks. Stippled area = period of darkness. N = 6 for weeks 1-3 and 5 for weeks 4-10.

amount of intertubular tissue in their testes, other members of the Cebidae (*Lagothrix*, *Pithecia*) also had larger amounts of intertubular tissue than the Callitrichid species examined. The seminiferous tubules of the owl monkey were smaller in transverse section than those of other species. However, this was not an absolute distinction for the cebids also tended to have smaller cross-sectional areas to their tubules than the callitrichids. There are insufficient data at present to be sure whether these findings represent a taxonomic difference but the possibility is worthy of further study. It is also relevant to suggest that when comparative studies of testicular size in primates are carried out, investigators should attempt to measure the various compartments of the testis rather than employing only gross measurements such as testicular weight or volume.

GESTATION AND INTERBIRTH-INTERVALS

Estimates of the gestation period in the owl monkey vary considerably (126 days[61], 133 days[21], 148-159 days[15,16]). Although the estimate of 133 days by Hunter *et al*[21] refers to one female, it is based on a single timed mating and is therefore accurate. Female owl monkeys have given birth as little as 138 days after being paired with males for the first time. Hence earlier estimates of five months for the gestation period, which were derived from data on inter-birth intervals, are

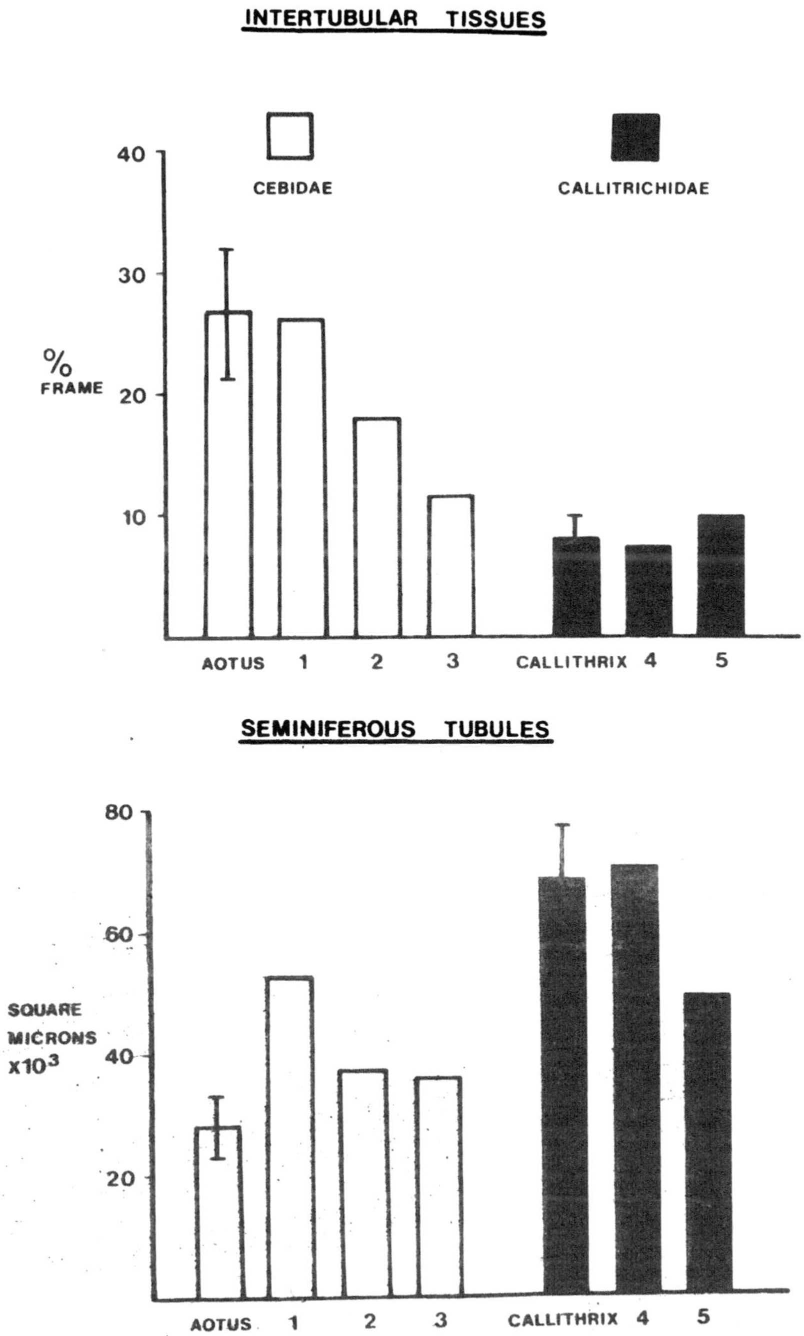

Fig. 7. Cross sectional areas of intertubular tissue and seminiferous tubules in transverse sections of testes from *Aotus* and six other species of New World monkeys. Data for *Aotus* and *Callithrix jacchus* are means (± standard deviation) for nine specimens of each genus. The remaining data refer to a single specimen of 1) *Cebus apella*, 2) *Lagothrix lagotricha*, 3) *Pithecia pithecia*, 4) *Saguinus fuscicollis*, and 5) *Leontopithecus rosalia*. Three scans were made on each section using an image analyser and the percentage area of each scan occupied by intertubular tissue was calculated. 90 tubules were also measured on each section and the mean cross sectional area calculated.

probably incorrect.

Chorionic gonadotrophin is detectable in the urine of owl monkeys from 16 weeks pre partum until birth (Fig. 8). Hall and Hodgen[61] found that a subhuman primate pregnancy test kit (developed by NIH in the USA) was 94% accurate in diagnosing pregnancy in the owl monkey between the 14th week pre partum and the final week of gestation. We have found this kit to be most useful in the management of a captive breeding programme for owl monkeys. However, urine samples should be treated in a fresh condition; if they are frozen and stored prior to testing then faint false positive results may occur.

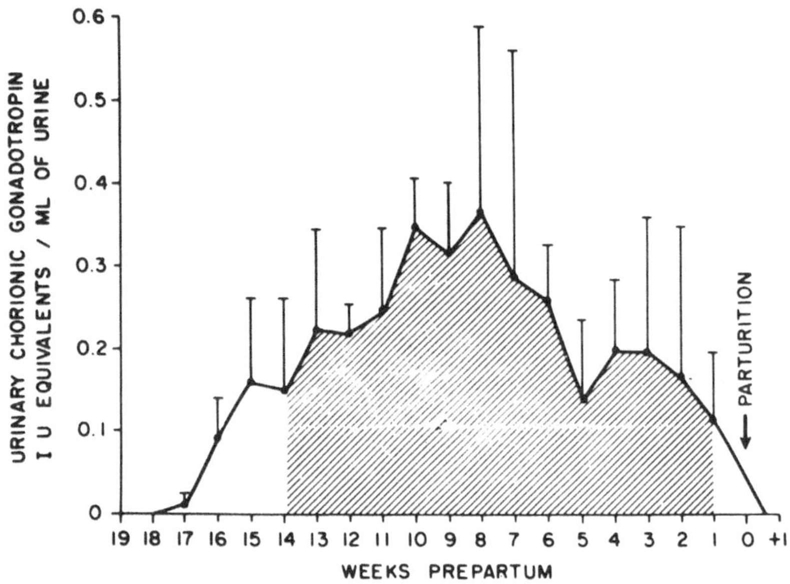

Fig. 8. Urinary gonadotrophin measurements during pregnancy in five owl monkeys. 94% of subhuman primate pregnancy tests were positive over the time interval indicated by cross-hatching.
After Hall and Hodgen[61], with the permission of the American Association for Laboratory Animal Science.

Inter-birth intervals for the owl monkey are shown in Fig. 9 and range from 166-419 days. The mean inter-birth interval is 253 days. Thus, in captivity, a female owl monkey will produce one offspring every 8 months on average. There is no obvious pattern in the distribution of inter-birth intervals, such as would be expected if a post-partum "oestrus" occurred. Detailed behavioural observations on eight groups of owl monkeys during 4 months after birth of an infant confirm that there is no post partum "oestrus". In the common marmoset, by contrast, there is an "oestrus" at 7-10 days post partum[33,62].

Under conditions of controlled lighting and heating, owl monkeys show no apparent annual birth peak or birth season (Fig. 9). Reports from the wild are fragmentary and it is not know whether the owl monkey is a seasonal breeder under natural conditions[7].

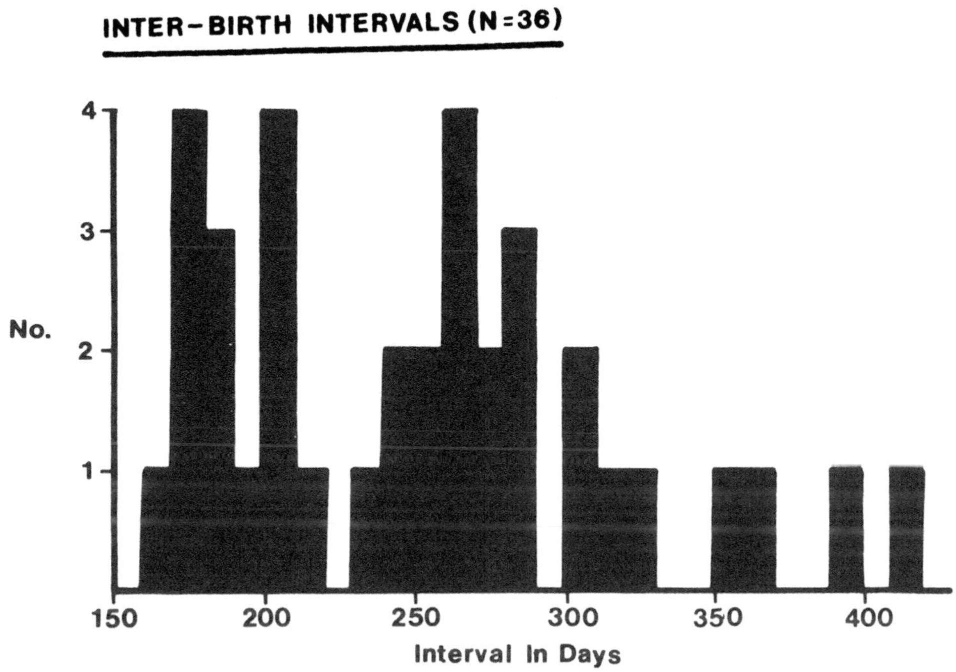

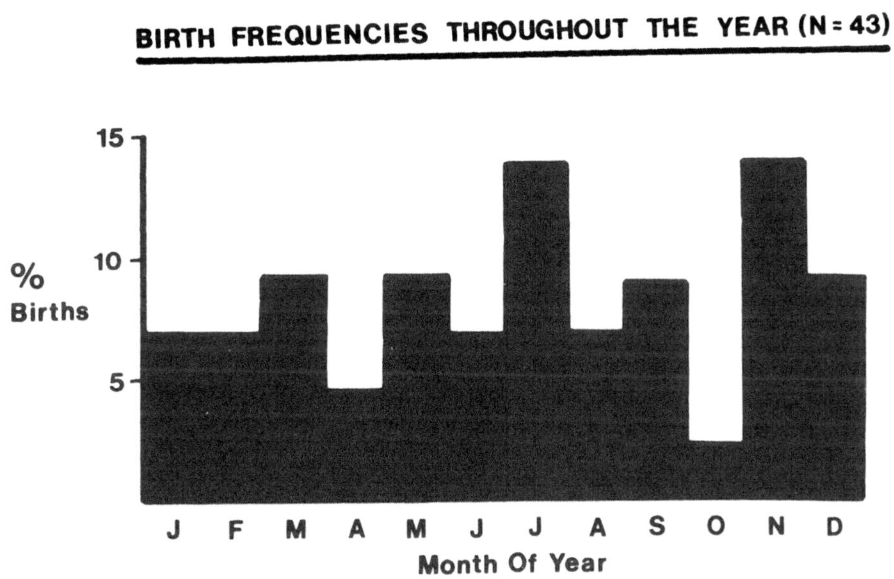

Fig. 9. Inter-birth intervals and birth frequencies throughout the year in a captive colony of Colombian owl monkeys. All data refer to animals kept under controlled conditions of heating and lighting as described in the text.

PARENTAL BEHAVIOUR AND DEVELOPMENT OF THE OFFSPRING

Newborn owl monkeys weigh between 90-105 grammes (N = 4, mean body weight = 96.5g). The pelage is well-developed at birth except that the abdomen and inner surfaces of the limbs are sparsely covered with fine hair. The black tri-radiate markings on the infant's head join to form a single stripe which extends across the scalp and down the centre of the back. These markings are quite conspicuous as the infant clings against the pale ventral side of its parent. The newborn clings to the parent in a distinctive ventro-lateral posture (Plate I) which Meritt[16] has aptly termed the "thigh-hip position". Distinctive infant clinging positions occur in a number of primates (eg. transversely on the mother's ventrum in Lemur fulvus but longitudinally in L. catta[63]). In Chiropotes albinasus the infant may rest in the flexure of the mother's thigh but with its head pointing inwards towards her abdomen[64], and the same is true of Pithecia pithecia (author's observations). The clinging posture used by young owl monkeys is to some degree innate or subject to rapid learning within the first 24 hours after birth. In experiments in which the mother was tranquilized on the day of giving birth and restrained in an upright position infants were still able to move into a ventro-lateral clinging position (Fig. 10 and Plate II). Three infants were

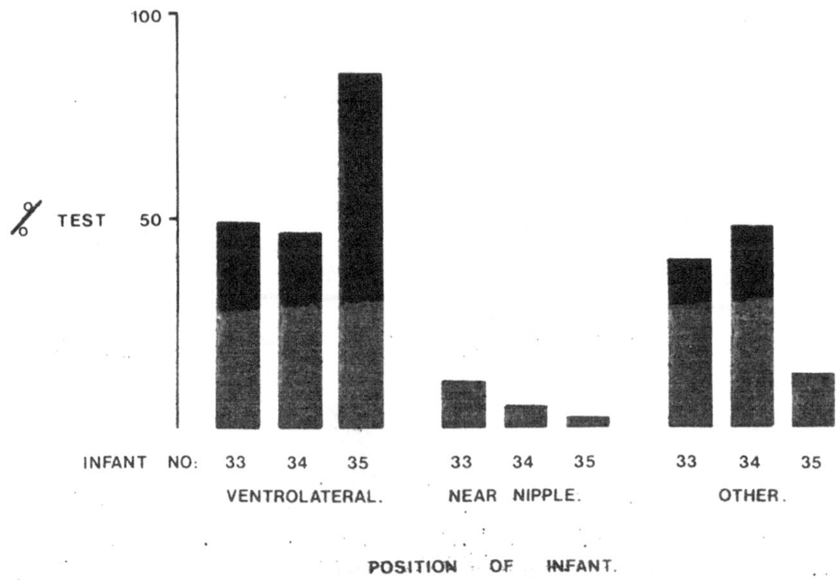

Fig. 10. Positional behaviour by infant owl monkeys after tranquillization of the mother. Data are expressed as percentages of the total observation time (4 x 5 minute trials, infants 33 and 35; 5 x 5 minute trials, infant 34).

studied and four or five consecutive trials each lasting 5 minutes were conducted, during which the infant was removed from the mother's body and immediately replaced at shoulder level. Infants showed a strong upward climbing response (Plate IIa) but spent relatively little time near the nipple, although rhythmic side to side head movements were observed when in this area (Plate IIb). A large portion of each test was spent in a ventro-lateral clinging posture (Plate IIc, d). Whereas infants were very mobile and vocal when in other positions they tended to remain immobile or to sleep when in the ventro-lateral position. Since infants failed to reach a ventro-lateral position during some trials, or climbed upwards persistently and gave distress calls, it seems that the mother also plays an important role in positioning the newborn.

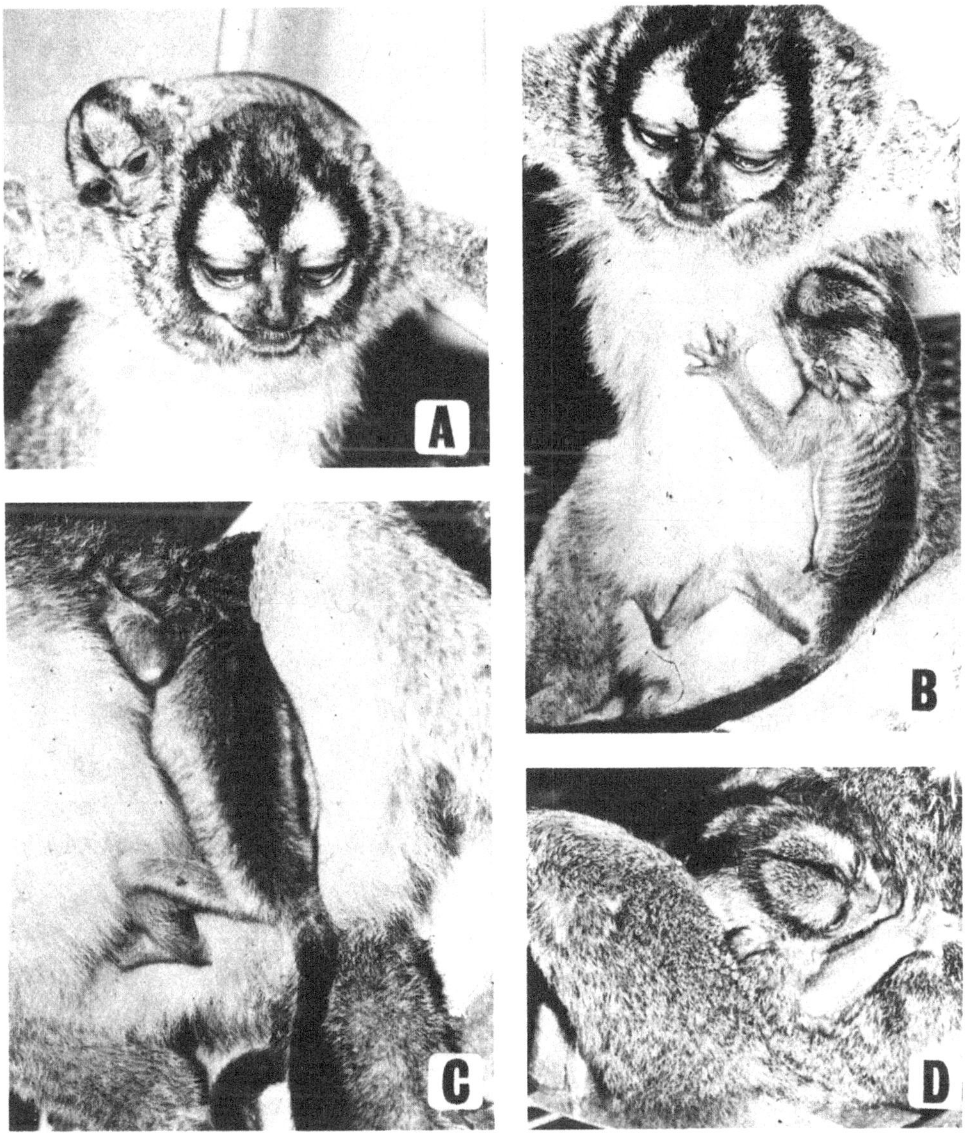

Plate II. Positional behaviour in newborn owl monkeys after tranquillization of the mother. A. Infant shows a strong upward climbing response and comes to rest clinging laterally to the mother's neck. B. Suckling behaviour. C. Infant moving into a ventro-lateral clinging position. D. Ventro-lateral clinging posture to show orientation of infant's head.

Male owl monkeys, as well as females, play a major role in carrying and caring for their offspring. Such involvement of the male has been described in various callitrichid species (Callithrix jacchus[65]; Leontopithecus rosalia[66]; Saguinus fuscicollis[67]) and some other monogamous primates such as the siamang[68]. Detailed observations of parental behaviour and infant development were made on 7 captive groups of owl monkeys containing 10 infants, and supplementary data were collected on a further 6 groups and 23 offspring[25]. The first observed occurrences of selected behaviours in infant owl monkeys are shown in Table 3.

Table 3. Age of first observed occurrence of selected behaviours in 10 infant owl monkeys

Infant No.	Sex	Day of first observation	Transfers	Clings dorsally	Gets off	Eats solid food	"Urine-washes"
2	M	5	5	5	40	45	101
3	M	6	6	6	35	35	70
4	F	1	3	3	22	35	63
5	M	1	2	2	26	48	105
12	M	2	2	2	23	37	62
13	M	1	1	1	37	47	109
14	M	2	2	2	27	48	109
15	M	1	2	1	26	39	76
CZ_1	M	3	3	6	46	60	141
CZ_2	F	1	1	1	34	42	48
	Range		1-6	1-6	22-46	35-60	48-141
	Median		2	2	30.5	43.5	88.5

Development is rapid and the offspring may transfer from the female to the male parent on the day of birth in some groups. Dorsal clinging may be observed as early as the first day but it is not until the offspring is between 3 and 4 weeks of age that dorsal clinging begins to replace the ventro-lateral posture as the major position in which the infant rests on the parent. The offspring first begins to get off the parent between 22 and 46 days and it begins to eat solid food at between 35 and 60 days. The growth of independence of the offspring is a complex process, in which the parents play different roles. As can be seen in Fig. 11A there is an obvious sex difference in carrying behaviour; females carry their offspring most of the time during the first post-natal week but therefore the male performs this function and the infant transfers to its mother mainly in order to suckle. Time spent on the male peaks during week 3 and then shows a gradual decline. This correlates with the fact that from week 4 or 5 onwards infants spend increasing amounts of time off their parents (Fig. 11B). The number of "time off" episodes is greatest between weeks 7 and 11 but then declines as the infant spends progressively longer periods without returning to its parents. By the 18th week, offspring move independently of their parents most of the time, but should any disturbance occur, they invariably return to the adult male and attempt to re-establish contact.

Female owl monkeys suckle their offspring for periods lasting from 7 seconds to 2 minutes 40 seconds (146 cases: mean bout duration = 27 seconds). In owl monkeys, as in other New World primates, the nipples are axillary in position

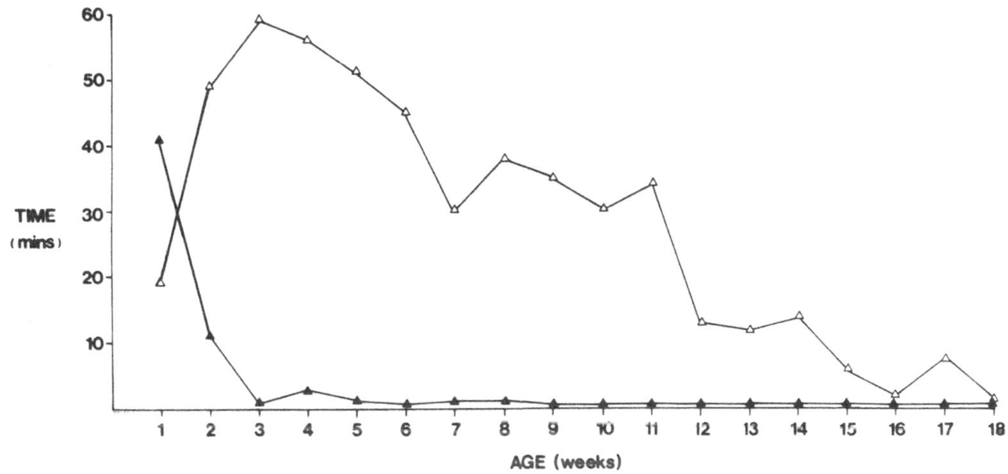

Fig. 11A. Time spent by infant owl monkeys on each parent: ▲ on female parent; Δ on male parent

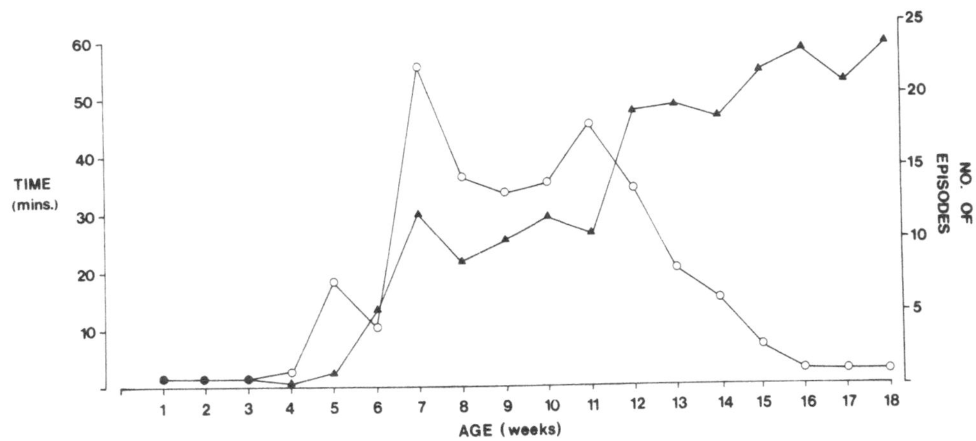

Fig. 11B. Time spent "off" parents by infant owl monkeys: ▲ time off; O number of time off episodes. Data are median values for seven family groups containing a single offspring.

and the female usually lifts her arm slightly in order to facilitate the infant's attempts to suckle. The infant makes rapid side to side head movements as it seeks the nipple and it may shift from one nipple to the other a number of times during each suckling bout (range 1-9, mean 1.57). Owl monkeys rarely remain on the nipple except to suckle, in contrast to many Old World monkey species (eg. rhesus monkeys[69]; baboons[70]). Fig. 12 shows that suckling frequencies decline from an average of 1.0 bouts/hour in weeks 1-3 to a mean of 0.27/hour during weeks 16-18. Forty of the 146 suckling bouts (ie. 27%) were followed immediately by maternal rejections which consisted of biting the infant's tail, hands and feet. The infant promptly transferred to the male parent after 90% of such rejection episodes. The patterning of post-suckling rejection behaviour varies according to the infant's age and is highest (65%) at between 4 and 6 weeks of age (Fig. 12). This is the period when the offspring

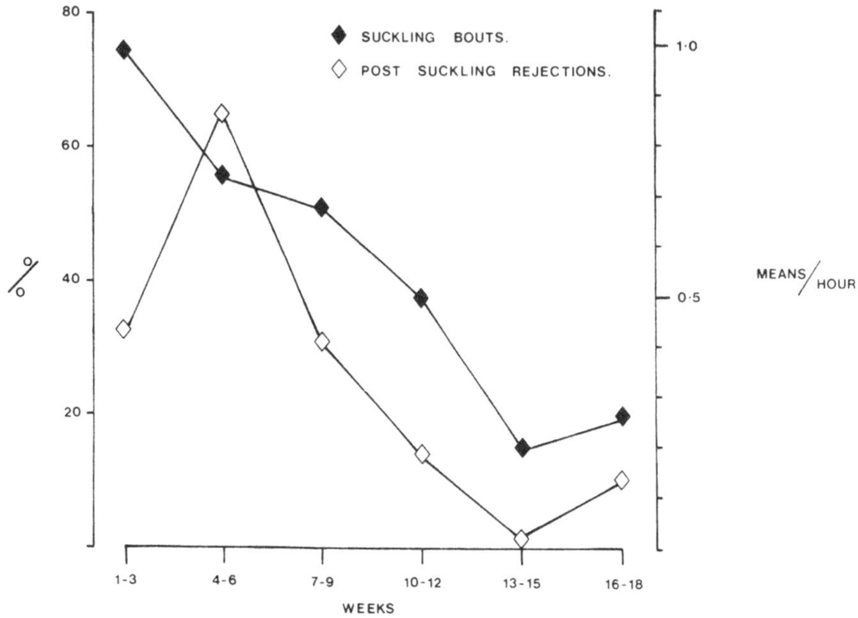

Fig. 12. Frequencies of suckling (◆) and of maternal rejection after suckling (◇) in owl monkeys. Data for 10 infants in 7 family groups. Data on suckling bouts expressed as mean frequencies/hour/week. Post suckling rejections are expressed as percentages.

begins to take solid food, so it is possible that the mother's punitive behaviour plays some role in the weaning process. In Harlow's[71] studies of maternal-infant attachment in rhesus monkeys, one classic experiment provided infants with a choice between two "surrogate mothers", which offered them tactile comfort or a supply of milk. Infants spent more time clinging to surrogates which were covered with soft material rather than to wire mesh surrogates which possessed a milk supply. In a sense, the parental system of owl monkeys provides a natural parallel to this experimental situation. Female owl monkeys provide their offspring with milk but reject them more frequently than males when they are between 2 and 8 weeks of age (Fig. 13A). The infant transfers actively to the male, which provides tactile comfort, warmth, etc., and moves to the female only to suckle. Males rarely reject their offspring before they are 8 weeks old, but then frequencies of paternal rejections increase and exceed the maternal values (Fig. 13A). Many of these rejections occur in response to the infant's attempts to re-establish contact with the male after a "time off" episode. The male's behaviour may be important in encouraging the offspring to spend longer periods on its own and hence may contribute to the growth of its independence.

Hinde and Spencer-Booth[69] and Hinde[72] have employed a method of measuring maintenance of proximity between parent and offspring which is useful when applied to the owl monkey. The formula $\%AP-\%L_{inf}$ refers to the percentage of approaches (AP) and leavings (L) which are due to the offspring rather than its parent. The results in Fig.13B show that during weeks 5 and 6 (when there are negative values for the equation) it is principally the adult male which is responsible for maintaining proximity between itself and the offspring. From week 7 or 8 onwards the situation is reversed and negative values are replaced by positive or occasional zero values.

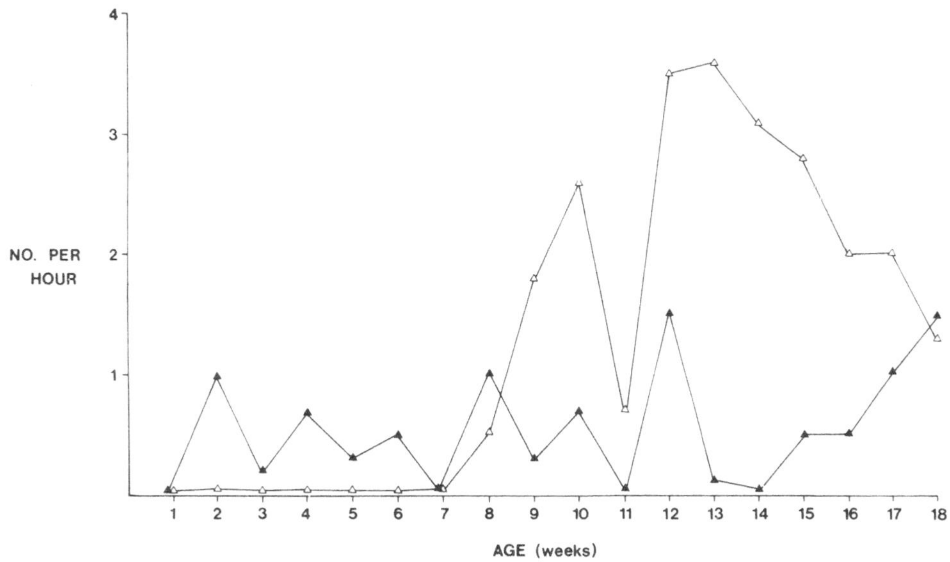

Fig. 13A. Rejection of infant owl monkeys by their parents: ▲ female rejects infant; Δ male rejects infant

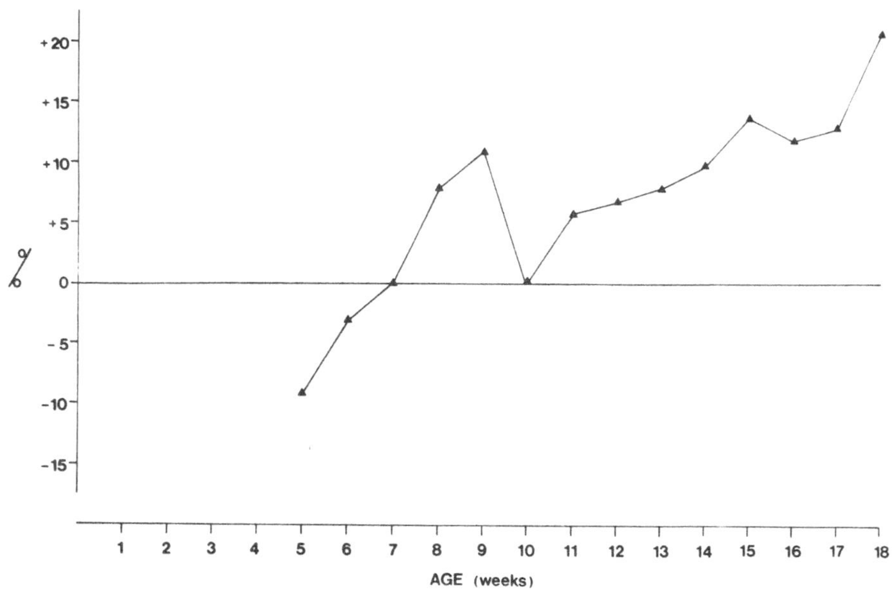

Fig. 13B. %AP-Linf for infant owl monkeys and their male parents. Data are mean frequencies/hour/week. Median values for 7 family groups containing a single offspring

The greater development of paternal behaviour among monogamous primates is consistent with a higher degree of "parental investment" by males of these species[73]. In the marmoset, which may produce two sets of twins annually and which has a post-partum "oestrus", male and female parents exhibit quite similar curves for carrying and rejection behaviour[65]. In the owl monkey, which normally produces a single offspring and has a longer interbirth interval with no post-partum matings, each male sires less offspring than does his counterpart in a marmoset group. It is tempting to speculate that the greater degree of paternal behaviour in the owl monkey has been selected for on the basis of sociobiological factors. However, it is the case that some monogamous primates exhibit very little paternal behaviour (*Indri indri*[74]; *Hylobates lar*[75]). If parental investment is such a powerful selective force it is hard to explain the above facts, even if it is argued that the male indri or gibbon expresses the majority of his "investment" in offspring in some other fashion, such as by territorial defence. Male and female owl monkeys are very similar in size and a five week old infant weighs as much as 200 grammes, which is 20% of maternal body weight. Paternal carrying behaviour is probably adaptive in this context as well, particularly since the species has a low basal metabolic rate[76,77] and females might be unable to carry the infant full time, lactate, and search for food. Older siblings also carry infants occasionally but such behaviour is less frequent than in some callitrichid species (eg. *Callithrix jacchus*[78]; *Leontopithecus rosalia*[66]; *Saguinus fuscicollis*[79]).

Sassenrath *et al*[80] have reported that in some male Callicebus monkeys testosterone levels decrease during the period when they are transporting offspring. We have measured levels of testosterone and prolactin in adult male owl monkeys. These males were either transporting offspring aged less than 10 weeks or had no infants at the time blood samples were taken. Fig. 14 shows that testosterone levels in males carrying offspring averaged 19.2 ± 1.93 ng/ml (mean ± s.e.m.) and prolactin levels were 2.3 ± 0.32 ng/ml. In males not transporting young infants testosterone levels were 15.21 ± 1.25 ng/ml and prolactin 1.7 ± 0.23 ng/ml. The slight elevation of prolactin and testosterone levels in males with young offspring is not statistically significant, however. The prolactin assay employed has been validated for use on the common marmoset[81] but not on other New World primates. Further, in the present study, blood samples were collected from tranquillized monkeys and the process of capturing or tranquillizing animals (using ketamine hydrochloride) might have affected prolactin levels. The results shown in Fig. 14 therefore represent preliminary findings.

Maynard-Smith[82] points out that it is interesting that male lactation has not developed in association with paternal behaviour in mammals since males could then share the burden of feeding offspring as well as carrying them. However, such changes would involve central dopaminergic mechanisms and might severely affect the male's sexual behaviour. Thus, when hyperprolactinaemia occurs in human males, it is associated not only with breast activity but with infertility and impotence[83].

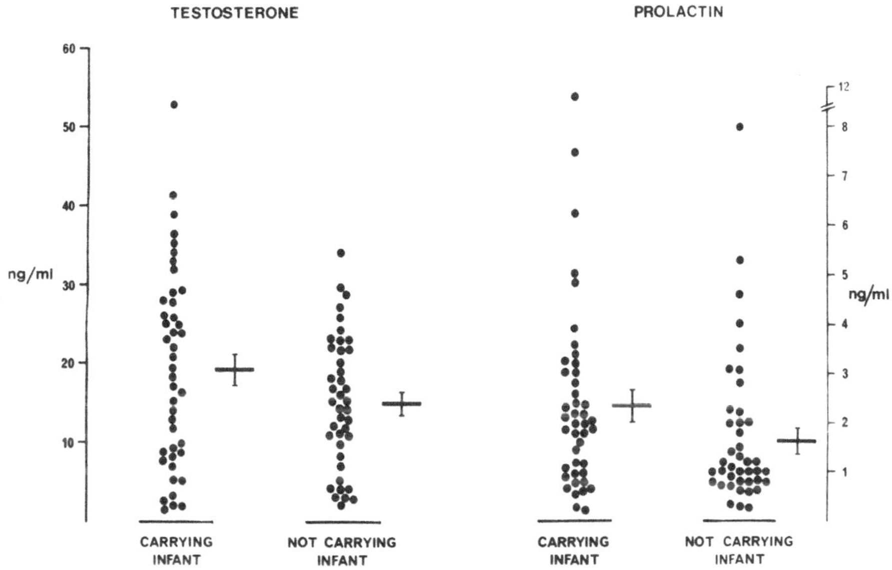

Fig. 14. Plasma testosterone and prolactin levels in male owl monkeys which are either carrying infants aged less than 10 weeks or have no infant offspring in their groups. Horizontal bars = means, vertical bars = standard errors of means.

PHYSICAL AND HORMONAL CHANGES DURING PUBERTY

Measurements of circulating testosterone provide a sensitive indicator of the age of onset of puberty in males, since hormone levels begin to rise before secondary sexual characteristics develop and before spermatogenesis is completed. Longitudinal measurements of plasma testosterone during development in six male owl monkeys are shown in Fig. 15. Data on testicular growth, body weight and development of the subcaudal glandular complex were also obtained from the same animals[23]. Testosterone was first detected in the plasma of males when they were between 211 and 337 days of age (median 313 days). Larger rises in levels of the hormone were measurable between 300 and 400 days. Male owl monkeys enter puberty at a surprisingly early age, particularly when it is considered that in common marmosets, which weigh half as much, puberty begins at about 250 days[84]. In man, the first increases in plasma testosterone during puberty occur at night[85]. All the blood samples from male owl monkeys were collected during the illuminated phase of the lighting cycle, when these nocturnal animals were resting or asleep. It is possible that the earliest rises in pubertal testosterone were detected, rather than the later general increases which are measurable in plasma from active monkeys.

Figs. 16 and 17 show data on growth in testicular volume and body weight in young males as compared to sexually mature animals. Even in adulthood the testes of the owl monkeys are very small (range 378-673mm^3, median 514mm^3) and errors of measurement can lead to incorrect calculations of testicular volumes during development. This may account for the fact that although testicular

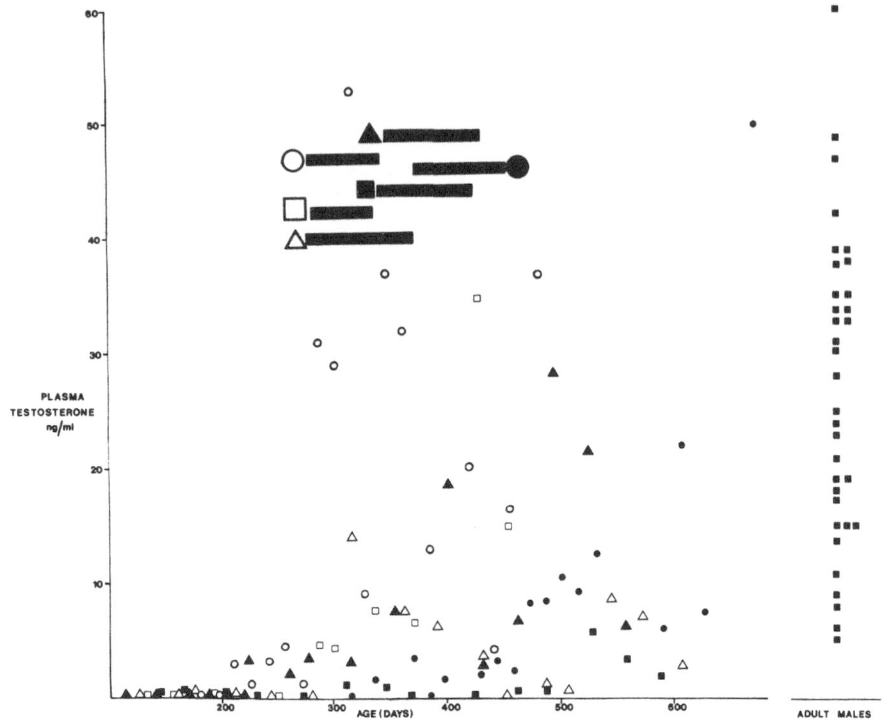

Fig. 15. Plasma testosterone levels and growth of the subcaudal gland in six male owl monkeys aged between 114 and 711 days. Male 2 (▲), male 3 (△), male 5 (□), male 7 (■), male 4829 (O), male 4465 (●). Values for adult males are shown on the right (■) for comparative purposes. Horizontal bars indicate the time which elapsed between the first appearance and the complete development of specialized subcaudal hairs in each male.

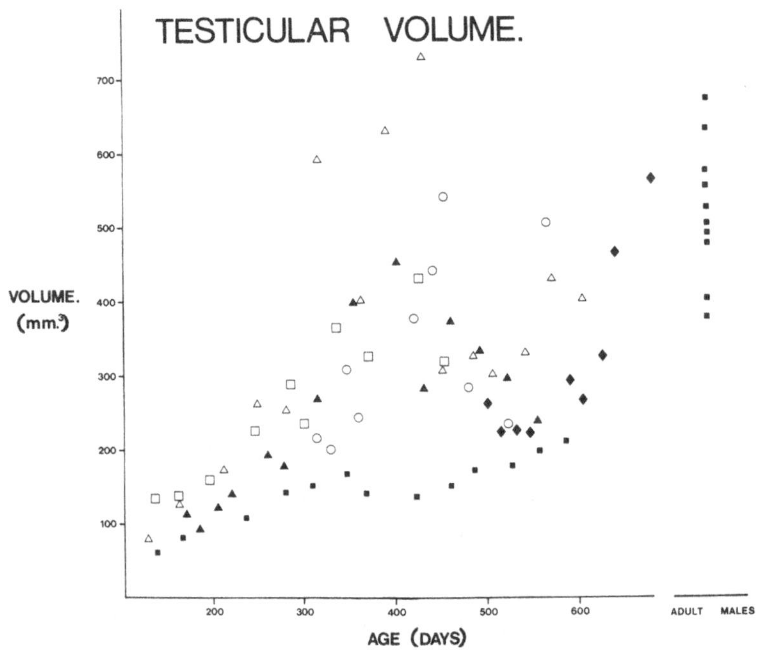

Fig. 16. Mean testis volume in six male owl monkeys aged between 114 and 711 days. Symbols as in Fig. 15. Individual values for adult males are shown on the right.

volume increased in all subjects, consecutive measurements fluctuated considerably and there were no pronounced changes during puberty.

Males first entered the body weight range for adults (800-1080g) when they were between 370 and 520 days of age (median 472 days). Since owl monkeys are monomorphic it is not surprising that no obvious adolescent "growth spurt" occurred (Fig. 17), such as has been reported for various catarrhine primates.

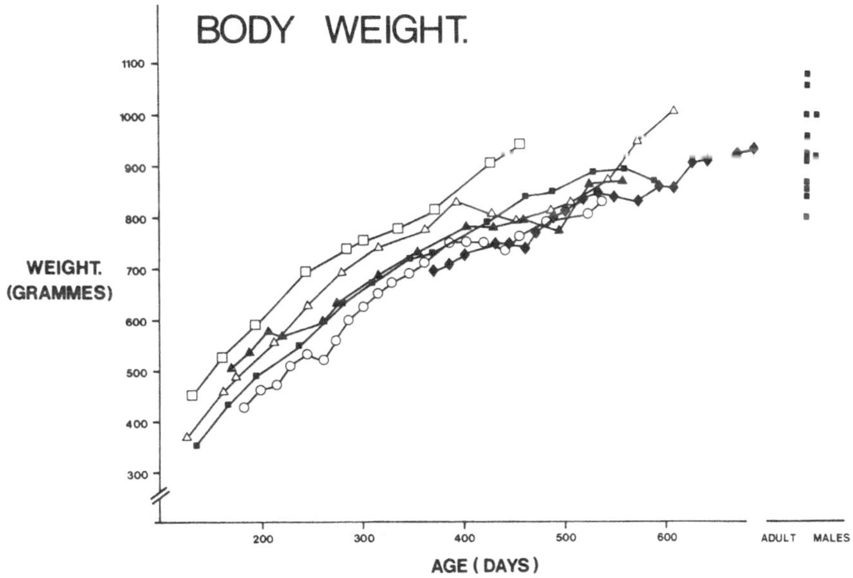

Fig. 17. Body weights of six owl monkeys aged between 114 and 711 days. Symbols as in Fig. 15. Individual values for adult males are shown on the right.

A more useful external indicator of pubertal development was provided by growth of the subcaudal scent-marking gland. This subcaudal complex was not present in juvenile males (Plate IIIa) but at between 282 and 370 days (median 316) the hairs in the subcaudal region began to stiffen and turn brownish in colour (Plate IIIb). A fully mature appearance of the gland (Plate IIIc) was apparent when six males were aged between 336 and 442 (median 397 days). As can be seen in Fig. 15 development of the gland correlates with increasing levels of testosterone during puberty. Administration of testosterone to one prepubertal male caused the gland to develop prematurely and it had reached adult appearance by 278 days. The external appearance of the gland remains unchanged after castration in adulthood (Plate IIId) as is the case with the circumgenital-suprapubic glands of *Saguinus fuscicollis*[86], although no studies have been conducted to examine histological changes in either species. The subcaudal gland consists of numerous sebaceous and apocrine components[87] and these are poorly developed in the prepubertal animal[88].

Although no quantitative studies have been carried out it seems that female owl monkeys grow at a similar rate to males and that the subcaudal gland

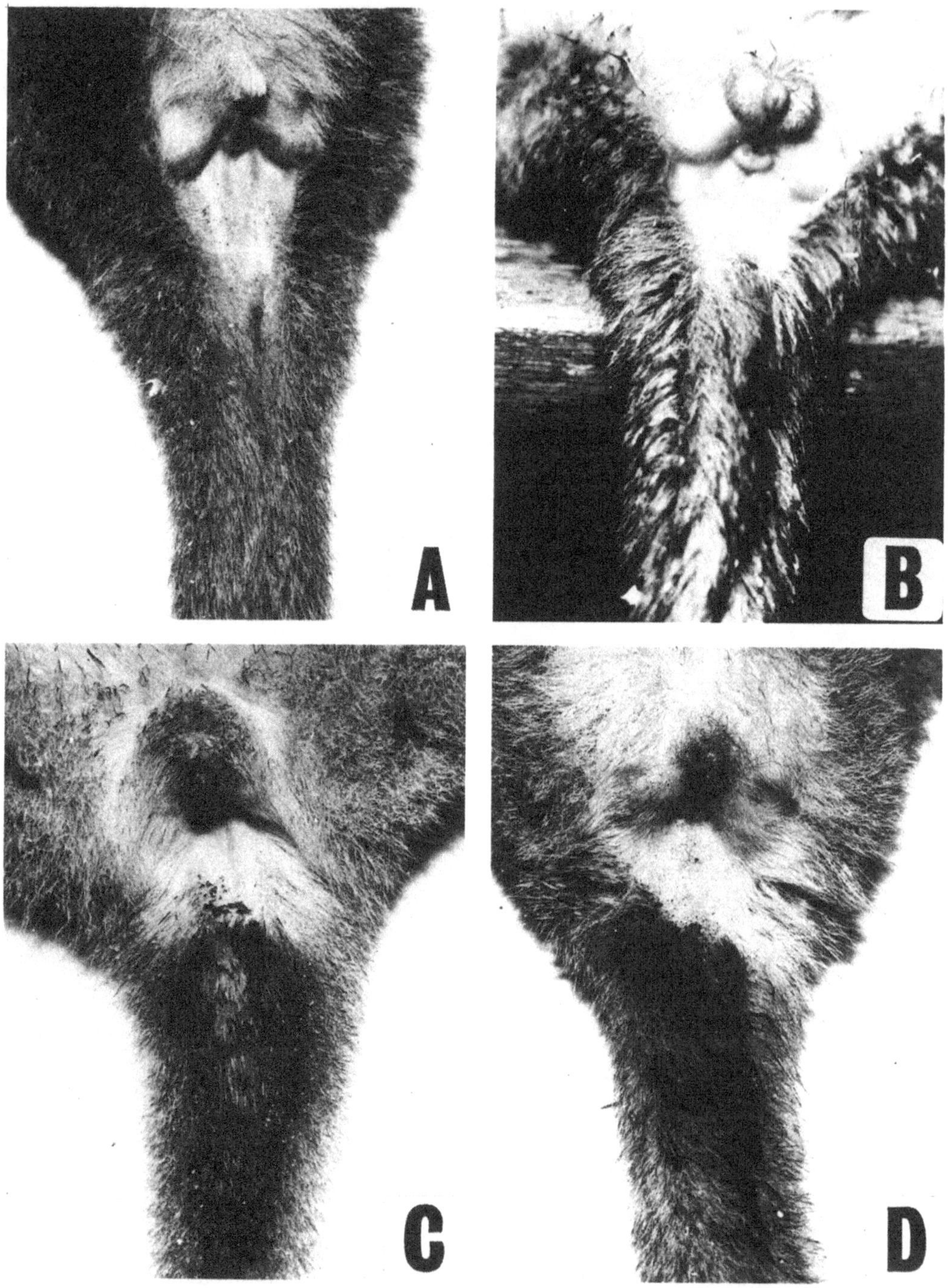

PLATE III. The subcaudal gland of the owl monkey. A. Juvenile male: no glandular development. B. Pubertal male with a partially developed gland. C. An adult male with a fully developed gland. D. An adult male 3 years after castration; the stiff, dark hairs of the subcaudal gland are still obvious. Note that in all males the external genitalia are inconspicuous.

develops at the same age in both sexes. By comparison with data on other monogamous species (eg. Callithrix jacchus[84]) it may be inferred that sexual maturity is attained at a similar age in males and females. Four captive born animals from our colony have produced offspring so far and although there is no precise information on the age of first fertile matings it is probable that owl monkeys are reproductively mature by 18-24 months.

CHANGES IN SOCIAL ORGANIZATION DURING PUBERTY

In some monogamous New World primates it has been found that only one pair of adults in a group is reproductively active[84]. In the owl monkey, maturing offspring rarely show any signs of sexual activity. In over 500 hours of observations on 7 captive groups there were no copulations which involved offspring of mature age. One male was seen to make thrusting movements against branches on a single occasion but no attempts at mounting were recorded. Concentrations of plasma testosterone in such males were apparently normal (Fig. 15: males 3, 5 and 7) and did not differ from males caged outside family groups (males 2, 4829 and 4465). There was no indication that puberty was in any way retarded in males which remained in their natal groups. We have not studied levels of circulating or urinary steroids in maturing female offspring so it is not known whether any repression of development occurs in the female owl monkey. It should be borne in mind that, quite apart from endocrine mechanisms, there may be social factors which inhibit sexual activity between closely related animals. Inhibition of son-mother matings have been reported for rhesus monkeys[89]. One would expect social factors to play an important role in the choice of sexual partners in species, like the owl monkey, which live in small family groups.

These problems naturally lead to the question of how new family groups arise in the owl monkey and other monogamous primate species. Male and female offspring may become peripheralized as they reach sexual maturity (eg. Hylobates lar[90,91]; Symphalangus syndactylus[68,92]; Callithrix jacchus[65]). Carpenter[90] suggested that as young gibbons mature, their parents become aggressive towards them and drive them from the group. However, various field-workers have suggested that the offspring itself plays an active role in the process of peripheralization[91,92]. In captive family groups of owl monkeys there is no evidence that levels of aggression increase between parents and offspring when the latter pass through puberty. Data on three maturing males and their parents are shown in Fig. 18. Aggression in such groups is infrequent (usually less than one occurrence per hour) and consists of pushing or nipping conspecifics rather than severe attacks. Similar results were obtained from three groups containing female offspring and there was no indication of increasing aggression between adults and mature offspring of the same sex. However, measurements of aggressive interactions alone provide a poor indicator of social relationships in these

TESTOSTERONE AND AGGRESSIVE BEHAVIOUR DURING PUBERTY IN MALES.

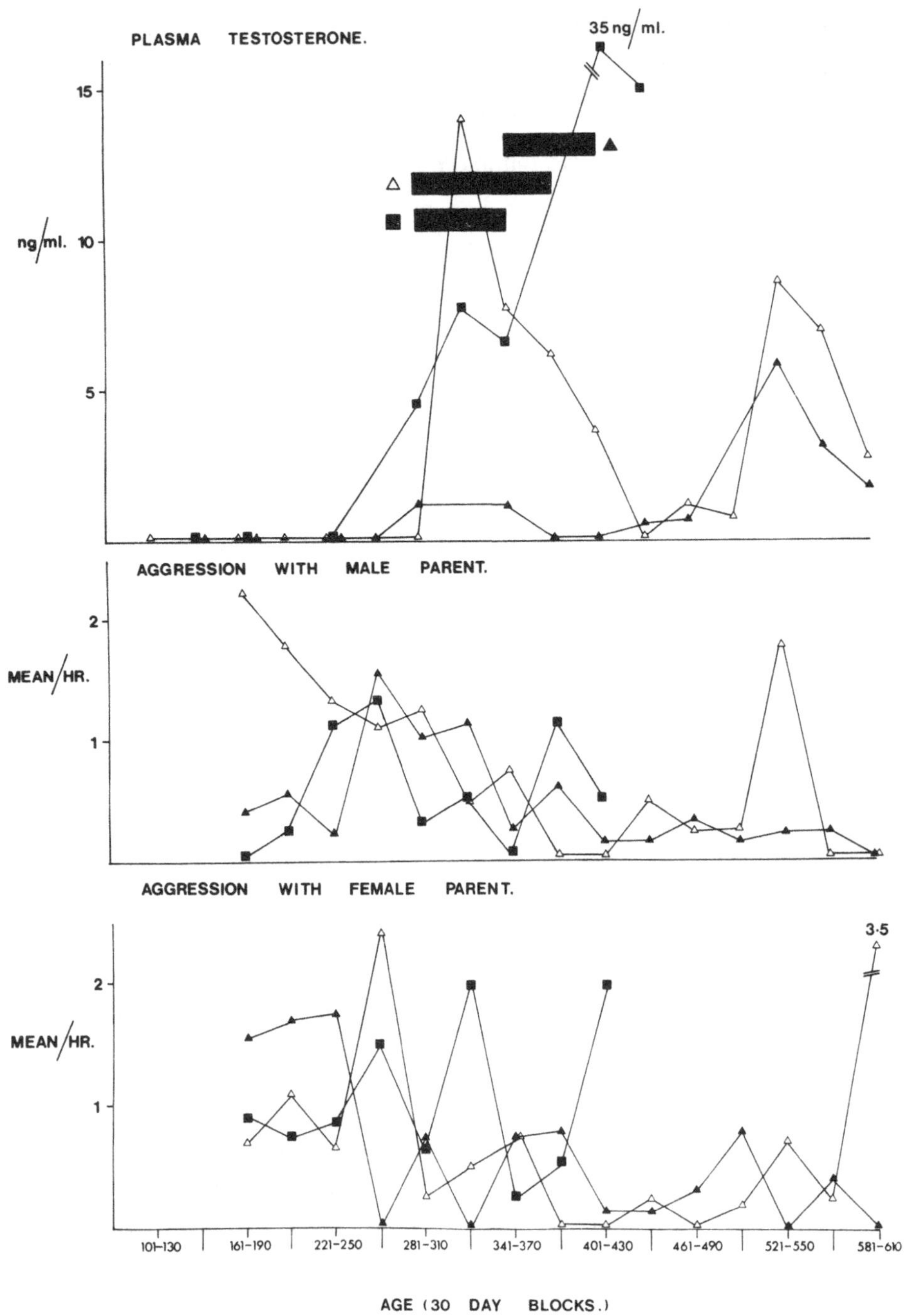

Fig. 18. Frequencies of aggression between young male owl monkeys (No.3 △, No.5 ■, No.7 ▲) and their parents, compared with repeated measures of circulating testosterone during puberty. Horizontal bars indicate the timing of rapid growth of the subcaudal gland in each male. Behavioural data were collected during 166 hours of observation on three family groups. Data are expressed as means/hour during consecutive 30-day periods.

family groups. Data were also collected on frequencies of play, grooming, food-sharing and proximity between parents and their offspring. None of these behaviours showed consistent changes as young animals in the groups passed through puberty. As can be seen in Fig. 19 male parents showed a tendency to interact with their offspring more than did female parents, particularly in the case of grooming behaviour. Thus it appears that the closer relationship established between adult males and infants continues to some extent when the latter approach maturity.

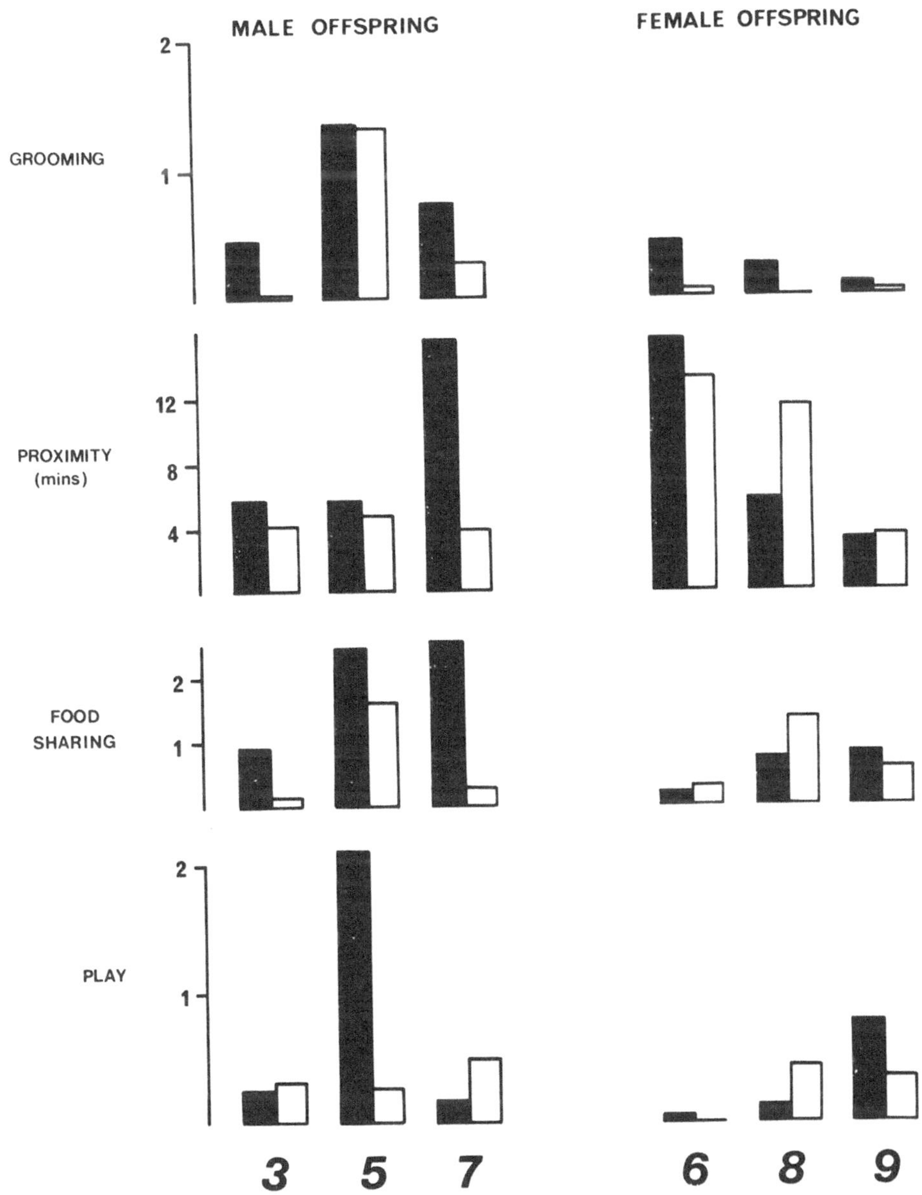

Fig. 19. Behavioural interactions between adult owl monkeys and their offspring aged between 160 and 550 days. Six family groups were studied containing three male offspring (3, 5, 7) and three females (6, 8, 9). ■ adult male-offspring interactions; □ adult female-offspring interactions. Data on male 5 were only collected until 430 days of age.

Fights between parents and older offspring do occasionally occur in captive owl monkey groups, particularly in groups containing three or more offspring. It is possible that under normal circumstances owl monkeys emigrate from their natal groups before they reach two years of age. It seems probable that emigration would be an active process and not simply an expulsion of maturing animals by their parents. In *Saguinus oedipus* juvenile animals sometimes interchange between groups in the wild[93]. Although adult owl monkeys are highly aggressive towards strange adult conspecifics of the same sex, they do not attack juveniles (Hunter and Dixson, unpublished observations). The possibility that immature owl monkeys interchange between groups in the wild should be investigated.

OLFACTORY COMMUNICATIONS AND REPRODUCTION

Most New World monkeys and prosimian primates employ scent-marking displays to deposit urine or the secretions of specialized cutaneous glands[94-96]. The possibility that olfactory communication plays an important role in the reproductive biology of New World primates has often been raised and there is experimental evidence to support this view. Epple's experiments on *Callithrix jacchus* and *Saguinus fuscicollis* have shown that odour cues can convey information about an individual's identity, sex, breeding condition and "dominance" within a family group[95]. Only the "dominant" male and female in groups of these callitrichid species are reproductively active and they also show higher frequencies of scent-marking than other group members. In the case of *S. fuscicollis* it is the female partner which shows the highest frequencies of marking behaviour (using the suprapubic glands) and which is most aggressive towards strange conspecifics[97]. There appear to be interspecific variations in these behaviours, however. Fig. 20 shows frequencies of scent marking behaviours in six captive family groups of owl monkeys. Adults of both sexes and immature offspring frequently mark using a stereotyped "urine washing" display. The ipsi-lateral hand and foot are placed together under the genital area and a few drops of urine are voided whilst the animal rubs the palm and sole together. This distinctive marking pattern occurs in some prosimian species (eg. *Galago crassicaudatus*, *Microcebus murinus*) as well as in certain Cebids (eg. *Cebus*, *Saimiri*, *Aotus*) and was probably present in the common ancestors of both groups. Urine washing may have non-communicatory functions such as in thermoregulation[98,99], but in the squirrel and Cebus monkeys, females may mark more frequently when they are sexually receptive and males pay additional attention to these cues[99-101]. This is not the case in captive owl monkeys, however. Immature animals of both sexes as well as adults usually employ the behaviour in non-sexual contexts. The display appears very early in ontogeny; at between 48-141 days in 10 captive born specimens (Table 3). By contrast, marking with the subcaudal glandular complex is much more frequent in adults than in immature animals. It is possible that this type of marking is influenced by gonadal hormones since it is rarely observed prior to puberty when the subcaudal gland enlarges. Even mature offspring in captive family groups show tail rubbing behaviour infrequently and it appears that the behaviour is repressed in non-breeding group members. Breeding males usually show the highest frequencies of tail rubbing (Fig. 20) although this is not an absolute rule and females in some groups may mark more often than their male partners.

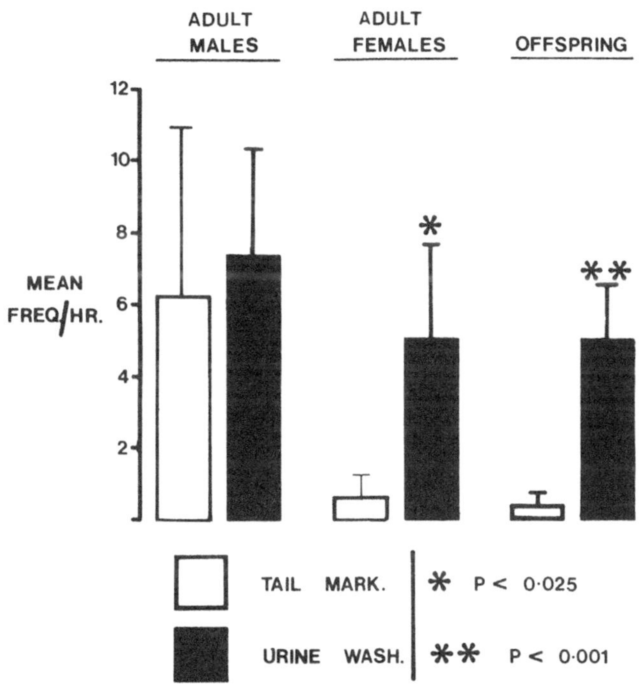

Fig. 20. Scent marking in six captive family groups of owl monkeys: frequencies of urine washing and tail marking. Adult males mark frequently by both methods whereas adult females and offspring urine wash significantly more frequently. Offspring in these groups (3 males, 3 females) were between 160 and 550 days old when behavioural data (333 hours) were collected.

In order to investigate the importance of olfactory cues in the sexual and aggressive behaviour of owl monkeys we have employed a reversible anosmia technique similar to that used by Michael and Keverne[102] in their studies of sexual communication in rhesus monkeys. Swabs of optical gauze impregnated with Bismuth-iodoform paste were inserted via the nares into the nasal cavity. Radiography was used to check the position of the plugs which were placed just below the cribriform plate (Plate IV). Two sets of behavioural experiments were performed[88]. In the first experiment, four males were tested for sexual behaviour under three conditions: 1, the males were untreated; 2, males were rendered partially anosmic using the procedure described above; and 3, males were retested after removal of the plugs. Eight tests were conducted under each condition and each male was always paired with the same female partner. Blocking input to the main olfactory bulbs had little influence on the males' sexual behaviour (Fig. 21). A significant decrease in anogential inspections by males

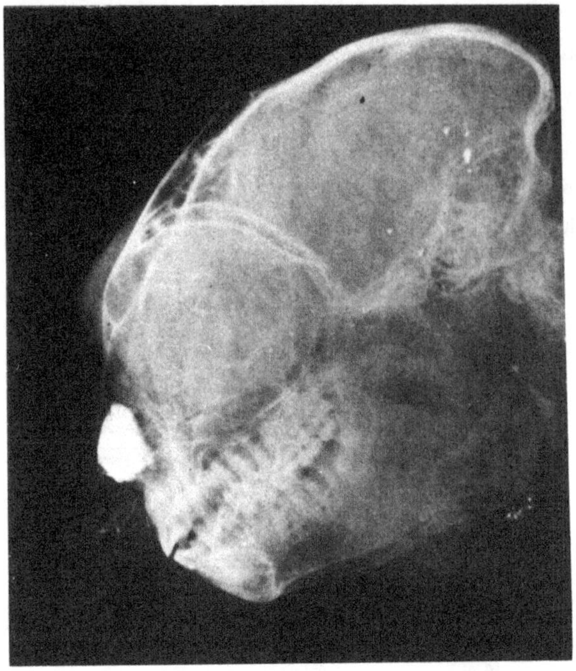

PLATE IV. Radiograph of the head of a male owl monkey in lateral view to show plugs containing bismuth iodoform paste which were inserted into the nasal passages. The effects of this method of inducing anosmia upon sexual and aggressive behaviour are described in the text.

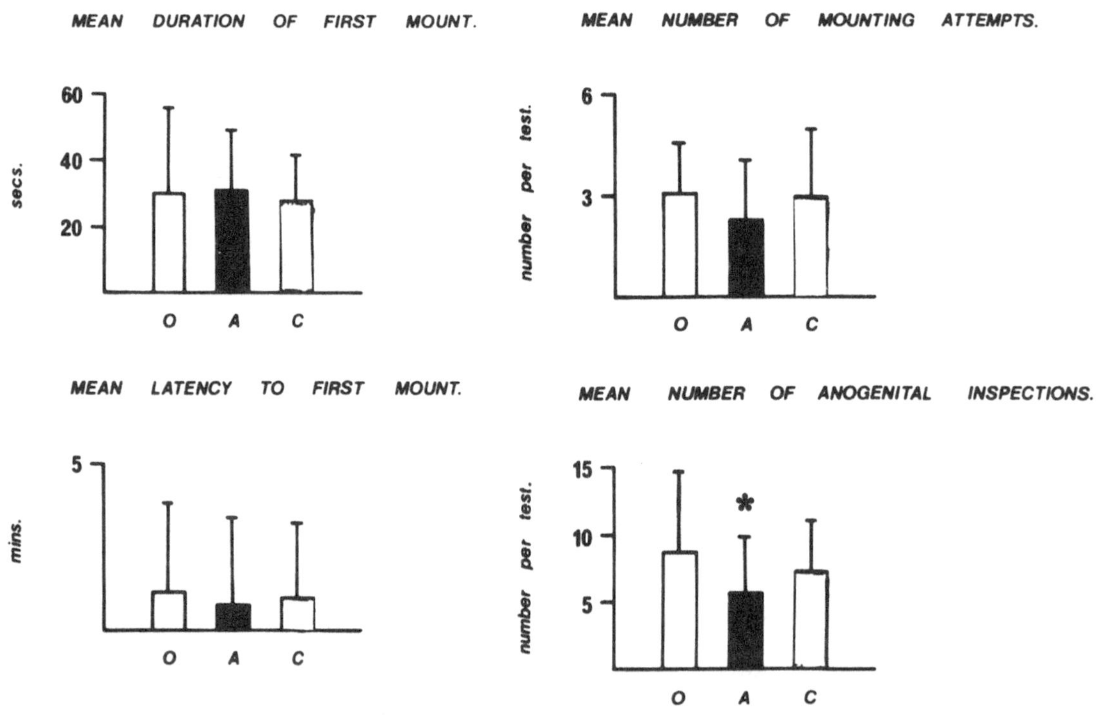

Fig. 21. Effects of partial anosmia upon sexual behaviour in four adult male owl monkeys. Males were rendered anosmic by inserting plugs containing anaesthetic paste into the nasal passages (see Plate 4 and text for explanation). Each male was tested 8 times with the same female; O = when untreated, A = when anosmic, and C = after removal of the plugs. Data are means ± s.e.m. for various behaviours by the male. A significant decrease in olfactory inspections (*$p<0.05$) occurred in anosmic males.

did occur. Latencies to first mount, frequencies and duration of mounts did not alter significantly, however. Sexual arousal and copulatory mechanisms were apparently not greatly influenced by the procedure. Some individual variations did occur; thus one male mounted the female during 63% of tests when anosmic as compared with 100% of tests prior to treatment and 88% after removal of the plugs. It is also the case that different results might have been obtained if males had been paired with unfamiliar females or if males in family groups had been studied since copulations are infrequent in that context. The technique used to induce anosmia did not block input to the accessory olfactory bulb via the vomeronasal organ, which is present in owl monkeys as in most New World monkeys and prosimian primates. The importance of the vomeronasal system in neuroendocrine function has been amply demonstrated in research on rodents[103,104], but there have been no studies on primates.

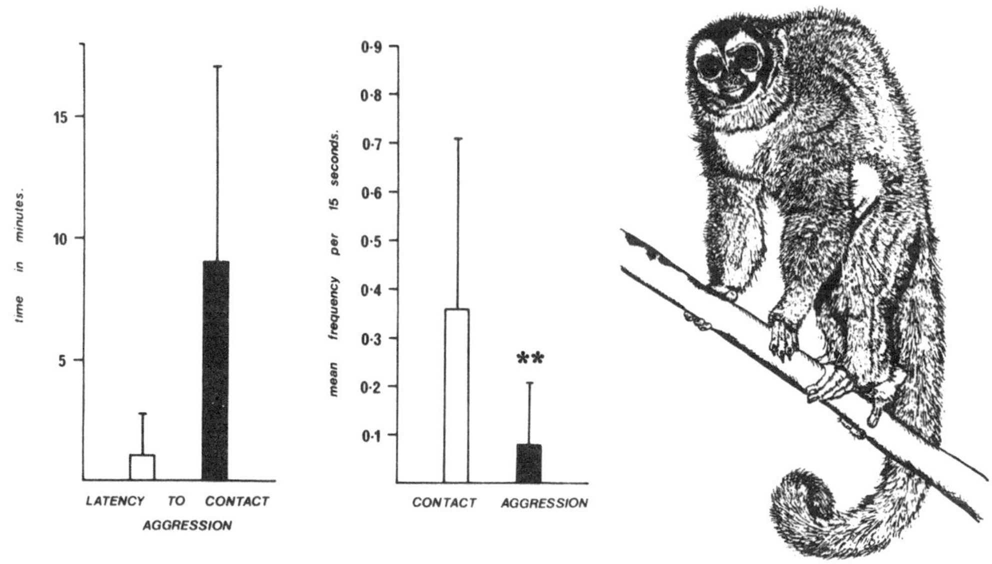

Fig. 22. The "arching display" of a male owl monkey which occurs frequently during aggressive encounters is shown on the right. The effects of partial anosmia upon frequencies of inter-male aggression are shown on the left. Data refer to 5 pairs of males which were either untreated (open bars) or rendered anosmic (solid bars) using anaesthetic plugs placed in the nasal passages. Frequencies of contact aggression were significantly lower in anosmic males. (** $p < 0.05$: 1 tail related t-test). For further explanation see text.

A second experiment was conducted in order to investigate the effects of anosmia upon inter-male aggression in the owl monkey. Owl monkeys show a sex difference in aggressiveness when paired with strange conspecifics; members of the same sex indulge in frequent "arching displays" (Fig. 22) and contact aggression, whereas members of the opposite sex arch infrequently and do not fight. The effects are most pronounced where males are concerned and olfactory cues play some role in this behaviour. Thus males take longer to initiate contact aggression and show lower frequencies of such aggression if they are first rendered anosmic (Fig. 22). The results are not due to some non-specific effect of anosmia or to discomfort occasioned by inserting the anaesthetic plugs. If a non-specific effect was responsible one would expect to see disruption of other behaviours, such as sexual patterns, but this is not the case. In control tests, where only one plug was inserted and no anaesthetic paste was used no effects upon inter-male aggression were observed. In a second control test it was shown that after insertion of plugs into the nasal cavity males were no longer able to discriminate conspecific odours (gauze pads impregnated with urine and subcaudal gland secretions) from saline[88].

Whilst other cues besides olfactory stimuli must be involved in sexual recognition and aggression in owl monkeys it is clear that olfaction does play an important role in these processes. Epple[95] has suggested that olfactory cues may be important in sexual recognition, courtship and pair-bonding in callitrichid species. Owl monkeys, like other monogamous primates, are monomorphic and it is extremely difficult for a human observer to distinguish the sexes without a close examination of their genitalia. The nocturnal habits of this monkey have inevitably led to a reduction of visual displays and it is quite possible that scent-marking and olfaction are most important in pair formation and maintenance of the "pair bond". Such problems would undoubtedly repay further study in the laboratory for at the present time we have few insights into the mechanisms which control pair formation in monogamous primates.

CONCLUSIONS AND SUGGESTIONS FOR FUTURE RESEARCH

Studies of the reproductive physiology and behaviour of any primate species in captivity depend upon a sound knowledge of its biology under natural conditions. Many of the observations described in this review require further amplification from studies in the field if they are to be interpreted correctly. This would apply to quantitative work on parent-infant behaviour, olfactory communication and social interactions between adults and maturing offspring as well as to the possible effects of seasonal and nutritional factors upon reproduction. Conversely, one may hope that detailed investigation of owl monkeys in the laboratory will assist field workers who attempt to study this nocturnal primate. Much has been achieved by using radio-tracking techniques to study nocturnal prosimians [105,106]. Preliminary work in our laboratory indicates that owl monkeys may be fitted with radio-transmitter harnesses and will tolerate them without showing signs of discomfort. Thorington, Muckenhirn and Montgomery[107] attached a transmitter to one owl monkey and were able to track the animal for 12 nights in the forest. If owl monkey groups are trapped in future, in the course of such field studies, it would also be valuable to collect blood samples for work on genetics. In this way it might be possible to assess whether juveniles transfer between family groups in the manner described for *Saguinus oedipus*[93].

Wright[6] has found that an owl monkey group may occupy a small home range (3.1

hectares) and that there are extensive areas of overlap between the home ranges of neighbouring groups. Since Aotus is hypometabolic[76,77] it is possible that this aspect of physiology may have important effects upon ecology and ranging behaviour. It would be of interest to enquire how, under nocturnal conditions, these animals maintain a monogamous social system rather than a non-gregarious system such as occurs in the majority of nocturnal prosimians. Observations and experiments on captive Aotus lead one to suggest that communication between breeding groups in the wild may entail a complex system of scent-marking displays, arch postures and vocalizations.

Estimates of population sizes for Aotus vary tremendously, as was pointed out in the introduction to this chapter. It would be valuable to obtain more accurate information on this subject, particularly because so many owl monkeys are removed from the wild for biomedical research. Although Aotus has a vast distribution range and is not yet endangered, some populations such as those in Colombia are under pressure and require conservation.

Owl monkeys play a vital role in malarial research, particularly the Colombian form, since it will act as a host for Plasmodium falciparum[11,13]. The occurrence of drug-resistant strains of P. falciparum and the search for a suitable anti-malarial vaccine make it likely that requirements for Aotus will continue in future. Owl monkeys have also been used in large numbers as experimental subjects for the vital induction of cancer[14,108], trachoma research [109] and for studies of the visual and auditory systems[110,111].

The owl monkey offers certain advantages, as compared with Old World monkeys, for research on reproduction. It breeds rapidly and attains sexual maturity in half the time span required by macaque or baboon species. Since Aotus rarely produces twins and does not exhibit a post-partum "oestrus" it is not feasible to breed this monkey in such large numbers as marmosets or tamarins. However, in investigations where body size is a limiting factor the owl monkey is preferable to callitrichid species. It is possible to draw blood samples for hormone radioimmunoassays or to obtain cerebro-spinal fluid from the cisterna magna much more readily and frequently from Aotus, which weighs 1 kilogramme, than from callitrichids weighing 350-450 grammes. If owl monkeys are to be used in neuroendocrine investiations, more research will be required to validate radioimmunoassays for the measurement of the gonadotrophins, prolactin and other pituitary hormones. It is our intention to use owl monkeys for experimental work on the neuroendocrine control of primate sexual and aggressive behaviour. All the necessary monkeys for this work will be produced by captive breeding. Owl monkeys are not difficult to breed in captivity and there would seem to be little justification for removing still more animals from the wild. However, despite the importance of this species in a range of biomedical research projects there have been relatively few attempts to set up large scale captive breeding programmes or to study its reproductive biology. It is important to solve this problem because the annual requirement for owl monkeys in the USA alone totals 1465 animals (National Primate Plan, US Department of Health, Education and Welfare, 1978) and wild stocks of Aotus are not inexhaustible.

ACKNOWLEDGEMENTS

The investigations reported in this chapter received financial support from the Wellcome Trust (UK) and the malaria component of the UNDP/World Bank/WHO Special Programme for Research and Training in Tropical Diseases. I am extremely grateful for this assistance and also wish to thank the following colleagues who collaborated on various studies: Dr R.D. Martin, Dr R.C. Bonney, Mr D. Fleming, Dr J. Hunter, Dr J.S. Gardner and Ms L. George. My thanks to Mrs B. Murrill and her staff for excellent care of the Aotus breeding colony, to Mr T. Dennett for photographic assistance and to Mrs A. McGlashan who prepared the manuscript for publication.

REFERENCES

1. Reumer, J.W.F. and De Boer, L.E.M. (1980) Standardization of Aotus chromosome nomenclature, with descriptions of the 2n = 49-50 karyotype and that of a new hybrid. J.Human Ecol., 9, 461-482.
2. Ma, N.S.F., Jones, T.C., Miller, A.C., Morgan, L.M. and Adams, E.A. (1976) Chromosome polymorphism and banding patterns in the owl monkey (Aotus). Lab.Anim.Sci., 26, 1022-1036.
3. Elliott, D.G. (1913) Descriptions of new species of monkeys of genus Seniocebus and Aotus from Colombia, South America. Bull.Amer.Mus.Nat.Hist., 32, 251-253.
4. Herschovitz, P. (1948) Mammals of Northern Colombia, preliminary report 4: monkeys (primates) with taxonomic revisions of some forms. Proc.U.S.Nat. Mus., 98, 323-427.
5. Yunis, E., Torres de Caballero, O.M. and Ramirez, C. (1977) Genus Aotus Q and G band karyotypes and natural hybrids. Folia Primatol., 27, 165-177.
6. Wright, P.C. (1978) Home range, activity pattern and agonistic encounters of a group of night monkeys (Aotus trivirgatus) in Peru. Folia Primatol., 29, 43-55.
7. Wright, P.C. (1981) The night monkeys, genus Aotus. In: Coimbra-Filho, A.F. and Mittermeier, R.A. (eds.) Ecology and Behaviour of Neotropical Primates, pp.211-240. (Academio Brasilera de Ciencias : Rio de Janeiro).
8. Rathbun, G.B. and Gache, M.J. (1977) The status of Aotus trivirgatus in Argentina. Centro Argentino de Primates and National Institutes of Health Report, Washington, DC.
9. Heffner, P.G. (1977) Census of Aotus in the north of Colombia. Report on PAHO project AMRO-3171 Pan American Health Organization, Washington, DC.
10. Green, K.M. (1978) Primate censusing in Northern Colombia: a comparison of

two techniques. Primates, 19, 523-530.

11. Geiman, Q.M. and Meagler, M.J. (1967) Susceptibility of a New World monkey to Plasmodium falciparum from Man. Nature (Lond), 215, 437.

12. Voller, A., Green, G.I. and Richards, W.H.G. (1973) Cross immunity studies with East and West African strains of Plasmodium falciparum in owl monkeys (Aotus trivirgatus). J.Trop.Med.Hyg., 76, 135-139.

13. Schmidt, L.H. (1978) Plasmodium falciparum and Plasmodium vivax infections in the owl monkey (Aotus trivirgatus). I. The course of untreated infections. II. Responses to chloroquine, quinine and pyrimethamine. III. Methods employed in the search for new schizonticidal drugs. Am.J.Trop. Med.Hyg., 26, 671-737.

14. Epstein, M.A. (1976) E.B. virus in the owl monkey (Aotus trivirgatus). Lab.Anim.Sci., 26, 1127-1130.

15. Elliott, M.W., Sehgal, P.K. and Chalifoux, L.V. (1976) Management and breeding of Aotus trivirgatus. Lab.Anim.Sci., 26, 1037-1040.

16. Meritt, D.A. Jr. (1976) The owl monkey, Aotus trivirgatus: husbandry, behavior, and breeding. Proc.Natn.Conf.AAZPA, 107-123.

17. Cicmanec, J.C. and Campbell, A.K. (1977) Breeding the owl monkey (Aotus trivirgatus) in a laboratory environment. Lab.Anim.Sci., 27, 512-517.

18. Dixson, A.F., Martin, R.D., Bonney, R.C. and Fleming, D. (1980) Reproductive biology of the owl monkey (Aotus trivirgatus griseimembra). In: Anand Kumar, T.C. (ed.) Non-Human Primate Models for Study of Human Reproduction, pp.61-68. (Karger : Basel).

19. Bonney, R.C., Dixson, A.F. and Fleming, D. (1979) Cyclic changes in the circulating and urinary levels of ovarian steroids in the adult female owl monkey (Aotus trivirgatus). J.Reprod.Fert., 56, 271-280.

20. Bonney, R.C., Dixson, A.F. and Fleming, D. (1980) Plasma concentrations of oestradiol-17β, oestrone, progesterone and testosterone during the ovarian cycle of the owl monkey (Aotus trivirgatus). J.Reprod.Fert., 60, 101-107.

21. Hunter, A.J., Martin, R.D., Dixson, A.F. and Rudder, B.C.C. (1979) Gestation and inter-birth intervals in the owl monkey (Aotus trivirgatus griseimembra). Folia Primatol., 31, 165-175.

22. Dixson, A.F. (1980) Androgens and aggression in primates: a review. Aggressive Behavior, 6, 37-67.

23. Dixson, A.F., Gardener, J.S. and Bonney, R.C. (1980) Puberty in the male owl monkey (Aotus trivirgatus griseimembra): a study of physical and hormonal development. Int.J.Primatol., 1, 129-139.

24. Dixson, A.F. and Gardner, J.S. (1981) Diurnal variations in plasma testosterone in a male nocturnal primate, the owl monkey (Aotus trivirgatus). J.Reprod.Fert., 62, 83-86.

25. Dixson, A.F. and Fleming, D. (1981) Parental behaviour and infant development in owl monkeys (Aotus trivirgatus griseimembra). J.Zool.(Lond), 194, 25-39.

26. Meritt, G.F. and Meritt, D.A. Jr. (1979) Hand-rearing techniques for douroucoulis. Int.Z.Yrbk., 18. 201-204.
27. Jarosz, S.J., Kuehl, T.J. and Dukelow, W.R. (1977) Vaginal cytology and gestation in the squirrel monkey (Saimiri sciureus). Biol.Reprod., 16, 97-103.
28. Nagle, C.A., Denari, J.H., Riarke, A., Quiroga, S., Zarate, R., Germino, N.I., Merlo, A. and Rosner, J.M. (1980) Endocrine and morphological aspects of the menstrual cycle in the cebus monkey (Cebus apella). In: Anand Kumar, T.C. (ed.) Non-Human Primates for Study of Human Reproduction, pp.69-81. (Karger : Basel).
29. Hearn, J.P., Abbott, D.H., Chambers, P.C., Hodges, J.K. and Lunn, S.F. (1978) Use of the common marmoset, Callithrix jacchus, in reproductive research. In: Goldsmith, E.J. and Moor-Jankowksi, J. (eds.) Primates in Medicine, 10, pp.40-49. (Karger : Basel).
30. Hill, W.C.O. (1960) Primates: Comparative Anatomy and Taxonomy, Vol. 4. (Edinburgh University Press : Edinburgh).
31. Koering, M.J. (1974) Comparative morphology of the primate ovary. Contrib.Primatol., 3, 38-81.
32. Hertig, A.T., Barton, B.R. and Mackey, J.J. (1976) The female reproductive tract of the owl monkey (Aotus trivirgatus) with special reference to the ovary. Lab.Anim.Sci., 26, 1041-1067.
33. Hearn, J.P. and Lunn, S.F. (1975) The reproductive biology of the marmoset monkey, Callithrix jacchus . Lab.Anim.Handbooks, 6, 191-202.
34. Channing, C.P., Fowler, S., Engel, B. and Vitek, K. (1977) Failure of daily injections of ketamine HCl to adversely alter menstrual cycle length, blood oestrogen and progesterone levels in the rhesus monkey. Proc.Soc.Exp.Biol.Med., 155, 615-619.
35. Koyama, T., de la Peria, A. and Hagino, N. (1977) Plasma estrogen, progestin and luteinizing hormone during the normal menstrual cycle in the baboon: role of luteinizing hormone. Am.J.Obstet.Gynecol., 127, 67-72.
36. Hodges, J.K., Gulick, B.A., Czekala, N.M. and Lasley, B.L. (1981) Comparison of urinary oestrogen excretion in South American primates. J.Reprod. Fert., 61, 83-90.
37. Bonney, R.C. and Setchell, K.D.R. (1980) The excretion of gonadal steroids during the reproductive cycle of the owl monkey (Aotus trivirgatus). J.Steroid Biochem., 12, 417-421.
38. Shackleton, C.H.L. (1974) Progesterone and oestrogen metabolism in the pregnant marmoset (Callithrix jacchus). J.Steroid Biochem., 5, 597-600.
39. Shackleton, C.H.L. (1975) The excretion of steroids by the adult marmoset monkey (Callithrix jacchus). J.Steroid Biochem., 6, 1429-1432.
40. Wilson, M.I. (1977) Characterization of the oestrous cycle and mating

season of squirrel monkeys from copulatory behaviour. J.Reprod.Fert., 51, 57-63.

41. Eaton, G.G., Slob, A. and Resko, J.A. (1973) Cycles of mating behaviour, oestrogen and progesterone in the Thick-tailed bushbaby (Galago crassicaudatus crassicaudatus) under laboratory conditions. Anim.Behav., 21, 309-315.

42. Evans, C.S. and Goy, R.W. (1968) Social behaviour and reproductive cycles in captive Ring-tailed lemurs (Lemur catta). J.Zool.(Lond), 156, 181-197.

43. Scruton, D.M. and Herbert, J. (1970) The menstrual cycle and its effect on behaviour in the Talapoin monkey (Miopithecus talapoin). J.Zool.(Lond), 162, 419-436.

44. Michael, R.P., Herbert, J. and Welegalla, J. (1967) Ovarian hormones and the sexual behaviour of the male rhesus monkey (Macaca mulatta) under laboratory conditions. J.Endrocrinol., 39, 81-98.

45. Eaton, G.G. and Resko, J.A. (1974) Ovarian hormones and sexual behaviour of Macaca nemestrina. J.Comp.Physiol.Psychol., 86, 919-925.

46. Rowell, T.E. and Chalmers, N. (1970) Reproductive cycles of the mangabey Cercocebus albigena. Folia Primatol., 12, 264-272.

47. Saayman, G.S. (1970) The menstrual cycle and sexual behaviour in a troop of free-ranging chacma baboons (Papio ursinus). Folia Primatol., 12, 81-110.

48. Young, W.C. and Orbison, W.D. (1944) Changes in selected features of behaviour in pairs of oppositely-sexed chimpanzees during the sexual cycle and after ovariectomy. J.Comp.Psychol., 37, 107-143.

49. Nadler, R.D. (1975) Sexual cyclicity in captive lowland gorillas. Science N.Y., 189, 813-814.

50. Nadler, R.D. (1977) Sexual behaviour of captive orang-utans. Arch.Sex. Behav., 6, 457-475.

51. Everitt, B.J. and Herbert, J. (1969) The role of ovarian hormones in sexual preference in rhesus monkeys. Anim.Behav., 17, 738-746.

52. Dixson, A.F. and Herbert, J. (1977) Gonadal hormones and sexual behaviour in groups of adult Talapoin monkeys (Miopithecus talapoin). Hormones & Behav., 8, 141-154.

53. Kleiman, D.G. (1977) Monogamy in mammals. Quart.Rev.Biol., 52, 39-69.

54. Epple, G. (1980) Paper read at the VIIIth Congress of the International Primatological Society, Florence, July 1980.

55. Moynihan, M. (1964) Some behaviour patterns of platyrrhine monkeys. I. The night monkey (Aotus trivirgatus). Smithson.Misc.Coll., 146, 1-84.

56. Hunt, R.D., Chalifoux, L.V., King, N.W. and Trum, B.F. (1975) Arrested spermatogenesis in owl monkeys (Aotus trivirgatus). J.Med.Primatol., 4, 399-400.

57. King, N. (1975) Morphological observations on the owl monkey testicles.

Primate Record, 6, 13.

58. Goodman, R.L., Hotchkiss, J., Karsch, F.J. and Knobil, E. (1974) Diurnal variations in serum testosterone concentrations in the adult male rhesus monkey. Biol.Reprod., 11, 624-630.

59. Mukka, V., Prahalda, S. and Moudgal, N.R. (1976) Effect of constant light on nyctohemeral variations in serum testosterone in male Macaca radiata. Nature (Lond), 260, 778-780.

60. Van Horn, R.N., Beamer, N.B. and Dixson, A.F. (1976) Diurnal variations of plasma testosterone in two prosimian primates (Galago crassicaudatus crassicaudatus and Lemur catta). Biol.Reprod., 15, 523-528.

61. Hall, R.D. and Hodgen, G.D. (1979) Pregnancy diagnosis in owl monkeys (Aotus trivirgatus): Evaluation of the haemagglutination inhibition test for urinary chorionic gonadotrophin. Lab.Anim.Sci., 29, 345-348.

62. Epple, G. (1970) Maintenance, breeding and development of marmoset monkeys in captivity. Folia Primatol., 12, 56-76.

63. Klopfer, P.H. and Boscoff, K.J. (1979) Maternal behavior in prosimians. In: Doyle, G.A. and Martin, R.D. (eds.) The Study of Prosimian Behavior, pp.123-156. (Academic Press : New York).

64. Roosmalen, M.G.M. van, Mittermeier, R.A. and Milton, K. (1981) The bearded sakis, genus Chiropotes. In: Coimbra-Filho, A.F. and Mittermeier, R.A. (eds.) Ecology and Behavior of Neotropical Primates, pp.419-441. (Academio Brasilera de Ciencias : Rio de Janeiro).

65. Ingram, J. (1977) Interactions between parents and infants and the development of independence in the common marmoset (Callithrix jacchus). Anim.Behav., 25, 811-827.

66. Hoage, R.J. (1977) Parental care in Leontopithecus rosalia rosalia: sex and age differences in carrying behavior and the role of prior experience. In: Kleiman, D.G. (ed.) The Biology and Conservation of the Callitrichidae, pp.293-305. (Smithsonian Institute Press : Washington).

67. Epple, G. (1975) Parental behavior in Saguinus fuscicollis spp. Folia Primatol., 24, 221-238.

68. Chivers, D. (1974) The Siamang in Malaya. Contrib.Primatol., 4, 1-335.

69. Hinde, R.A. and Spencer-Booth, Y. (1968) The study of mother-infant interaction in captive group-living rhesus monkeys. Proc.Roy.Soc.Lond. Ser.B. 169, 177-201.

70. Rowell, T.E., Din, N.A. and Omar, A. (1968) The social development of baboons in their first three months. J.Zool.(Lond), 155, 461-483.

71. Harlow, H.F. (1971) Learning to Love. (Ballantine Books : New York).

72. Hinde, R.A. (1971) Development of social behavior. In: Schrier, A.M. and Stollnitz, F. (eds.) Behavior of Non Human Primates, Vol.3, pp.1-68. (Academic Press : New York).

73. Trivers, R.L. (1972) Parental investment and sexual selection. In: Campbell, B. (ed.) Sexual Selection and the Descent of Man, pp.136-179. (Heinemann : London).
74. Pollock, J. (1975) The Social Behaviour and Ecology of Indri indri. PhD Thesis : University of London.
75. Chivers, D.J. (1972) The siamang and the gibbon in the Malay peninsula. In: Rumbaugh, D. (ed.) The Gibbon and Siamang, pp.103-135. (Karger : Basel).
76. Goffart, M. (1977) Hypometabolisme chez Aotus trivirgatus (Primates, Platyrrhini Cebidae). C.R.Seances Soc.Biol.Filiales, 171, 1149-1152.
77. Whittow, G.C., Guernsey, D.L. and Morishige, W.K. (1977) Thyroid activity in a hypometabolic primate, the owl monkey (Aotus trivirgatus). Arch.Int. de Physiol. et de Biochimie, 87, 963-967.
78. Box, H. (1977) Quantitative data on the carrying of young captive monkeys (Callithrix jacchus) by other members of their family groups. Primates, 18, 475-484.
79. Vogt, J.L., Carlson, H. and Menzel, E. (1978) Social behaviour of a marmoset (Saguinus fuscicollis) group. I. Parental care and infant development. Primates, 19, 715-726.
80. Sassenrath, E.N., Mason, W.A., Fitzgerald, R.C. and Kenney, M.D. (1980) Comparative endocrine correlates of reproductive status in Callithrix (Titi) and Saimiri (Squirrel) monkey. Antrop.Contemp., 3, 265 (Abstract).
81. McNeilly, A.S., Abbott, D.H., Lunn, S.F., Chambers, P.C. and Hearn, J.P. (1981) Plasma prolactin concentrations during the ovarian cycle and lactation and their relationship to return of fertility post-partum in the common marmoset (Callithrix jacchus). J.Reprod.Fert., 62, 353-360.
82. Maynard-Smith, J. (1977) Parental investment : a prospective analysis. Anim.Behav., 25, 1-9.
83. Thorner, M.O., Edwards, C.R.W., Hanker, J.P., Abraham, G. and Besser, G.M. (1977) Prolactin and gonadotrophin interaction in the male. In: Troen, P. and Nankin, H. (eds.) The Testis in Normal and Infertile Men. (Raven Press: New York).
84. Abbott, D.H. and Hearn, J.P. (1978) Physical, hormonal and behavioural aspects of sexual development in the marmoset monkey (Callithrix jacchus). J.Reprod.Fert., 53, 155-166.
85. Judd, H.L., Parker, D.C., Siller, T.M. and Yen, S.S.C. (1974) Nocturnal rise of plasma testosterone in pubertal boys. J.Clin.Endocr.Metab., 38, 710.
86. Epple, G. (1980) Relationships between aggression, scent marking and gonadal state in a primate, the tamarin Saguinus fuscicollis. In: Muller-Schwarze, D. and Silverstein, R.M. (eds.) Chemical Signals : Vertebrates and Aquatic Invertebrates, pp. 85-105. (Plenum : New York).

87. Hill, W.C.O., Appleyard, H.M. and Anber, L. (1959) The specialized area of skin glands in Aotus Humboldt (Simiae platyrrhini). Trans.Roy.Soc.Edin., 63, 535-551.

88. Hunter, A.J. (1981) Chemical communication, aggression and sexual behaviour in the owl monkey (Aotus trivirgatus griseimembra). PhD Thesis : University of London.

89. Sade. D.S. (1968) Inhibition of son-mother mating among free-ranging rhesus monkeys. Science and Psychoanalysis, 12, 18-37.

90. Carpenter, C.R. (1940) A field study in Siam of the behaviour and social relations of the gibbon. Comp.Psychol.Monogr., 16, 1-212.

91. Ellefson, J.O. (1974) A natural history of white-headed gibbons in the Malayan peninsula. In: Rumbaugh, D.M. (ed.) The Gibbon and the Siamang, Vol. 3, 2-136. (Karger : Basel).

92. Mackinnon, J. and Mackinnon, K. (1977) The formation of a new gibbon group. Primates, 18, 701-708.

93. Dawson, G.A. (1977) Composition and stability of social groups of the tamarin Saguinus oedipus geoffroyi in Panama: ecological and behavioural implications. In: Kleiman, D.G. (ed.) Biology and Conservation of the Callitrichidae, pp.23-37. (Smithsonian Institution Press : Washington).

94. Epple, G. and Lorenz, R. (1968) Vorkommen, morphologie und funktion der sternaldruse bei den Platyrrhini. Folio Primatol., 7, 98-126.

95. Epple, G. (1976) Chemical communication and reproductive process in non-human primates. In: Doty, R.L. (ed.) Mammalian Olfaction, Reproductive Processes and Behavior, pp.257-282. (Academic Press : New York).

96. Schilling, A. (1979) Olfactory communication in prosimians. In: Doyle, G.A. and Martin, R.D. (eds.) The Study of Prosimian Behavior, pp.461-542. (Academic Press : New York).

97. Epple, G. (1978) Lack of effects of castration on scent marking displays and aggression in a South American primate (Saguinus fuscicollis). Horm. Behav., 11, 139-150.

98. Welker, C. (1973) Ethologische Bedeutung des Harnwaschens von Galago crassicaudatus E. Geoffroy, 1812 (Lorisfornes: Galagidae). Folia Primatol., 20, 429-452.

99. Robinson, J.G. (1979) Correlation of urine washing in the wedge-capped capuchin Cebus nigrivittatus. In: Eisenberg, J.F. (ed.) Vertebrate Ecology in the Northern Neotropics, pp.137-143. (Smithsonian Institution Press : Washington).

100. Latta, J., Hopf, S. and Ploog, D. (1967) Observations on mating behavior and sexual play in the squirrel monkey (Saimiri sciureus). Primates, 8. 229-246.

101. Baldwin, J.D. (1970) Reproductive synchronization in squirrel monkeys (Saimiri). Primates, 11, 317-326.

102. Michael, R.P. and Keverne, E.B. (1968) Pheromones in the communication of sexual status primates. Nature (Lond), 218, 746-749.

103. Johns, M.A. (1980) The role of the vomeronasal system in mammalian reproductive physiology. In: Muller-Schwarze, D. and Silverstein, R.M. (eds.) Chemical Signals: Vertebrates and Aquatic Invertebrates, pp.341-364. (Plenum : New York).

104. Meredith, M. (1980) The vomeronasal organ and accessory olfactory system in the hamster. In: Muller-Schwarze, D. and Silverstein, R.M. (eds.) Chemical Signals: Vertebrates and Aquatic Invertebrates, pp.303-326. (Plenum : New York).

105. Charles-Dominique, P. (1977) Ecology and Behaviour of Nocturnal Primates. (Duckworth : London).

106. Bearder, S.K. and Martin, R.D. (1979) The social organization of a nocturnal primate revealed by radio tracking. In: Amlaner, C.J. and MacDonald, D.W. (eds.) A Handbook of Biotelemetry and Radiotracking. pp.633-648. (Pergamon Press : Oxford and New York).

107. Thorington, R.W. Jr., Muckenhirn, N.A. and Montgomery, G.C. (1976) Movements of a wild night monkey (Aotus trivirgatus). In: Thorington, R.W. and Heltne, P.G. (eds.) Neotropical Primates, pp.32-34. (National Academy of Science : Washington DC).

108. Hunt, R.D., Baharona, H. and Daniel, M.D. (1978) Herpes virus ateles malignant lymphona in owl monkeys. In: Bentvelzer, P., Hilgers, J. and Yohn, D.S. (eds.) Advances in Comparative Leukemia Research, pp.198-200. (Elsevier : Amsterdam).

109. Fraser, C.E.D. (1976) The owl monkey (Aotus trivirgatus) as an animal model in trachoma research. Lab.Anim.Sci., 26, 1138-1141.

110. Jacobs, G.H. (1977) Visual capacity of the owl monkey Aotus trivirgatus. I. Spectral sensitivity and colour vision. Vision Res., 17, 811-820.

111. Beecher, M.D. (1976) Studies on the hearing of the owl monkey (Aotus trivirgatus). Lab.Anim.Sci., 26, 1068-1072.

Chapter 4

The Saddle Back Tamarin and other Tamarins

G. Epple & Y. Katz

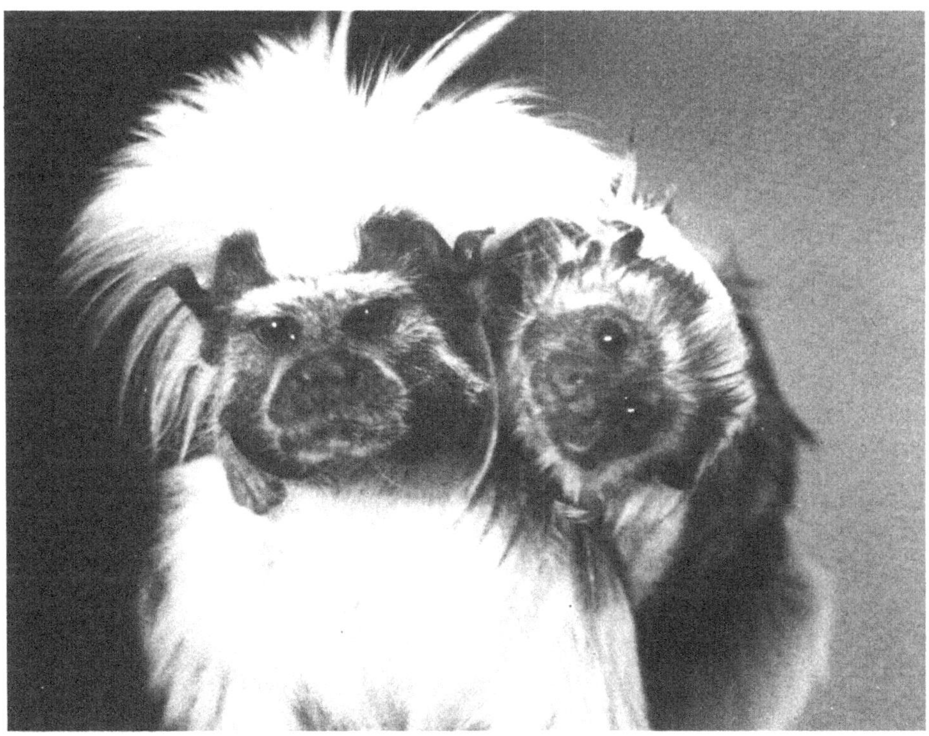

Saguinus oedipus oedipus

THE SADDLE BACK TAMARIN AND OTHER TAMARINS

Gisela Epple and Yair Katz
Monell Chemical Senses Center
3500 Market Street
Philadelphia, PA U.S.A.

INTRODUCTION

For many decades, various species of marmosets and tamarins, members of the family Callitrichidae, have been kept in captivity. Early on these animals were mostly kept as pets or were exhibited in zoological gardens[1]. Although early attempts to maintain and breed marmosets and tamarins for extended periods of time under captive conditions met with limited success, they have gradually increased our knowledge of the behavior and of the dietary and environmental requirements of callitrichids. More recently, biomedical and behavioral researchers have become interested in these small monkeys and in their potential as laboratory primates. As a result of their studies, our expertise in the maintenance of callitrichids in captivity has increased considerably[2-8].

The low purchase price of these monkeys, their small size and the fact that they regularly produce twins who become sexually mature within approximately two years (see below) provide many advantages over larger, more expensive laboratory primates. They enable the researcher to acquire, house and breed a large number of animals at relatively low cost. However, while great progress toward this goal has been made in the maintenance of the common marmoset, *Callithrix jacchus*[9,10], maintenance and husbandry procedures for the various tamarin species have not yet been fully established.

During the relatively short time for which callitrichids have been used in biomedical research, they have proven their value as model species in a number of areas. It appears, however, that different species differ in the degree to which they represent suitable models for medical research. While the common marmoset, for example, is used in reproductive research, teratology and periodontal disease studies[10], tamarins of the genus *Saguinus* have become increasingly important in immunology, virology and oncology. In callitrichids, fraternal twinning is characterized by the development of placental vascular anastomoses between the fetuses. This condition leads to hemopoietic chimerism and immunological tolerance between twins, making these primates unique subjects for immunology research[4,5,11,12]. These studies are mainly conducted on the saddle back tamarin, *Saguinus fuscicollis*, and the cotton top tamarin, Saguinus oedipus oedipus. Both of these species are also widely used in virology, oncology and cancer research. In a recent overview of the use of callitrichids in these areas of research, Wolfe and Deinhardt[13] have pointed out that "marmosets have proven more susceptible to a broader range of viruses than any other monkey species available". Marmoset cell lines also are valuable resources for viral carcinogenesis studies[13].

The cotton top tamarin shows a strong tendency to develop spontaneous colonic adenocarcinomas, a trend apparently not present to the same degree in other callitrichids[14]. Saguinus species are also of vital importance for the study of viral hepatitis, particularly hepatitis A[15]. Here, two closely related species of moustached tamarins, Saguinus mystax and Saguinus labiatus, are the most suitable species, showing a higher susceptibility to hepatitis A virus than other callitrichids[16]. In addition to their usefulness in medical research, callitrichids are becoming increasingly important in endocrine and behavioral research, and the literature reviewed later in this chapter documents their use in these areas of science. Although the examples of the utility of callitrichids as laboratory primates given here are by no means exhaustive, they sufficiently document their importance. Unfortunately, the increasing demand for marmosets and tamarins in biomedical research has met with an ever decreasing supply. Several species, among them the golden lion tamarin (Leontopithecus rosalia) and the cotton top tamarin (Saguinus oedipus oedipus) are threatened or endangered and the countries of origin are placing restrictions on the exportation of all callitrichids. On the other hand, no decisive breakthrough has been made in breeding large numbers and successive generations of any Saguinus species under laboratory conditions, although this appears to have been accomplished for the common marmoset (Callithrix jacchus)[9,10]. In this chapter we attempt to summarize some of the biological and behavioral information relevant for the maintenance and husbandry of Saguinus species and thus make a contribution toward the continuing use of these primates in the laboratory.

SOCIAL AND REPRODUCTIVE BIOLOGY

The social organization of tamarin groups

During recent years, several field studies of tamarin species have appeared in the literature. These studies suggest that most tamarins live in relatively small groups, each containing a stable nucleus consisting of a breeding female, her dependent young and a male with whom she probably has a monogamous pair bond. Although small groups predominate, group size and stability vary within and among species. Single individuals, small groups of 2-12 and occasionally quite large groups of up to 40 individuals, the latter probably representing temporary aggregations of several groups, were seen[17-27]. Although most of the field studies do not include many data on social behavior, a few deal in some detail with social organization. Preliminary studies on Saguinus mystax in Peru indicate that this species lives in small families, consisting of the parents, and one or a few sets of twin offspring. Interestingly, the groups regularly associate with Saguinus fuscicollis groups at this locality[17]. In a study of Saguinus oedipus geoffroyi in the dry forests of the Panama Canal Zone, Dawson[19,20] found groups varying in size between 1 and 19, with groups of 7 being the most frequent. The groups contain adult and juvenile males and females, plus one set of infant twins. Only one female appears to be reproductively active and from laboratory studies, one may infer that it is the dominant one. Similar to what is seen in the laboratory, males and females maintain parallel dominance hierachies and there seems to be a relatively high level of intra-group aggression. Animals emigrate from groups and immigrate into other groups to the extent that the group membership is quite unstable. Immature males and females tend to emigrate from groups more frequently than mature individuals. It appears that juveniles may change group affiliation often and with a minimum of interference from the residents, while the breeding pair may be much less likely to emigrate from the group. Thus, the social organization of Saguinus oedipus geoffroyi is quite flexible. The nucleus of the groups consist of a dominant male, a dominant female and their dependent offspring. In addition, a variable number of more or less temporary group members, mostly juveniles and young adults are present. Although kinship relations between the breeding pair and these temporary group members are unknown, immigrants into a group may well be kin of the breeding pair. The size and stability of these groups, as well as the size of their home ranges, is also affected by ecological factors. Thus, a group living in the moist lowland occupied and aggressively defended a territory of 26 ha while a group occupying the dry upland area used a much larger home range, which was not defended as a territory[19,20].

Neyman[25] studied Saguinus oedipus oedipus in the coastal lowlands of Columbia. Here, groups consist of 3-13 individuals. In this species, also, there appears to be only one reproductively active female per group. Similar to Saguinus oedipus geoffroyi[19,20], the cotton top tamarin groups are rather unstable, with animals leaving groups and joining others. Apart from established groups which are clearly attached to a home range, transient individuals and groups occur. In contrast to Saguinus oedipus geoffroyi, females appear to be in transit more frequently than males. Juveniles, however, are not preferentially involved in these transits. There was evidence that the tamarins occupy and defend territories, 7.8-10 ha in size. Contacts between neighbors occur irregularly and are accompanied by mild aggression. The behavior of encountering groups suggests the recognition of mutual territorial boundaries[25].

Saguinus nigricollis was observed by Izawa[23] in the Rio Caqueta basin in Columbia. There, the sizes of stable groups range between 4 and 8. One adult, bonded pair seems to form the social nucleus of each group and the existence of a pair bond is readily apparent in the close spatial and behavioral association between the mates. The pair bonded female is the only one who reproduces. While the bonded pair of each group forms a stable nucleus, nonbonded members appear to leave their original group and to join others. The home ranges of the groups overlap and there is little evidence of territorial defense. On the contrary, two or more groups are frequently seen to associate for short periods of time in overlapping areas, forming troops of up to 40 individuals. During these periods, the bonded nuclear pair of each group avoids the bonded pairs of other groups, while the other group members interact, apparently engaging in play[25].

Saguinus fuscicollis has been studied intensively by Terborg in Southeastern Peru and these studies will shortly be published in book form[26]. At this locality, Saguinus fuscicollis groups are small and quite stable, defending territories which each group shares with one group of Saguinus imperator. The groups usually contain only one adult breeding female but there is evidence that this female may mate with more than one male. Young females disperse as they reach maturity, i.e., earlier than males. However, there is little evidence that dispersing animals immigrate into other groups to the extent shown by the Saguinus oedipus subspecies[26].

In summarizing the few field studies reviewed above, it becomes evident that there is considerable variability in social organization among Saguinus species. On one hand, all Saguinus species share with other callitrichids the reproductive strategy of limiting breeding to a single female in the group. On the other hand, adherance to a strictly monogamous mating system, and the extent of intra- and inter-group aggression, which influence group stability, territoriality and the mode of dispersal vary among species. Group size, group stability and spacing behavior, in turn, are strongly influenced by a variety of ecological factors.

In the laboratory, tamarins, like most callitrichids, establish monogamous pair bonds and are characterized by high levels of aggression directed at nonrelated adult conspecifics[28,29]. In laboratory families of Saguinus fuscicollis developing naturally from an adult pair and its progeny, as well as in groups containing several nonrelated males and females, only one female ever bears offspring[1]. In families, the mother remains the only reproductively active female and there is little sexual activity among her adult offspring. In groups containing several nonrelated adults, one female usually establishes dominance over all other females, pairs bonds to a dominant male and inhibits bonding and reproduction in the other females, although these may engage in sexual activity[28,30].

The establishment of a pair bond may be an important factor in determining the social status and reproductive success of males and particularly of females. Our understanding of the mechanisms involved in the establishment and maintenance of the pair bond in callitrichids, however, is incomplete. Preference for the mate, expressed in spatial proximity, a number of "affectionate behaviors" and close socio-sexual association between mated partners may be involved in these processes[28-32]. In addition to these associative behaviors, saddle back tamarins apparently utilize aggressive rejection of potential challengers to a bond to enforce monogamy[28]. Pair bonded adults violently attack nonrelated adult group members with relative frequency, making necessary the removal of the recipient of such aggression from the group. Overt aggression is also used to prevent friendly social contact with adult conspecifics not belonging to the same social group[28,33]. Females tend to be more aggressive than males and the predominant targets of their aggression are other females[28,33]. It is obvious that overt aggression may be more frequent in the laboratory, where the animal eliciting such behavior has no chance to avoid it by retreating.

The fact that in the laboratory females are more aggressive than males makes it practically impossible to maintain saddle back tamarin groups containing more than one adult, nonrelated female. While mothers and daughters may cohabit peacefully for years in large, stable families, groups containing several nonrelated adult females usually break up due to vicious fighting among females shortly after group formation, and deaths due to fighting are not uncommon. Males, on the other hand, are more compatible and laboratory groups consisting of several nonrelated males and one female may be stable for extended periods of time. These findings are in accordance with the field observations on this species[26].

Sexual Behavior

In most marmosets and tamarins a permanent pair bond exists between the breeding male and breeding female of families and between the α-♂ and α-♀ of heterosexual groups containing nonrelated adults[1,28,29,30,31,32,34,35]. In natural families of *Saguinus fuscicollis*, sexual interactions involving full copulation are practically limited to the bonded pair, the parents. In our large families, almost no sexual behavior is shown by adult offspring and the removal of one parent from the family results in cessation of all breeding, even though adults of both sexes may be present[36]. This suggests that this species normally observes a behavioral incest tabu, possibly caused by the familiarity between family members. If this is true, one may expect close kin to produce offspring with each other provided they did not grow up together. Wolfe *et al.*[8] report brother-sister breeding but the social history of these pairs is not mentioned. In heterosexual groups of nonrelated adults, sexual behavior is usually shown by all members. The existence of a pair bond between the α-♂ and the α-♀ does not necessarily prevent sexual interactions between non-bonded partners[6,30,37]. However, quantitative as well as qualitative differences in the sexual and associated social behaviors of the various individuals within a group exist.

In a study of Saguinus fuscicollis trios consisting of two adult, nonrelated males and one adult female, the pair bond between the female and one of the males was apparent in the close social and sexual association between the female and this male. However, the non-bonded male also mated with the female, though much less frequently[30]. The fact that the bonded male mates more frequently with the female may confer reproductive priviledges to this male, i.e., it may increase his chance to inseminate the female. It does not, however, mean that all other males are completely deprived of this chance. This is suggested by Terborg's[26] observation of a wild female mating with two males and by the results of a laboratory experiment investigating pair bonding of castrated males when in competition with intact males[36]. In this experiment, five trios, each consisting of an intact male, a sexually experienced castrate and a female were observed. In two of the trios, a pair bond between the female and the castrate was established but infants were born in all five trios[36]. In contrast to Saguinus fuscicollis, non-bonded golden lion tamarin males (Leontopithecus rosalia) may have much fewer chances to reproduce. Kleiman[31] found that in trios of golden lion tamarins one of the two males was sexually inhibited and concluded from her studies that there is mating exclusivity in the species.

In contrast to many other simian primates, callitrichids show no easily detectable signs of ovarian cyclicity, such as changes in vaginal cytology, perineal swellings or menstrual bleeding. Even possible changes in sexual and associated behaviors are so subtle that they cannot easily be used as indices of cyclicity. This is true for all genera of marmosets and tamarins. However, while Callithrix jacchus usually shows an immediate post partum estrus[10,35,67], Saguinus species do not do so predictably, and it is therefore even more difficult to assess the reproductive state of the female.

In established pairs of Saguinus fuscicollis, copulations are relatively infrequent and there is no reliable cyclicity of copulatory activity. Epple[36] studied the sexual behavior of five established pairs, each composed of a vasectomized male and an intact, nonpregnant female. Each subject was observed for 10 minutes five times weekly for approximately 6 months. At the same time, vaginal smears were taken from the females 5 times per week. There were no reliable changes in vaginal cytology which could be used to evaluate the females' cycles. The average copulatory score of the pairs was 0.2 per 10 minutes and the copulatory activity of the pairs did not reveal any detectable cyclicity of mating behavior indicative of an estrus cycle. Moreover, some of the females were remated with fertile males after completion of the experiment and sperm was recovered in vaginal smears well into early pregnancy, showing that copulatory behavior extends into pregnancy.

These results suggest that in established pairs of Saguinus fuscicollis, estrus is usually "silent". Nevertheless, behavioral estrus activities sometimes and rather unpredictably occur, but in our colony they appear to be limited to groups containing more than one male and it may be possible that they become evident only when the bonded male has to compete for the female. Interestingly, it is the behavior of the male rather than that of the female which suggests that the female may be in estrus. In groups containing nonrelated males, or in families containing mature sons, the pair bonded males sporadically show a behavior which we have termed "follow-guard female". It is characterized by increased sexual activity of both bonded partners, a strong increase in sniffing of the female by the male and continuous attempts by the male to maintain contact with the female and to prevent contact between the female and all other males. These behaviors, and the fact that conception of several term babies in our colony could be dated back to these periods, suggest that the female is ovulating. Since "follow-guard female" is almost exclusively shown in larger groups and hardly ever in single pairs, the male's behavior may be caused not only by the attractiveness of the female during this period of time but primarily by the presence of potential competitors for access to the female. Even in large groups, however, "follow-guard female" is a sporadic behavior which does not occur reliably or predictably.

In Saguinus oedipus oedipus, female scent marking behavior may be a useful tool to evaluate cyclicity. French and Snowdon[38] report that anogenital marking (but not suprapubic marking) is increased during periods in which the female may have been in estrus. In this study, estrus was backdated from the birth of term infants using a gestation period of 150 days. In Leontopithecus rosalia there seems to be a relatively clearcut behavioral estrus cycle reflected in a peak in copulatory activity, male attention to the female (approaching, sniffing and grooming of the female) and a drop in the female's scent marking activity[39].

Steroid levels and reproductive cyclicity

In the absence of reliable morphological and behavioral indices of female cyclicity, monitoring of the female's sex hormone and/or gonadotropin levels is one alternative for the study of the reproductive cycle. While the endocrine events during the reproductive cycle of Callithrix jacchus have been studied quite extensively by Hearn and his co-workers[10], comparatively little is known about Saguinus and the only endocrine data on cyclicity are provided by Preslock and co-workers[40,41] for Saguinus oedipus oedipus (5 females) and Saguinus fuscicollis (1 female).

In our laboratory, we have started to look at plasma steroid levels in male and female *Saguinus fuscicollis* of different age classes. To obtain pilot data on which further experimental work could be based, blood samples from a number of young and adult, intact and castrated males and females were analyzed in a cross-sectional approach. In addition, plasma and urine estradiol were monitored in a number of adult females in an effort to characterize the reproductive cycle[42].

Since these studies have not yet appeared in press, our methods will be briefly described here. All blood samples were collected by venipuncture under slight ketamine-HCl sedation between 10 and 12 a.m. Blood from 2 adult females living with castrated males was collected twice weekly for 2 months. Plasma was separated within 30 min and stored at -18°C. One hundred microliter aliquots of the thawed plasma were extracted once with 10 ml acid-washed, peroxide-free diethyl ether and once with 10 ml light petroleum ether. The combined extracts were dried under nitrogen, concentrated and subjected to a 2.5 gr Sephadex LH-20 separation column, eluted according to Zamečnik *et al.*[43]. Control plasma pool samples, containing known amounts of various steroids, were processed in the same fashion for determination of procedural precision (Table 1). The collected fractions were dried, their contents dissolved in steroid RIA buffer and aliquots were analyzed for their steroid contents using specific steroid RIA systems.

Table 1. Elution pattern and recovery values of tritiated steroids on a 2.5 g (8.0 ml) Sephadex LH-20 column.

Fraction No.	Fraction ml eluted	Steroid	Percent recovery
1	0-2.5	-	
2	2.5-5.5	Progesterone (4-pregnene-3,20-dione)	98
		DOC (4-pregnene-21-ol-3,20-dione)	25
		Androstenedione (4-androstene-3,17-dione)	96
		DHA (5α-androstane-3,17-dione)	97
3	5.5-9.5	DOC (4-pregnene-21-ol-3,20-dione)	67
		DHEA (5-androstene-3β-ol-17-one)	91
		Testosterone (4-androstene-17β-ol-3-one)	94
		DHT (5α-androstane-17β-ol-3-one)	87
4	9.5-14.0	Corticosterone (4-pregnene-11β,21-diol-3,20-dione)	96
		estrone (1,3,5(10)-estratriene-3β-ol-17-one)	86
5	14.0-24.0	-	
6	24.0-33.0	Cortisol (4-pregnene-11β,17α,21-triol-3,20-dione)	72
		Estradiol (1,3,5(10)-estratriene-3β,17β-diol)	94

In addition to monitoring plasma steroid levels, urinary estradiol levels were monitored in parous adult females over extended periods of time. Each female lived permanently with a castrated male. An attempt was also made to establish whether or not nonbreeding adult females, living in their natal families containing a reproductively active mother, exhibit cyclicity. In this study, we monitored urinary estradiol cyclicity in four adult females while each lived in her natal family and after each had been removed from the family and paired with a vasectomized adult male[42]. Five overnight urine samples per week were collected from each of the females, while the donor was confined in view of her mate or family to a metabolism cage between 4 p.m. and 9 a.m. the following day. Fifty microliter aliquots of the filtered urine were used for estradiol-17β RIA. A trace amount of estradiol-17β-glucuronate* was added to the samples, which were allowed to equilibrate at room temperature. A mixture of 1500 Fishman Units of Helix pomatia β-glucuronidase/aryl sulfatase in 35 μl water and 15 μl 1.0 M acetate buffer (pH 4.8) was added; the hydrolysis was then carried out in a constant temperature bath for two hours.

After hydrolysis, the samples were chilled and extracted with 10 ml acid-washed diethyl ether. The extracts were dried under nitrogen in a warm sand bath and redissolved in 2 ml steroid RIA buffer. The combined efficiency and recovery rate of the hydrolysis and extraction steps were estimated by counting the radioactivity in 1 ml of the extract in steroid RIA buffer. In our RIA system, urinary estrone does not cross-react with estradiol.

Aliquots (25-100 μl) of the final extract in steroid RIA buffer were assayed in a manner similar to that described for the blood samples. To provide an internal standard, 20 microliter aliquots of filtered urine were analyzed for their creatinine contents, using an alkaline picric acid - sodium borate - SDS reagent, modified after Heinegård and Tiderström[44]; the readings were acid-corrected for the presence of non-specific, creatinine-like compounds. All our results are expressed in μg steroid per mg of creatinine in the urine sample.

Table 2 lists some of the values recorded in our laboratory. Of special interest are the lack of radioimmunoassayable 5α-dihydrotestosterone, the high androstenedione and estrone levels (even in castrates), and the very high cortisol titers. Comparable cortisol concentrations were recorded also by Yamamoto et al.[45]. The preponderance of androstenedione and estrone over testosterone and estradiol, respectively, may reflect the conclusion by Preslock and Steinberger[46-49] that the delta-4 pathway of marmoset steroidogenesis is prevalent over the delta-5 alternative.

---

* The steroid conjugate was synthesized in our laboratory, using the same ^{3}H-estradiol-17β employed in the RIA, the sodium salt of uridine-5'-diphosphoglucuronic acid and uridine-5'-diphospho-glucuronyl transferase from rabbit liver microsomes.

Table 2. Steroid hormone levels in plasma samples of intact and gonadectomized adult male and female *Saguinus fuscicollis*. Values are mean ± S.E.M.; the number of samples is given in parentheses. Please note different concentration units.

	males		females	
Steroid	intact	gonadectomized	intact	gonadectomized
progesterone, ng/ml	3.41 ± 0.97 (9)	1.40 ± 0.40 (4)	28.84 ± 3.27 (26)	0.63 ± 0.12 (19)
androstenedione, ng/ml	127.78 ± 14.65 (10)	68.81 ± 20.12 (14)	15.33 ± 1.59 (26)	2.38 ± 0.32 (22)
testosterone, ng/ml	26.41 ± 6.02 (10)	1.23 ± 0.16 (29)	4.87 ± 0.45 (28)	1.56 ± 0.32 (26)
DHT	0 (10)	0 (29)	0 (21)	0 (19)
estrone, ng/ml	5.60 ± 1.69 (5)	6.13 ± 1.18 (7)	20.89 ± 2.85 (7)	16.12 ± 5.99 (7)
estradiol, pg/ml	175 ± 51 (7)	0 (7)	630 ± 140* (26)	0 (15)
cortisol, ng/ml	1.70 ± 0.30 (14)	3.29 ± 0.41 (31)	1.86 ± 0.26 (7)	2.94 ± 1.11 (6)

* peaks: 1693 ± 205 (7); nadirs: 350 ± 51 (13); 6 zeros.

The ratio of estrone to estradiol in our studies is quite different from that reported by Preslock *et al.*[40]. These authors quote immunoassayed estradiol peak values of 6.2 ng/ml, which probably contained high amounts of cross-reacting estrone. This is suggested by their statement that "the thin-layer chromatography step was omitted so that rapid measurement of total serum estrogen concentrations was obtained". Our results, on the other hand, indicate that plasma estrone is a high-titer product of extragonadal aromatization of androstenedione, probably of adrenal origin. Preslock *et al.*[40] also report that "serum progestins" (measured as progesterone, using canine corticosterone binding globulin as a ligand) peak at an average value of either 272 ng/ml (according to their Table 3) or 140 ng/ml (according to their Figure 3). Again, methodological differences appear to be responsible for the differences between their findings and those reported here (Table 2). It is likely that the purification technique used by Preslock *et al.*[40] was not sufficient to remove all the cortisol from the ether-extracted serum. Since *Saguinus fuscicollis* have high cortisol titers (Table 2), the progestin levels reported by Preslock *et al.*[40] may have been inflated by corticosteroids.

Table 3 shows the mean plasma and urinary levels of the parous, pair-living females. The cycle length is defined as the mean number of days between estradiol peaks (the first day after the estradiol peak is defined as day 1). It is obvious, of course, that progesterone and LH levels have to be monitored in order to obtain information on ovulatory events during these cycles. Such work is presently in progress in our laboratory. As seen in the table, the urinary estradiol peak values varied between an individual mean of 3.28 μg/mg creatinine in ♀ 142 and 8.47 μg/mg in ♀ 147. Even twin sisters, represented by ♀ 142 and ♀ 143, show different levels. Similar variability is reflected in the baseline levels. It should be pointed out, however, that even the baseline levels are about 50-fold over the average woman's preovulatory phase.

Table 3. Plasma and urinary estradiol cyclicity in adult, parous females cohabiting with castrated males. Mean ± S.E.M.; plasma values in pg/mg, urinary values in μg/mg creatinine.

				estradiol levels	
I.D. no.	Age, years	Source	Mean cycle length (days*)	Peaks	Baseline
147	7	plasma	16.0 ± 1.0 (3)	1819 ± 162	261 ± 90
304	4		noncyclic	685 ± 260	
118	6	urine	18.2 ± 1.7 (4)	7.93 ± 0.55	2.44 ± 0.22
119	6		15.2 ± 0.6 (9)	4.44 ± 0.23	1.19 ± 0.13
142	4		16.4 ± 0.8 (7)	3.28 ± 0.43	0.87 ± 0.07
143	4		21.8 ± 1.1 (4)	5.34 ± 0.26	1.64 ± 0.16
147	4		16.6 ± 1.0 (7)	8.47 ± 0.69	2.97 ± 0.54

* The number of cycles monitored given in parentheses.

The average length of the cycle (17.3 ± 0.97) is in the same range as that of the common marmoset (16.4 ± 1.7 days between plasma estradiol peaks as determined by Hearn and co-workers[10]) and the cotton top tamarin (15.9 ± 1.0 days between plasma estradiol and progesterone peaks as determined by Preslock and co-workers[40,41]). The data also agree well with the average cycle length of 15.2 ± 1.6 days in Saguinus oedipus oedipus and 14.6 ± 1.4 days in Saguinus fuscicollis which were obtained during determinations of levels of neutrophilic granulocyte alkaline phosphatase in these species by Preslock and co-workers[40,41].

Table 4 shows the urinary estradiol levels of 4 adult females while living in their families, containing both parents, and after each female was removed from her family and permanently paired with an adult, vasectomized male. All females were at least 21 months of age at the beginning of the monitoring period, an age at which they are capable of delivering term offspring if paired earlier with a fertile male[50]. The twin sister of ♀ 194, paired earlier, was indeed raising her first set of infants while her sister remained in the family.

Table 4. Urinary estradiol patterns in adult females while living in their families and after pairing with castrated males. Mean ± S.E.M.; estradiol values in μg/mg creatinine.

I.D. no.	age (in months) sampling period covered	at time of pairing	in family estradiol levels (non-cyclic)	paired with adult male mean cycle length (days*)	estradiol levels peaks	baseline
194	24-31	28	0.240 ± 0.011	16.5 ± 1.5(4)	2.04 ± 0.13	1.00 ± 0.11
230	22-27	24	0.152 ± 0.011	15.7 ± 1.7(3)	1.26 ± 0.07	0.43 ± 0.06
236	23-29	25	0.109 ± 0.006	13.5 ± 0.7(7)	0.78 ± 0.04	0.27 ± 0.03
252	22-30	27	0.346 + 0.018	19.0 + 1.3(4)	1.17 + 0.06	0.38 + 0.02

* The number of cycles monitored given in parentheses.

All females displayed low, noncycling urinary estradiol levels as long as they remained members of their natal families. In all of them, pairing with adult, vasectomized males resulted in an almost immediate increase in estradiol levels. This was followed by the appearance of estradiol peaks at an average interval of 14.9 ± 0.7 days. The mean estradiol peak values of the females after pairing and their baseline values are lower than the corresponding values of the older, parous females shown in Table 3. Whether this is the result of differences in age, sexual experience or reproductive history cannot be determined at this time.

The present study suggests that mature Saguinus fuscicollis daughters do not experience regular reproductive cycles and are characterized by low estrogen levels as long as they live in their natal families, containing both parents. This may be indicative of an inhibitory influence exerted by the mother or by both parents. The presence or absence of siblings in the groups does not appear to be involved in this effect, since ♀ 230 lived only with her parents while the other females were members of large families. Removal from the family and pairing with an adult male results in estrogen increase and onset of cyclicity. This may be the result of a removal of parental suppression and/or stimulation by the adult male.

In common marmosets, suppression of cyclicity in all but the α-female appears to occur only when nonrelated females cohabit in one group, but is not seen in daughters living in their families[10]. It is not clear whether this is species specific. Moreover, it remains to be seen whether or not suppression of cyclicity in family living tamarins is a uniform phenomenon or whether this happens only in some families but not others. It is also possible that our data illustrate a delay in the onset of cyclicity and that daughters will eventually start cycling as they age in the families.

Pregnancy and Parturition

The Callitrichidae are the only simian primates in which multiple births are the rule rather than an exception and the regular production of heterozygous twins in an approximately 1:1 sex ratio is well documented. While in species of Callithrix triplets or even quadruplets are relatively frequent[10], twins are predominant in most species of Saguinus studied so far[5,8,11,12,51-57]. Although most sets of twins are heterozygotic, extensive placental vascular anastomoses develop early in pregnancy and result in sharing of the blood supply between the fetuses. This, in turn, leads to blood chimerism and immunological tolerance between twins but apparently does not cause the previously suspected funtional germ cell chimerism[4,11,12,52,53,58].

The gestation period varies among tamarins between 128 days in Leontopithecus rosalia[31,59] and 150 days in most species of Saguinus[3,5,6,8,34,36]. Infants are born in any month of the year but several species are seasonal breeders under natural conditions and tend to show a birth peak in the laboratory[6,8,18,24,26,39,51,56,57]. Several methods for the early detection and for the monitoring of pregnancy are now available. The appearence and disappearence of radioimmunoassayable urinary chorionic gonadotropin in the course of pregnancy has proven to be a valuable tool, although it cannot be used to time conception and parturition with great accuracy. Hearn[10] discusses the work on chorionic gonadotropin in Callithrix jacchus. In a study including several species of Saguinus (Saguinus fuscicollis, Saguinus nigricollis, Saguinus oedipus oedipus) urinary gonadotropin was detectable approximately 2 weeks after conception as defined by back dating from term deliveries. Peak levels were found between the seventh and ninth week after conception, declining thereafter. During the final month of pregnancy, chorionic gonadotropin levels were below detection[60].

In a study on Leontopithecus rosalia, urinary chorionic gonadotropin appeared in measurable quantities about 4 weeks after the estimated day of conception, remained at detection levels up to nine weeks before birth and then fell below detection levels[61]. A hemagglutination inhibition test can also be used to diagnose pregnancy. Hodgen et al.[60] obtained positive results using the Subhuman Primate Pregnancy Test Kit* with several species of Saguinus as early as 15-20 days after conception and were able to diagnose pregnancy more reliably by 25-30 days. During the final six weeks of pregnancy, all specimens gave negative results again.

Uterine palpation is also an excellent tool to diagnose pregnancy and predict delivery. Since it requires regular handling of the pregnant female, however, it may not be advisable for highly excitable individuals. Using abdominal palpation, trained observers not only can confirm pregnancy by 25-30 days, but are also able to detect the number of fetuses and follow their physical development[62,63].

---

* Available from the Contraceptive Development Branch, National Institute of Child Health and Human Development.

Parturition in callitrichids usually takes place during the night. Because of this, very few descriptions of the actual birth process and associated behaviors are available. The behavior of mother and neonates during the birth process are of critical importance for infant survival and therefore there is a great need for more information. The only studies dealing in some detail with parturition have been performed in Callithrix jacchus, and give information on physical and behavioral changes during pregnancy, on diurnal distribution of births, the course of labor and delivery and the immediate post partum behavior of mother, neonates and other group members[64-68]. Information of comparable detail is not available for any Saguinus species but some data on the physical condition of Saguinus neonates and other physical and behavioral development can be found in a number of papers[3,6,8,34,69-73,76-78].

Two observations emerging from the studies on parturition in common marmosets may be of relevance for the maintenance of callitrichid breeding colonies and therefore shall be discussed briefly. From his observations on parturition in family groups of Callithrix jacchus, which were living in relatively large enclosures, Rothe[64-67] concludes that in this species females normally separate from the group for the purpose of giving birth. He reports that the pregnant female leaves the sleeping box at the onset of labor. She gives birth at a locality up to five meters away from the rest of the group and stays away from the common sleeping quarters for the rest of the night, sleeping and resting with the neonates. In contrast to Rothe's observations, Stevenson[68] did not see females withdraw from the rest of the group prior to parturition. This might reflect individual variability or differences between the living quarters of Rothe's and Stevenson's colonies.

Another important finding emerging from Rothe's[64-67] and Stevenson's[68] work is that neonates depend almost entirely on their own efforts to gain access to their mother's body and nipples. Therefore, their chance of surviving the first hours of extrauterine life is dependent upon the vigor of the neonates. As soon as they have been expelled far enough, the babies grasp their mother's fur with both hands, performing rowing and rotating movements. After establishing contact with the mother's body, they orient themselves toward her head. Immediately after being expelled fully, even if still attached to the unborn palacenta, the neonates start to climb along the mother's abdomen or back toward her nipples. In doing so, they receive no manual support from the mother who only licks the neonates and may cup one or both hands under their heads. This possibly aids the babies in their initial orientation on the mother's body. Neonates who are too weak to move and vocalize are neglected by the mother after a short period of initial licking. Moreover, they are in great danger of being eaten by the group, particularly if they assume unnatural postures and do not vocalize[65,67].

We have observed a few birth episodes in our colony of Saguinus fuscicollis and Saguinus labiatus. In the cages in which these tamarins are housed (see below), parturient females cannot withdraw from the rest of the group, even if they should normally do so. Therefore, it may be an artifact that during those deliveries we observed, the mother was attended by her mate. During one Saguinus fuscicollis delivery, the mother expelled the single infant while standing on a branch. One of the two adult males living with her immediately retrieved the neonate which had fallen to the floor of the cage, and carried it for about 1/2 hour while the mother rested. During this time, the infant was licked dry by the second male living with the pair. In a Saguinus labiatus family, we again observed the male actively assisting the parturient female. In this case, twins were born in rapid succession. The mother expelled the first infant while standing on a branch. The neonate, still attached to the unborn placenta, was hanging down. The father approached and supported the neonate with both arms. The baby crawled onto the male's body, rupturing the umbilical cord. The father carried the infant while the mother expelled the second neonate which then crawled onto her body. During the delivery, the father repeatedly threatened the other family members who tried to approach the parturient female.

Similar to Callithrix jacchus, neonatal tamarins mount the body of their carrier by their own effort. The carrier may partially support the infant by holding its head with both hands and by pulling it close, in this way directing it toward his own body. However, infants are never picked up and fully supported as seen, for example, in macaques. Neonates or older dependent infants which are too weak to mount their carrier and cling to its body during normal locomotion will invariably fall. Although experienced tamarin parents do not usually neglect a fallen infant, but hover over it, attempting to facilitate remounting by the baby, repeated falls weaken the infant. After repeated attempts at retrieval, the parents finally neglect the babies.

Care of infants

During the first month of life, young tamarins are always carried by a group member. Even on the first day, the infants are capable of supporting themselves on the body of their carrier during the normal activities of the group. The infants are usually carried dorsally, riding on the back of their carrier, often draped across its shoulders. Ventral carrying only occurs when the infants nurse.

Data on the care and on the physical and behavioral development of infants have been provided for Saguinus midas[34], Saguinus oedipus oedipus and Saguinus oedipus geofroyi[3,6,37,70,71,72,73,74], Saguinus fuscicollis[1,75,76] and Leontopithecus rosalia[77,78]. To review these studies in detail would go beyond the scope of this chapter. However, one important observation emerging from all of the papers, the strong participation of the father and other group members in the care of the offspring, has to be discussed. In contrast to the majority of primate species, transport of the young and other care-giving behaviors are performed by all group members. Usually, mother, father, nonrelated adults and even juveniles participate in infant care. Although the parents, and particularly the father, tend to perform most of the care giving at least for very young infants, the degree to which the various group members are involved is subject to considerable interindividual and interspecies variability[34,37,70-74,76-80]. Several authors have recently pointed out that participation in infant care by juveniles not only benefits the parents but might be important in preparing the juveniles for their future role as parents[10,79,81].

Our observations on Saguinus fuscicollis and Saguinus labiatus show that this experience is absolutely essential for the development of adequate parental behavior, particularly in females of these species. Animals who have been removed from their natal family before they have had a chance to participate in the care of younger siblings almost always neglect and often even kill their infants. We reported previously that in our colony the neonates of 76.5% of all Saguinus fuscicollis primiparas who had never participated in the care of younger siblings were found dead or severely mutilated[*80,81]. Similar observations were subsequently made in our Saguinus labiatus. There is evidence that most of these infants were born alive and healthy and were killed by the mother or both parents[80,81]. Eighty percent of all experienced primiparas, on the other hand, took adequate care of their offspring. These data demonstrate that participation in the care of infants prior to becoming a parent is essential for the development of adequate parental care. This experience is probably important for both parents, but may be more crucial for the mother than for the father. This is suggested by our observation that all Saguinus fuscicollis pairs consisting of parentally experienced pluriparas and parentally inexperienced males give adequate care to their first offspring sired by the male. In pairs with parentally naive fathers, the mothers seemed to receive less help in infant care from their mates during the first few days postpartum than in pairs where both parents were experienced. This indicates that previous parental experience is more crucial for the mother than for the father, perhaps because she is the one who has first access to the neonates[80,81].

The parental inadequacy of naive animals seems to correct itself somewhat as successive sets of infants are born. However, breeding pairs containing pluriparas who never participated in sibling care during their first year of life and have now had a large number of litters still tend to occasionally kill one or both of their twins, chew the tails off the neonates or bite them more or less severely. Thus, it appears that a permanent deficiency exists which can

* Since parturition was not observed, stillbirths, perhaps caused by unknown blood factors[8,82] cannot be excluded.

only be partly corrected as experience with their own offspring increases over the years. Similar observations have been made in Leontopithecus rosalia[79,83]. According to our experience, the tendency to aggress against neonates is enhanced in a densely populated colony room. Removing "killer" pairs from our colony room of 1,000 square feet, housing 30 groups, and placing them into isolation shortly before parturition reduced the likelihood of the neonates being killed but did not eliminate it.

Physical and reproductive development

Little is known about the development of Saguinus species. Some information on birth weights and their relationship to the number of neonates, on dentition, ossification, infant mortality and behavioral development is given by Chrisren[34], Glaser[84], Epple[3], Hampton et al.[55] and Wolfe et al.[8].

Females maturing in their families do not reproduce and there is little sexual activity among adult, family living offspring. Therefore, the age when sexual maturity is reached is hard to determine in animals living in their parental groups. Abbott and Hearn[85] studied endocrine and behavioral parameters in male and female common marmosets which were removed from their families prior to puberty. In this species a period of puberty (400-500 days of age) when gametes are produced and copulations occur, but female cycles may be anovulatory, is followed by sexual maturity at the age of 500 to 600 days, when most first conceptions occur. No comparably detailed data are available for any Saguinus species. However, some histological data on the gonadal development of Saguinus oedipus oedipus and Saguinus fuscicollis from fetal stages to adulthood are provided by Hampton and Taylor[86]. According to these authors, the testes are abdominal at birth, become inguinal at 2-3 months and descend to the scrotum at 8-11 months. At that age, the tubule diameter increases to a prepubertal width of 100-110 μm. Prepubertal changes in the testes begin at 14 months of age when the tubules are open and their diameter has increased to 120-130 μm, but mature sperm is not seen until 16 months of age. The adult testis shows a tubule diameter of 220-230 μm.

In neonatal females, primordial follicles extend almost to the gonadal surface. Oogenesis ceases shortly after birth, when all oocytes reach the diplotene stage of meiosis. At four months of age, the number of granulosa cells increases, forming primary follicles and follicular enlargement forming secondary and tertiary follicles is seen at 8 months. No pubertal ovaries were available for study. The adult ovary possesses a large amount of permanent tissue which shows the histological characteristics of luteal tissue. This appears to be derived from artretic follicles and is present in addition to the corpus luteum of ovulation. Its functional significance is, to date, unknown.

In our Saguinus fuscicollis, the testes are abdominal at birth but reliably appear high in the inguinal canal on the third day after birth. They remain inguinal for approximately 70 days, when they begin to descend into the scrotum. Descensus proceeds slowly and is completed by 90-150 days of age. Individual variability however, is present. We have no histological data on pubertal changes in the gonads of either sex, but in one 13 month old male (living with an adult female), whose testes were sectioned, the epididymis contained a large amount of mature sperm.

The observations reviewed above as well as reproduction records from several colonies suggest that *Saguinus* species reach sexual maturity at approximately the same age as *Callithrix jacchus*. However, the results of a recent study[50] suggest that, depending on social living conditions, *Saguinus fuscicollis* may reach sexual maturity considerably earlier than expected. Epple and Katz[50] recorded the age at which young females experienced their first evident pregnancy and at which young males caused their first evident pregnancy, in animals which were removed from their families and cohabited from 6 months of age with either an adult or a young nonrelated sex partner. The following pair combinations and trios were studied: 1) one young male and one young female (8 pairs); 2) one young male and one adult female (7 pairs); 3) one adult male and one young female (5 pairs); 4) one adult male, one young male and one young female (5 trios). In this study, only those pregnancies confirmed by abortion or term birth were recorded and no efforts were made to detect early pregnancies.

Table 5 shows the ages at which the juveniles were removed from their families, the number of females in whom pregnancies were observed, the ratio of aborted to term pregnancies and the mean age at which young females conceived and young males sired offspring.

Table 5. Reproduction in juvenile females (f) and juvenile males (m) grouped with juvenile or adult (M,F) mates of the opposite sex. Means and standard errors are given. Conception dates were estimated from a gestation period of 150 days. Abortions were assumed to have taken place at midterm.

Subject	Partner	Age (days) when placed in group	Ratio of: subjects to pregnancies	Ratio of: births to abortions	Age (days) at conception for: all pregnancies	Age (days) at conception for: term pregnancies
f	m	181.4±7.1	8:6	3:3	631.0±25.9	633.7±44.7
f	M	188.0±4.3	5:5	5:0	398.4±56.8	398.4±56.8
f	mM	196.2±10.6	5:5	4:1	400.8±63.1	405.0±81.3
m	f	187.5±5.6	8:6	-	627.0±27.8	632.0±50.7
m	F	184.1±3.7	7:7	-	444.1±45.5	453.8±64.1

As the table shows, young females living with adult males in pairs and trios conceived at a significantly earlier age than young females living with young males. Young males living with adult females sired offspring at a significantly earlier age than young males living with females of their own age. The data seem to suggest that young females can conceive at an earlier age than males are able to impregnate. However, there was no significant difference in the ages at which young females cohabiting with adult males conceived and young males cohabiting with adult females sired offspring. A more clear cut difference might have emerged if a larger number of subjects had been used.

All young females cohabiting with adult males reproduced. Two of the eight young females living with young males, on the other hand, showed no evidence of pregnancy up to an age of over 3 years. Moreover, the percentage of pregnancies progressing to term was higher in young females living with adult males (90%) than those living with a male of their own age (75%). The study discussed above suggests that in the saddle back tamarin the age at puberty is, in part, dependent on social cues. Monkeys of both sexes are capable of producing offspring at an earlier age when they cohabit with an adult mate than when they cohabit with a partner of their own age. This effect may not be unique to Saguinus fuscicollis. Abbott and Hearn[85]. also reported early reproductive success in juvenile common marmosets paired with adults of the opposite sex. Whether these effects are the result of a behavioral process, a physiological process, or both, remains to be seen.

The studies reviewed above show that early removal from the family and pairing with an adult sex partner can advance the age at which tamarins will produce young. It is not advisable, however, to remove young tamarins from their parents in order to accelerate their reproductive performance before they have participated in the care of their siblings. Being deprived of this parental experience will result in inadequate care of infants once these animals breed and their offspring are unlikely to survive.

MANAGEMENT OF LABORATORY COLONIES

General Considerations

The monogamous mating system, participation of the father and older siblings in infant care, reproductive suppression in all but one female of each group and a tendency toward territoriality and strong aggressiveness against adult conspecifics not belonging to the same group are characteristics which set tamarins and marmosets apart from most other primates used in biomedical research. These characteristics have to be taken into account in the establishment and maintenance of successful laboratory breeding colonies. It is now generally accepted that for breeding purposes, all callitrichids should be maintained as permanently cohabiting male-female pairs and that each breeding pair and their progeny should be housed in a separate cage. In tamarins, adequate parental behavior develops only after animals have participated in the care of infants before becoming parents. Therefore, young tamarins designated to become breeders should remain with their parents at least until their younger siblings have been weaned. For the same reason, removal of the neonates from their parents for hand rearing is not recommended for animals selected as future breeders, although this may shorten interbirth intervals in the mother and result in a higher reproductive yield[8]. Many laboratories now are observing these general guidelines successfully. They have reported their husbandry procedures and have published reproduction statistics[3-10,34,54-57,59,80,81,87,88].

Although breeding success in many colonies has improved constantly during recent years, a variety of health disorders still pose problems in the maintenance and propagation in newly imported as well as colony born tamarins. One problem, which has appeared worldwide in tamarins and marmosets which have lived in a colony environment for months or years in apparently good health is "Wasting Marmoset Syndrome". The condition is characterized by chronically progressing emaciation and finally death. It is associated with a variety of symptoms such as hair loss, loss of muscle mass, skin lesions, chronic diarrhea and sometimes very selective eating habits and is often accompanied by anemia, malabsorption and chronic, recurrent colitis. Occasionally, the condition can be reversed by dietary changes such as increasing the protein content of the diet, but a clear relationship between wasting and dietary deficiencies has not been documented. Indeed, at present it is not at all clear whether all wasting symptoms have a common etiology or whether they are the result of a number of different disorders and deficiencies[89-92]. Efforts to identify nutritional and other possible causes for this disorder are presently under way in many laboratories, and the Veterinary Resources Branch of the National Institutes of Health* serves as a center for the collection and distribution of information about the "syndrome".

A variety of other health problems, such as the high susceptibility of callitrichids to several viruses, bacteria and parasites have to be dealt with in colony management. A detailed discussion of the papers concerned with these problems is beyond the scope of this article. Reviews by Cicmanec[93], Hunt et al.[94], Kingston[95] and Wagner[96] deal with the most frequently encountered parasitic, viral and bacterial infections and their clinical treatment. Further, detailed information can be found in the volume on marmosets in experimental medicine edited by Gengozian and Deinhardt[5].

Housing and maintenance of *Saguinus fuscicollis*

The considerations on callitrichid management outlined above are now taken into account by most researchers concerned with establishing breeding colonies[3-10,34,57,87,88]. Details of housing, feeding and health-care, however,

* Building 14 D, Room 331, Bethesda, MD 20205, U.S.A.

vary among colonies, and are determined not only by the physical facilities available but also by the kind of research problems addressed and, to a large degree, by the disposition of the particular callitrichid species maintained. Therefore, rather than discussing all the colony management procedures published previously, we shall describe our own procedures as an example and also present some reproduction statistics.

Our colony of callitrichids is maintained for the purpose of behavioral and endocrine research and contains approximately 200 Saguinus fuscicollis and a small number of Saguinus labiatus and Saguinus leucopus. All animals which are maintained as breeders live as permanently cohabiting male-female pairs, some as parents of large families of up to 12 members. Each pair or group inhabits a home cage. Cages housing pairs or small families (up to 4 animals) measure 0.6 x 1.2 x 1.8 m, large family cages 1.76 x 1.20 x 1.20 m. Although other laboratories have reported breeding success in smaller cages[4-10,87,88], a cage of this size provides the minimum amount of space necessary for the maintenance of larger groups and for the conduct of our behavioral studies. All our cages are constructed of aluminum sheeting and wire mesh and are mounted on casters. Each cage has a solid back and side walls of aluminum sheeting and a top, floor and front of 2.5 x 2.5 cm wire mesh. It is divided by a wire mesh wall into 2 compartments which are connected by a small sliding door. Both compartments are accessible to the animals and are equipped with natural branches, wire mesh shelves and a plastic nest box. The cage floors are 2 feet above the room floor. All refuse falls out of reach of the monkeys onto brown packing paper which is spread on the floor of the room and is exchanged daily. The cages are arranged in rows, each cage front facing the solid back of the previous row. Therefore, their inhabitants cannot see the animals in other cages. This provides a certain degree of isolation from neighboring groups, which we have found to be essential for the successful breeding of Saguinus fuscicollis in densely populated colony rooms.

The colony is housed entirely indoors and our animal rooms are maintained at a temperature of 27°C and at 50% relative humidity. They are equipped with Vita Lights*, a fluorescent light mimicking the full daylight spectrum, and are lighted for 12 hours a day. The animal rooms are cleaned daily. The cages are washed in a commercial cage washer, using hot water and a chlorinated detergent, followed by a clean water rinse. Since odor communication and scent marking behavior are of great importance in the social life of Saguinus fuscicollis[97], frequent sanitizing, leading to a constant disruption of the olfactory environment, is avoided. Therefore, the cages are washed only when necessary (usually once a month).

In their natural environment, tamarins are omnivorous, consuming a varied

* Duro Test, North Bergen, NJ, U.S.A.

diet. Izawa[23] for example, reports that Saguinus nigricollis eats fruit, sprouts, tree sap and a large variety of insects. In addition, this species spends a considerable amount of time hunting large grasshoppers, and Izawa[23] argues that insects and particularly large grasshoppers constitute its main food. Since the nutritional requirements of tamarins under laboratory conditions have not been well defined, we provide our animals with a varied diet as well. The animals are fed twice daily, receiving a choice of the following items [the code in parentheses indicates morning (M) and afternoon feeding (A) and the number of days per week on which the item is included in the diet]: canned marmoset diet* (M3), oatmeal made of rolled oats, milk and butter and supplemented with vitamin D_3 at 200 international units per animal (M4), banana (M7), apple (M5), lettuce (M1), cooked carrots (M1), hard boiled eggs (M7), Purina high protein monkey chow (A4), Purina cat chow (A3). Boiled chicken and live mealworms serve as occasional "treats". The daily addition of eggs to the diet has eliminated most cases of "Marmoset Wasting Syndrome" in the colony. Presently, our losses from wasting syndrome range between 1% and 3% of the resident population per year.

One full-time animal caretaker, assisted by 2-3 part-time students, handles the colony. In addition to the caretaking staff, two technicians, several researchers and a variable number of students conducting research projects enter the colony. All personnel fill out a health questionnaire when they enter the colony for the first time and are advised to report any illness of their own or of persons with whom they associate. Persons who have been exposed to diseases to which callitrichids are known to be susceptible will not enter the colony for several weeks. Each animal is checked daily by the author or her senior technician. Any loss of condition such as ruffled or dull hair coat, weight loss or inactivity are recorded and an effort is made to identify and correct its cause. It is worth noting here that not infrequently the cause for such loss of condition appears to be social stress, particularly in large families. These are the only routine health precautions taken. No particular clothing and no facial masks are worn around the animals. The colony is closed. Except for the purchase of a few Saguinus labiatus in 1977, we have not acquired any animals since 1971. No other primate species are housed in our building and the monkeys are not exposed to other laboratory animals. Under these conditions, we have had no major health problems in the colony.

Reproductive statistics

The colony presently contains 216 Saguinus fuscicollis, all but 9 individuals born in the colony. We maintain Saguinus f. illigeri, a few Saguinus f. fuscicollis and Saguinus f. nigrifrons, as well as hybrids between these subspecies and a single Saguinus f. lagonotus female. The colony was established from 40 wild born males and 24 wild born females, purchased between 1969 and 1971.

* Hills', PO Box 148, Topeka, KA 66001, U.S.A.

Forty-six of these animals survived quarantaine, and from among them, 17 females were selected as potential breeders. Twelve of the 17 females were successful and they and their offspring have produced a total of 504 term infants to date. In addition to our saddle back tamarins, we maintain several breeding groups of *Saguinus labiatus*, derived from three wild-caught pairs purchased in 1977.

Table 6. Reproductive history of the colony. I. *Saguinus fuscicollis* between November, 1969 and March, 1981. II. *Saguinus labiatus* between February, 1978 and March, 1981.

	I	II
A. Total # of term babies	504 (100%)	37 (100%)
B. # born alive (% of A)	397 (78.8%)	34 (91.9%)
C. # killed by parents (% of A)	76 (15.1%)	3 (8.1%)
D. # still born (% of A)	31 (6.1%)	0
E. # of abortions (incidents)	26	0
F. # reaching at least 1 year of age in colony (% of B)	389 (97.9%)	25 (71.4%)
G. # disposed of alive (% of B)		
under 1 year old	8 (2.0%)	
one year and older	70 (17.6%)	
H. # retained in the colony (% of B)	319 (80.4%)	

Table 6 shows the total number of offspring produced between 1969 and 1981, and their mortality and survival records. The space available to the colony is limited and because of this space limitation, we regularly dispose of our surplus animals, mostly adults, which are placed into breeding programs at other institutions. Table 7 summarizes the life statistics of only those animals who were permanently retained in our colony.

Table 7. Mortality and survival records of *Saguinus fuscicollis* born and retained in the colony between November, 1969 and March, 1981. Only animals born and retained in the colony are included here.

A. Total # of animals born and retained (%)	319	(100%)
B. Total # of animals who died (% of A):	112	(35%)
a. before 10 days of age (% of B)	49	(43.8%)
b. between 10 days and 1 year of age (% of B)	34	(30.4%)
c. between 1 and 2 years of age (% of B)	11	(9.8%)
d. after 2 years of age (% of B)	18	(16.0%)
C. Total # of animals presently alive (% of A)	207	(65%)
a. under 1 year of age (% of C)	52	(25%)
b. between 1 and 2 years of age (% of C)	32	(15.5%)
c. 2 years old or older (% of C)	123	(59.5%)

Table 8 shows the number of breeding *Saguinus fuscicollis* females maintained in the colony between 1969 and March, 1981, their genealogy, the average lengths of time they lived in a breeding situation (i.e., pair bonded to a fertile male*) and the average number of live babies produced per female. The genealogy of the females is encoded as follows: F_1 - both parents wild born; F_{1-2} - offspring of a wild born male and an F_1 female; F_{2-1} - offspring of an F_1 male and a wild born female; F_2 - both parents F_1; F_x - this category includes 3 daughters of an F_1 father and an F_{1-2} mother, 2 daughters of a wild born male and an F_{2-3} female, 2 daughters of an F_1 male and an F_{3-4} female and 1 daughter of an F_2 male and a wild born female.

Table 8. Origin and number of breeding females between 1969 and March, 1981, average number of years maintained in a breeding position and average number of term offspring produced per female. The number of term babies believed to have been born alive but killed by the parents is given in parentheses in addition to the number of live offspring.

	Wild born (n = 12)	F_1 (n = 18)	F_{1-2} (n = 10) F_{2-1} (n = 1)	F_2 (n = 6)	F_x (n = 8)
# of years spent as a breeder	5.3	4.8	2.9	1.5	2.9
# of term babies	10.9 (0)	8.6 (2.7)	5 (1.1)	1.8 (0.2)	5.4 (0.8)

Some of the breeding females lived in trios with 2 males at the same time or were consecutively paired with several males, one male at a time. A total of 22 wild born males, 18 F_1, 13 F_2, 9 F_{1-2}, 4 F_{2-1}, 2 F_{1-3}, 3 F_{2-3} and 2 F_{3-1} males lived in a breeding situation. Fourteen of the wild born and 12 of the laboratory born males lived in trios, each consisting of 2 males (both either wild or laboratory born) and one female and their genetic input into the female's offspring is unknown. No effort was made to pair wild born and laboratory born animals with mates of the same origin. However, once the impact of parental experience on raising performance was known, we tried to pair those animals who had never participated in the care of their siblings, and were therefore parentally inexperienced,with mates who had been helpers of their parents and therefore were experienced.

As Table 8 shows, the fecundity of wild born and laboratory born females is approximately the same, with 2 live infants produced on the average per year. However, there was considerable variability among individual females. Some wild born as well as some laboratory born females regularly delivered 4 infants per year, one F_1 even having 6 babies (triplets twice) in 1980. There was no

* Some of the females intermittently lived with sterile males for experimental purposes.

difference in fecundity between purebred and hybrid mothers with the exception of *Saguinus f. fuscicollis* females. One out of 3 wild caught females and 2 out of 3 laboratory born females of this subspecies, failed to reproduce. Since the number of females is so small, however, and since the 2 laboratory born nonbreeders are sisters, these data are inconclusive.

The longevity record in the colony is maintained by two wild-caught females, purchased in 1969. They are estimated to be 13 and 15 years old, have produced 25 and 26 term babies and are still breeding. The mother who produced most live offspring in the colony, however, is an F_1 female, presently 11 years of age, who has given birth to 28 live babies since November, 1971 and has raised 23 of them. In general, the survival rate of the offspring born in the colony was excellent. However, although 97.9% of all live born *Saguinus fuscicollis* survived to at least one year of age (Table 6-F), the offspring of a few females survived much less well than the offspring of others. The most unsuccessful mother for example, an F_{1-2} female, lost 7 of her 12 live born offspring before they were one year old. Although immunological blood factors, known to occur in this species[81], may be responsible for the death of some of the neonates, the deaths of older infants are unexplained.

In summarizing our husbandry procedures and reproduction statistics, it appears that there are no insurmountable difficulties in the long term maintenance of *Saguinus fuscicollis*. Taking into account some of the behavioral characteristics outlined above, providing the animals with a sufficient amount of visually shielded space and a varied diet and selecting parentally experienced breeders should enable a laboratory to produce these tamarins through successive generations. Our limited experience with *Saguinus labiatus* suggests that this tamarin is an even better candidate for successful laboratory breeding.

REFERENCES

1. Epple, G. (1975). The behavior of marmoset monkeys (Callithricidae). In: L.R. Rosenblum (ed.) *Primate Behavior*, *Vol. 4*, p . 195 (New York: Academic Press
2. Deinhardt, J.B., Devine, J., Passovoy, M., Pohlman, R. and Deinhardt, F. (1967). Marmosets as laboratory animals. I. Care of marmosets in the laboratory, pathology and outline of statistical evaluation of data. *Lab. Anim. Care*, *17*, 11
3. Epple, G. (1970). Maintenance, breeding and development of marmoset monkeys (Callithricidae) in captivity. *Folia primat.* *12*, 56
4. Gengozian, N. (1969). Marmosets: Their potential in experimental medicine. *Ann. N.Y. Acad. Sci.*, *162*, 336
5. Gengozian, N., Batson, J.S. and Smith, T.A. (1978). Breeding of marmosets in a colony environment. In: N. Gengozian and F. Deinhardt (eds.) *Marmosets*

in Experimental Medicine. Primates in Medicine, Vol. 10, p. 71 (Basel: Karger)

6. Hampton, J.K., Hampton, S.H. and Landwehr, B.T. (1966). Observations on a successful breeding colony of the marmoset Oedipomidas oedipus. Folia Primat. 4, 265

7. Ogden, J.D. and Wolfe, L.G. (1979). Reproduction of wild-caught marmosets (Saguinus labiatus labiatus) under laboratory conditions. Lab. Anim. Sci., 29, 545

8. Wolfe, L.G., Deinhardt, F., Ogden, J.D., Adams, M.R. and Fisher, L.E. (1975). Reproduction of wild-caught and laboratory born marmoset species used in biomedical research (Saguinus sp. Callithrix jacchus). Lab. Anim. Sci. 26, 802

9. Hiddleston, W.A. (1976). Large scale production of a small laboratory primate - Callithrix jacchus. In: T. Antikatzides, S. Erichsen and A. Spiegel (eds.) The Laboratory Animal in the Study of Reproduction, p.51 (Stuttgart: Gustav Fischer Verlag)

10. Hearn, J.P. (1974-81). See reference list of Chapter 6

11. Gengozian, N. (1978). Immunology and blood chimerism of the marmoset. In: N. Gengozian and F. Deinhardt (eds.) Marmosets in Experimental Medicine: Primates in Medicine, Vol. 10, p.173 (Basel: Karger)

12. Gengozian, N. (1979). The marmoset as a model for twinning, chimerism and immunologic tolerance. In: E.J. Andres, B.C. Ward and N.H. Altman (eds.) Spontaneous Animal Models of Human Disease, Vol. 1, p.222 (New York: Academic Press)

13. Wolfe, L.G. and Deinhardt, F. (1978). Overview of viral oncology studies in Saguinus and Callithrix species. In: N. Gengozian and F. Deinhardt (eds.) Marmosets in Experimental Medicine: Primates in Medicine, Vol. 10, p.96 (Basel: Karger)

14. Lushbaugh, C.C., Humason, G.L., Swartzendruber, D.C., Richer, C.B. and Gengozian, N. (1978). Spontaneous colonic adenocarcinoma in marmosets. In: N. Gengozian and F. Deinhardt (eds.) Marmosets in Experimental Medicine: Primates in Medicine, Vol. 10, p.119 (Basel: Karger)

15. Deinhardt, F. (1978). Hepatitis in marmosets: An introduction. In: N. Gengozian and F. Deinhardt (eds.) Marmosets in Experimental Medicine: Primates in Medicine, Vol. 10, p.277 (Basel: Karger)

16. Provost, P.J., Villarejos, V.M. and Hilleman, M.R. (1978). Tests in Rufiventer and other marmosets of susceptibility to human hepatitis A virus. In: N. Gengozian and F. Deinhardt (eds.) Marmosets in Experimental Medicine: Primates in Medicine, Vol. 10, p.288 (Basel: Karger)

17. Castro, R. and Soini, P. (1977). Field studies on Saguinus mystax and other callitrichids in Amazoniam Peru. In: D.G. Kleiman (ed.) The Biology and Conservation of the Callitrichidae, p.73 (Washington, D.C.: Smithsonian

Institution Press)

18. Coimbra-Filho, A.F. (1969). Mico-leão *Leontideus rosalia* (Linnaeus, 1766), situação atual de espécie no Brasil (Callithricidae, Primates). *An. Acad. Brasil Ciênc.*, *41*, 29
19. Dawson, G.A. (1977). Composition and stability of social groups of the tamarin *Saguinus oedipus geoffroyi* in Panama: Ecological and behavioral implications. In: D.G. Kleiman (ed.) *The Biology and Conservation of the Callitrichidae*, p. 23 (Washington, D.C.: Smithsonian Institution Press)
20. Dawson, G.A. (1979). The use of time and space by the Panamanian tamarin, *Saguinus oedipus*. *Folia primat.*, *31*, 253
21. Freese, C.H., Freese, M.A. and Castro, N. (1977). The status of callitrichids in Peru. In: D.G. Kleiman (ed.) *The Biology and Conservation of the Callitrichidae*, p. 118 (Washington, D.C.: Smithsonian Institution Press)
22. Hernandez-Camacho, J. and Cooper, R.W. (1976). Neotropical primates: aspects of habitat usage, population density and regional distribution in La Macarena, Columbia. In: R.W. Thorington and P.G. Heltne (eds.) *Neotropical Primates, Field Studies and Conservation*, p. 35 (Washington, D.C.: Natl. Acad. Sci.)
23. Izawa, K. (1978). A field study of the ecology and behavior of the black-mantle tamarin (*Saguinus nigricollis*). *Primates*, *19*, 241
24. Moynihan, M. (1970). Some behavior patterns of platyrrhine monkeys. II *Saguinus geoffroyi* and some other tamarins. *Smithson. Contrib. Zool.*, *28*, 1
25. Neyman, P.F. (1977). Aspects of the ecology and social organization of free-ranging cotton top tamarins (*Saguinus oedipus*) and the conservation status of the species. In: D.G. Kleiman (ed.) *Biology and Conservation of the Callitrichidae*, p. 39 (Washington, D.C.: Smithsonian Institution Press)
26. Terborg, J. (in press). *The Behavioral Ecology of Five New World Primates* (Princeton: Princeton University Press)
27. Thorington, R.W., Jr. (1968). Observations of the tamarin *Saguinus midas*. *Folia primat.*, *9*, 95
28. Epple, G. (1977). Notes on the establishment and maintenance of the pair bond in *Saguinus fuscicollis*. In: D.G. Kleiman (ed.) *The Biology and Conservation of the Callitrichidae*, p. 231 (Washington, D.C.: Smithsonian Institution Press)
29. Kleiman, D.G. (1977). Monogamy in mammals. *Quart. Rev. Biol.*, *52*, 39
30. Epple, G. (1972). Social behavior of laboratory groups of *Saguinus fuscicollis*. In: D.D. Bridwater (ed.) *Saving the Lion Marmoset, Proc. WAPT Golden Lion Marmoset Conference*, p. 50 (Oglebay Park, Wheeling, West Virginia: WAPT)
31. Kleiman, D.G. (1978). The development of pair preferences in the lion tamarin (*Leontopithecus rosalia*) male competition or female choice?

In: H. Rothe, H.J. Wolters and J.P. Hearn (eds.) Biology and Behavior of Marmosets, p. 203 (Göttingen: Eigenverlag Rothe)

32. Poole, T.B. (1978). A behavioral investigation of "pair bond" maintenance in Callithrix jacchus jacchus. In: H. Rothe, H.J. Wolters and J.P. Hearn (eds.) Biology and Behavior of Marmosets, p. 209 (Göttingen, W. Germany: Eigenverlag Rothe)
33. Epple, G. (1978). Lack of effects of castration on scent marking, displays and aggression in a South American primate (Saguinus fuscicollis). Horm. Behav., 11, 139
34. Christen, A. (1974). Fortpflanzungsbiologie und Verhalten bei Cebuella pygmaea und Tamarin tamarin. Fortschritte der Verhaltensforschung. Beih. Z. Tierpsychol., 14, 5
35. Rothe, H. (1975). Some aspects of sexuality and reproduction in groups of captive marmosets (Callithrix jacchus). Z. Tierpsychol., 37, 255
36. Epple, G. (unpublished)
37. Epple, G. (1967). Vergleichende Untersuchungen über Sexual- und Sozialverhalten der Kallenaffen (Hapalidae). Folia primat., 7, 37
38. French, J.A. and Snowdon, C.T. (in press). Sexual dimorphism in intergroup spacing behavior in the tamarin, Saguinus oedipus. Anim. Behav.
39. Kleiman, D.G. (1977). Characteristics of reproduction and sociosexual interactions in pairs of lion tamarins (Leontopithecus rosalia) during the reproductive cycle. In: D.G. Kleiman (ed.) The Biology and Conservation of the Callithricidae, p. 181 (Washington, D.C.: Smithsonian Institution Press)
40. Preslock, J.P., Hampton, S.H. and Hampton, J.K. (1973). Cyclic variations of serum progestins and immunoreactive estrogens in marmosets. Endocrinol., 92, 1096
41. Hampton, S.H. and Hampton, J.K., Jr. (1977). Detection of reproductive cycles and pregnancy in tamarins (Saguinus spp.). In: D.G. Kleiman (ed.) The Biology and Conservation of the Callitrichidae, p. 173 (Washington, D.C.: Smithsonian Institution Press)
42. Katz, Y. and Epple, G. (in preparation). Social influences on plasma and urinary estradiol cyclicity in saddle back tamarins (Saguinus fuscicollis)
43. Zamečnik, J., Barbe, G., Moger, W.H. and Armstrong, D.T. (1977). Radioimmunoassay for androsterone, 5α-androstane-3α,17β-diol and 5α-androstane-3β,17β-diol. Steroids, 30, 679
44. Heingård, D. and Tiderström, G. (1973). Determination of serum creatinine by a direct colorimetric method. Clin. Chim. Acta 43, 305
45. Yamamoto, S., Utsu, S., Tanioka, Y. and Ohsawa, N. (1977). Extremely high levels of corticosteroids and low levels of corticosteroid binding macromolecules in plasma of marmoset monkeys. Acta Endocr., 85, 398
46. Preslock, J.P. and Steinberger, E. (1976). Pathway of testosterone

biosynthesis in the testis of the marmoset Saguinus oedipus. Steroids, 28, 775

47. Preslock, J.P. and Steinberger, E. (1977). Testicular steroidogenesis in the common marmoset, Callithrix jacchus. Biol. Reprod., 17, 289

48. Preslock, J.P. and Steinberger, E. (1979). Metabolism of pregnenolone and progesterone by testicular microsomes of the baboon Papio anubis and the marmoset Saguinus oedipus. J. Steroid Biochem., 10, 75

49. Preslock, J.P. and Steinberger, E. (1979). Product-inhibition of testicular steroidogenic enzymes in the marmoset Saguinus oedipus. J. Steroid Biochem., 11, 1151

50. Epple, G. and Katz, Y. (1980). Social influences on first reproductive success and related behaviors in the saddle back tamarin (Saguinus fuscicollis, Callitrichidae). Int. J. Primatol., 1, 171

51. Dawson, G.A. and Dukelow, W.R. (1976). Reproductive characteristics of free-ranging Panamanian tamarins (Saguinus oedipus geoffroyi). J. Med. Primatol., 5, 266

52. Benirschke, K., Anderson, J.M. and Brownhill, L.E. (1962). Marrow chimerism in the marmoset. Science, 138, 513

53. Benirschke, K., Anderson, J.M. and Brownhill, L.E. (1963). Heterosexual cells in testes of chimeric marmoset monkeys. Cytogenetics, 2, 331

54. Hampton, J.K. and Hampton, S.H. (1965). Marmosets (Hapalidae): Breeding seasons, twinning and sex offspring. Science, 150, 915

55. Hampton, J.K., Jr., Hampton, S.H. and Levy, B.M. (1971). Reproductive physiology and pregnancy in marmosets. In: Medical Primatology, 1970, Proc. 2nd Conf. Exp. Med. Surg. Primates, p. 527 (Basel:Karger, 1971)

56. Hampton, S.H., Gross, M.J. and Hampton, J.K., Jr. (1978). A comparison of captive breeding performance and offspring survival in the family Callitrichidae. In: N. Gengozian and F. Deinhardt (eds.) Marmosets in Experimental Medicine: Primates in Medicine, Vol. 10, p. 88 (Basel:Karger)

57. Ogden, J.D., Wolfe, L.G. and Deinhardt, F.W. (1978). Breeding Saguinus and Callithrix species of marmosets under laboratory conditions. In: N. Gengozian and F. Deinhardt (eds.) Marmosets in Experimental Medicine: Primates in Medicine, Vol. 10, p. 79 (Basel:Karger)

58. Gengozian, N., Brewer, J.G., Preston, K.J. and Batson, J.S. (1980). Presumptive evidence for the absence of functional germ cell chimerism in the marmoset. J. Med. Primatol, 9, 9

59. Wilson, C.G. (1977). Gestation and reproduction in golden lion tamarins. In: D.G. Kleiman (ed.) The Biology and Conservation of the Callitrichidae, p. 191 (Washington, D.C.: Smithsonian Institution Press)

60. Hodgen, G.D., Wolfe, L.G., Ogden, J.D., Adams, M.R., Descalzi, C.C. and Hildebrand, D.F. (1976). Diagnosis of pregnancy in marmosets: Hemagglutination inhibition test and radioimmunoassay for urinary chorionic.

gonadotropin. Lab Anim. Sci. 26, 224

61. Kleiman, D.G., Garcey, D.W. and Hodgen, G.D. (1978). Urinary chorionic gonadotropin levels in pregnant golden lion tamarins. J. Med. Primatol., 7, 333
62. Gengozian, N., Smith, T.A. and Gosslee, D.G. (1974). External uterine palpation to identify stages of pregnancy in the marmoset Saguinus fuscicollis ssp. J. Med. Primatol., 3, 236
63. Phillips, J.R. and Grist, S.M. (1975). The use of transabdominal palpation to determine the cause of pregnancy in the marmoset (Callithrix jacchus). J. Reprod. Fert., 43, 103
64. Rothe, H. (1973). Beobachtungen zur Geburt beim Weissbüscheläffchen (Callithrix jacchus, Erxleben, 1777). Folia primat., 19, 257
65. Rothe, H. (1974). Further observations on the delivery behavior of the common marmoset (Callithrix jacchus). Z. f. Säugetierkd, 39, 135
66. Rothe, H. (1975). Influence of newborn marmosets' (Callithrix jacchus) on expression and efficiency of maternal and paternal care. In: S. Kondo, M. Kawai and A. Ehara (eds.) Contemporary Primatology, p. 315 (Basel:Karger)
67. Rothe, H. (1977). Parturition and related behavior in Callithrix jacchus (Ceboidea, Callitrichidae) In: D.G. Kleiman (ed.) The Biology and Conservation of the Callitrichidae, p. 193 (Washington, D.C.: Smithsonian Institution Press)
68. Stevenson, M.F. (1976). Birth and perinatal behaviour in family groups of the common marmoset (Callithrix jacchus jacchus), compared to other primates. J. Human Evol., 5, 365
69. Pook, A.G. (1978). A comparison between the reproduction and parental behaviour of the Goeldi's monkey (Callimico goeldii) and of the true marmosets (Callitrichidae). In: H. Rothe, H.J. Wolters and J.P. Hearn (eds.) Biology and Behaviour of Marmosets, p. 1 (Göttingen: Eigenverlag Rothe)
70. Graetz, E. (1968). Studien über das mittelamerikanische Krallenäffchen Oedipomidas spixi. Sitzungsber. Ges. naturforsch. Freunde Berlin, 8, 29
71. Muckenhirn, N.A. (1967). The behavior and vocal repertoire of Saguinus oedipus (Hershkovitz, 1966) (Callithricidae, Primates). Thesis, College Park: Univ. of Maryland)
72. Willig, A. and Wendt, S. (1970). Aufzucht und Verhalten des Geoffroyi-Perückenäffchens Oedipomidas geoffroyi Pucheran, 1845. Säugetierkdl. Mittlg., 18, 117
73. Wendt, H. (1964). Erfolgreiche Zucht des Baumwöllköpfchens oder Pincheäffchens, Leontocebus (Oedipomidas) oedipus (Linné, 1758), in Gefangenschaft. Säugetierkdl. Mittlg., 12, 49
74. Wolters, H.J. (1978). Some aspects of role taking behaviour in captive family groups of the cotton top tamarin Saguinus oedipus oedipus. In: H.

Rothe, H.J. Wolters and J.P. Hearn (eds.) Biology and Behaviour of Marmosets, p. 259 (Göttingen: Eigenverlag Rothe)

75. Cebul, M.S. (1980). The development of social behavior in captive Saguinus fuscicollis. Thesis (New Haven: Yale University)

76. Vogt, J.L., Carlson, H. and Menzel, E. (1978). Social behavior of a marmoset monkey group. I Parental care and infant development. Primates, 19, 715

77. Altmann-Schönberner, D. (1965). Beobachtungen über Aufzucht und Entwicklung des Verhaltens beim grossen Löwenäffchen, Leontocebus rosalia. Zool. Garten, 31, 227

78. Franz, J. (1963). Beobachtungen an einer Löwenäffchen-Aufzucht. Zool. Garten, 28, 115

79. Hoage, R.C. (1977). Parental care in Leontopithecus rosalia rosalia: Sex and age differences in carrying behavior and the role of prior experience. In: D.G. Kleiman (ed.) The Biology and Conservation of the Callitrichidae, p. 293 (Washington, D.C.: Smithsonian Institution Press)

80. Epple, G. (1975b). Parental behavior in Saguinus fuscicollis spp. (Callitrichidae). Folia Primatol., 24, 221

81. Epple, G. (1978). Reproductive and social behavior of marmosets with special reference to captive breeding. In: N. Gengozian and F. Deinhardt (eds.) Marmosets in Experimental Medicine: Primates in Medicine, Vol. 10, p. 50 (Basel:Karger)

82. Gengozian, N. (1972). A blood factor in the marmoset, Saguinus fuscicollis - its detection, mode of inheritance and species specificity. J. Med. Primatol. 1, 272

83. Coimbra-Filho, A.F. and Mittermeier, R.A. (1976). Hybridization in the genus Leontopithecus, L.r. rosalia (Linnaeus, 1766), L.r. chrysomelas (Kuhl, 1820) (Callithricidae, Primates). Rev. Brasil Biol., 36, 129

84. Glaser, D. (1970). Über die Ossifikation bei der Extremitäten neugeborenen Primaten (Mammalia). Z. Morph. Tiere, 68, 127

85. Abbott, D.H. and Hearn, J.P. (1978). Physical, hormonal and behavioral aspects of sexual development in the marmoset monkey, Callithrix jacchus. J. Reprod. Fert., 53, 155

86. Hampton, S.H. and Taylor, A.C. (1971). Gonadal development in marmosets. Proc. 3rd Int. Congr. Primatol., Zürich, 1970, Vol. 1, p. 246, (Basel:Karger)

87. Cicmanec, J.L. and Campbell, A.K. (1978). Notes on comparative reproduction of selected Callitrichidae in the laboratory. In: N. Gengozian and F. Deinhardt (eds.) Marmosets in Experimental Medicine: Primates in Medicine, Vol. 10, p. 84 (Basel:Karger)

88. Kingston, W.R. (1975). The breeding of endangered species of marmosets and tamarins. In: R.D. Martin (ed.) Breeding of Endangered Species in Captivity, p. 273 (New York: Academic Press)

89. Chadwick, D.P., May, J.C. and Lorenz, D. (1979). Spontaneous zinc deficiency in marmosets, *Saguinus mystax*. *Lab. Anim. Sci.*, *29*, 482

90. King, G.J. (1976). An investigation into "wasting marmoset syndrome" at the Jersey Zoo. *Thirteenth Ann. Rep. Extract from the Jersey Wildlife Preservation Trust*

91. Richter, C.B., Tankersley, W. and Webb, A. (1978). Chronic recurrent colitis: a wasting syndrome in marmosets and tamarins. *AALAS 29th Ann. Ses. Abstract No.* 77

92. Shimwell, M., Warrington, B.F. and Fowler, J.S.L. (1979). Dietary habits relating to wasting marmoset syndrome (WMS). *Lab. Anim.*, *13*, 139

93. Cicmanec, J.L. (1977). Medical problems encountered in a callitrichid colony. In: D.G. Kleiman (ed.) *The Biology and Conservation of the Callitrichidae*, p.331 (Washington, D.C.: Smithsonian Institution Press)

94. Hunt, R.D., Anderson, M.P. and Chalifoux, L.V. (1978). Spontaneous infectious diseases of marmosets. In: N. Gengozian and F. Deinhardt (eds.) *Marmosets in Experimental Medicine: Primates in Medicine*, *Vol. 10*, p.239 (Basel: Karger)

95. Kingston, W.R. (1972). Diseases of marmosets. In: E.J. Goldsmith and J. Moor-Jankowski (eds.) *Medical Primatology*, p. 68 (Basel: Karger)

96. Wagner, D. (1978). Anaesthesia and treatment of marmosets. In: H. Rothe, H.J. Wolters and J.P. Hearn (eds.) *Biology and Behaviour of Marmosets*, p.291 (Göttingen: Eigenverlag Rothe)

97. Epple. G. (1974). Olfactory communication in South American primates. *Ann. N.Y. Acad. Sci.*, *237*, 261

Chapter 5

The Squirrel Monkey *(Saimiri sciureus)*

W. R. Dukelow

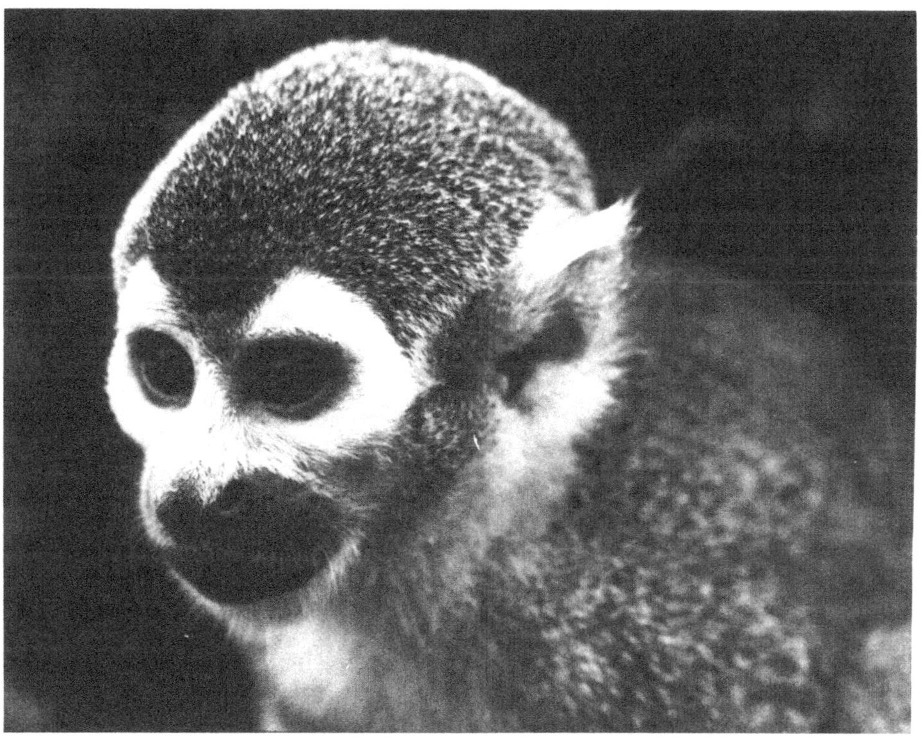

Saimiri sciureus

THE SQUIRREL MONKEY

W. Richard Dukelow
Endocrine Research Unit
Michigan State University
East Lansing, Michigan 48824 U.S.A.

INTRODUCTION

The squirrel monkey (Saimiri sciureus) is widely distributed in Central and South America between the 17°S and 10°N latitudes. They are particularly prevalent on the Pacific side of Central America and throughout the Amazon basin. For as long as 400 years they have been captured and traded as pets for the homes of the aristocracy of Europe and America. In their native environment squirrel monkeys are diurnal and arboreal. They inhibit tropical rain forests and prefer high canopy forests and forest edges. They are found in troops ranging from several dozen to several hundred animals.

Although some squirrel monkeys were used in behavioural research in the 1930's, the first captive births were in the early 1940's and it is even more recently that they have been extensively used in biomedical research. The rapid rise in their usage reflects their availability, ease of handling and adaptation to current medical problems ranging from reproduction and heart disease to modern space flight.

MANAGEMENT OF LABORATORY COLONIES

Social organisation and behaviour

Squirrel monkeys, even though arboreal, spend considerable time on the ground either in the forest or in captivity, playing and food-gathering. During the breeding season even more time is spent on the ground. When alarmed, however, they return immediately to the trees.

In resting animals two basic postures are assumed. These have been termed the 'huddle' and the 'sprawl'[1]. In the huddle the back is arched and the animal leans forward with weight on the arms. The tail is then wrapped around the body. This position is assumed during sleep or cold periods. The sprawl involves straddling a branch or perch with the limbs and tail hanging below. This is common in warm weather or when the animal is basking in the sun. It is associated with the lack of stress and with relaxation. Sick monkeys never assume the sprawl position. The huddle position will be assumed by sick monkeys and in the presence of more dominant animals.

The social behaviour of squirrel monkeys is characterised by single-sex groups during much of the year. Most females, after reaching puberty during their third year, will become pregnant annually and as a result they are either pregnant or lactating during much of the year[2]. Seasonal rainfall or a rainfall-induced change in vegetation or insect fauna appears responsible for the change and this is manifested both in the field and laboratory[3,4]. Throughout the year a definite dominance structure exists that persists throughout the yearly cycle. This dominance structure appears to be more the result of socialisation than endocrine-controlled[5], but some have suggested that the social organisation is strongly influenced by the endocrine state of the female[6]. Captivity does not seem to strongly alter such behaviour unless single caging is used in which case severe behavioural conditions can occur[7]. Characterisation of mating behaviour and sexual play has been studied with captive squirrel monkeys and can be compared with field observations[8]. Even surrogate raising of squirrel monkeys yields nearly normal behavioural responses[9]. Stress responses of removal of the infant from the surrogate closely correlates with similar separation of infants from their natural mother with regards to cortisol elevation but some behavioural differences in stress response are noted[10-12].

A male joining the troop during breeding season assumes a dominant position within the group heirarchy but the relative female positions do not change. These adjustments may be influenced by the degree of sexual dimorphism. Bolivian squirrel monkeys, with strong sexual dimorphism, exhibit a segregated form of social organisation whereas Guyanan squirrel monkeys, with lesser dimorphism, are more sexually integrated[13]. The younger animals begin to show the dominant heirarchy when assimilated into the adult social structure. When an adult female is transferred to an established group she will not be admitted to the established order but will tend to be accepted into groups of adult and juvenile males[14].

The reproductive readiness of the adult male usually coincides with the period of female receptivity and is characterised by an increase in body weight and the fatted-male phenomenon[15]. The relationship of this increased size with testicular size and androgen level has been shown[16]. During the rest of the year the adult males are the least social members of the troop. They seldom play with, groom or directly influence the activities of the females. When the birth season begins the females become aggressive towards the males and they are excluded from the central core group of the colony.

There is much more affiliative behaviour in the female subgroups although this is less than seen with some other primate species[17]. Once the birth season begins the younger nulliparous females associate themselves with mothers carrying infants. These animals have been termed 'aunts' and they often provide care for the newborn infant. In captivity breeding situations it is common practice to place an 'aunt' with an expectant mother to reduce stress. Throughout the wild birth season the females stay primarily in the trees. After birth the newborn clings to the mother's back and remains on the mother for several weeks. The mother pursues normal activities and when the infant wishes to nurse he merely moves forward on the mother, under an arm, and the mother raises slightly to allow nursing.

Infants will consume solid food at four to six weeks of age and natural weaning occurs at four to six months of age. Weaning is aided by behavioural actions of the mother to push her infant away when he tries to nurse and this encourages independence. Infants will form play groups at eight to ten weeks of age and this play is often rough and tumble. By one year of age juveniles are usually completely independent of their mothers even though they remain in peer groups with increasingly rough play and increasing interest in inanimate objects. At 36 months of age the female juveniles will enter the reproducing female group, initially as an 'aunt' during which time she may or may not get pregnant. Males must wait another two years before they will be allowed to enter the fatted male group during the mating season.

Breeding performance in captivity

The squirrel monkey has a very short cycle in comparison with other nonhuman primate species. It approximates eight to ten days. There is no bleeding associated with the cycle and vaginal cytology is not as regular an indicator of normal cyclicity as seen with other laboratory species. Because of these factors, timed mating is difficult. There is a definite breeding season, as previously discussed. If pregnancy does occur the gestation period is from 137 to 175 days in length with a mean of 150 days[18,19]. Squirrel monkeys have a high maternal weight to infant birth weight ratio (7:1). Twins have never been reported and it is unlikely that twins could occur in this species because of the weight ratio.

A conception rate from 50-70% can be expected after squirrel monkeys are acclimated to captivity but this is coupled with a relatively high incidence of stillborns or abortions (16.8%) and of neonatal death loss (34.3%)[20,21].

Normally males and females would be housed in group cages at a ratio of 1:10 or in smaller cage with a 1:3 ratio. The male need not be removed after mating and will not molest mothers or newborn infants. Despite the problems mentioned relative to vaginal cytology, some timed mating programs have been developed for squirrel monkeys[22]. Such procedures normally involve group housing and careful monitoring of vaginal lavages to determine the exact time of breeding.

There has been almost no research on selection systems for developing genetic lines of squirrel monkeys. This perhaps reflects the large size of the gene pool still available with this species and also the low numbers of animals born in captivity and the high abortion and neonatal death loss. In the future we will see such selection systems probably initially based on selection for birth weight and rate of gain (since these factors affect survival) but also for desirable traits relative to specific scientific research needs. Various subspecies of squirrel monkeys can be identified by karyotype and these subspecies will cross to produce hybrid individuals. No studies have yet been made to determine if heterosis occurs.

It is frequently assumed that colony-born animals will eventually prove to be more productive than feral-caught. Progress with squirrel monkey colonies to date have not shown this to be true as management and environmental factors can cause greater reproductive problems with these highly stressful primates. Recent progress has attempted to isolate the essential factors involved in a successful breeding program and in the future it is hopeful that captive born animals can reproduce at a level equal or better to feral animals (T. Clarkson, personal communication).

Housing and management

Single housing of squirrel monkeys should be avoided unless absolutely essential to the experimental design. They can be housed in small groups of three or four animals or in larger gang cages. Vertical height is important with this species and perches should be provided which will allow the animal to rest with its tail hanging and not touching the bottom of the cage. A minimum of 0.15 m^2 of floor space should be provided for each monkey and, more importantly, he should have access to at least 51 cm of vertical space. Normal standards of cleanliness for caging, bedding, feeders and water bottles (as pertains to other laboratory animals) should be maintained. Individual water bottles or automatic waterers can be used. An adult squirrel monkey will consume 50 to 100 ml per day. With automatic watering systems the pressure should be maintained at 150-300 gm/cm^2. Higher pressures will make it difficult for drinking.

Animal rooms should be maintained between 21 and 24°C with an approximate relative humidity of 55%. If the latter goes below 50% sneezing and sniffling may be observed and can lead to serious respiratory problems. Unfortunately many modern air conditioning systems are designed to lower the relative humidity below these levels and supplemental humidifying units must be provided. Automatic flush-type cages often provide sufficient moisture to prevent respiratory problems.

While commercially available cages are preferable, very adequate temporary caging can be provided from light wire mesh structures available in hardware stores. The cost of these is low but the basic requirements for floor space and vertical space, as well as the provision of perches, must be observed.

It is questionable if alteration of the photoperiod alters squirrel monkey cyclicity, however most animal rooms have controlled lighting to a 12:12 or 14:10 (light:dark) cycle.

Circulation of air in the colony is important and outtake fans or air conditioners should be adjusted to allow for eight to twelve air changes per hour keeping in mind the requirement for relative humidity mentioned above.

Squirrel monkeys are capable of inflicting severe bite wounds during capture and handling. While many colony handlers follow the practice of pulling, clipping or dulling the canine teeth this is not necessary if proper glove techniques and handling procedures are used. Careless cutting of the teeth can lead to dental abcesses[23,24]. Restraining devices of various kinds have been described and are applicable to squirrel monkeys[25].

Protective leather gloves of adequate size to protect the handler should be worn but these should not be so heavy as to endanger the monkey. Squirrel monkeys are easily trained to a variety of procedures and frequent handling will result in easier management of them. As few people as possible should be used in handling so that the animals become accustomed to the handlers. For simple transport of the monkeys they can be handled with the arms grasped behind the back similar to the procedure used for larger primates. Alternatively they can be grasped just under the arms with the fingers encircling the upper chest. This latter position is convenient for intramuscular or intraperitoneal injections since the injection site can be isolated by grasping the monkey's leg and holding it with the fourth and fifth fingers of the left hand while the thumb, index and middle fingers grasp the monkey under the arms. The arms and legs must be held tightly to prevent the animal from taking the syringe away from the handler.

Several methods of anesthesia can be used. Barbituates can be used by intra peritoneal administration at a level of 25 mg/kg (pentabarbitone-Na, Nembutal®, Abbott Laboratories, North Chicago, IL). Anesthesia will be complete within 10-15 minutes and lasts two to six hours. Barbituates reduce body temperature and therefore a heating pad should be provided during recovery. Pencyclidine-HCl (Sernylan®, Bioceutic Laboratories Inc., St. Louis, MO) can also be used with squirrel monkeys and is given intramuscularly as a dose of 0.5 to 1.5 mg/kg. Ketamine-HCl (Vetalar®, Parke-Davis, Inc., Detroit, MI), a dissociative anaesthetic, is also effective at a dose level of 13 mg/kg for chemical restraint and 25 mg/kg for surgical anaesthesia[26]. For short procedures thiamylal sodium can be used intravenously as a 2% solution administered at a level of 1.0 ml/kg. Inhalent anaesthetics (methoxyflurane, Metafane®, Pittman-Moore, Indianapolis, IN) can also be administered with a nose cone.

Blood sampling is easiest from the femoral vein in the small depression of the femoral triangle but can also be taken from the jugular vein. Excessive sampling can weaken the animal but up to five ml can be withdrawn at one time. No more than one ml blood should be withdrawn per 100 g body weight per month. Venipuncture sites have been described in the neck, arms, legs and tail for injection[27]. In the squirrel monkey the saphenous vein is located on the back of the leg and very near the surface. It is convenient for injections.

There are four main areas of concern relative to animal health and disease. The problems involved with low relative humidity have already been mentioned, and respiratory problems can result. Clinical tuberculosis is rare but the animals are susceptible to Mycobacterium tuberculosis. Tuberculosis testing is desirable on a six month basis but less critical then with Old World species. The most common organisms isolated from squirrel monkeys with respiratory distress are Klebsiella pneumoniae and Pasteurella multocida. After autopsy and examination of lung histology, Filaroides gordius is often found. This parasite causes little damage and is not a matter of major concern.

Squirrel monkeys also readily experience diarrhea caused by nutritional or environmental changes. This results in dehydration and should be treated with supplemental electrolytes as corrective fluid therapy. If prolonged or severe, protein replacement with an amino acid source (Aminosol®, Abbott Laboratories, North Chicago, IL) should be carried out.

Many endoparasites have been isolated from squirrel monkeys. Some of these are detrimental whereas others seem to live symbiotically with the monkey. These include cestodes, acanthocephalans, tremetodes and nematodes. Most of the gastrointestinal parasites can be controlled with Thiabendazole® (Merck, Sharp and Dohme, West Point, PA) at a dose rate of 100 mg/kg. Often at surgery or laparoscopy several types of abdominal filarial worms will be noted. These appear to be endemic to the squirrel monkey and fortunately do little harm.

The fourth major category of health problems relates to dental care. This is particularly important for monkeys maintained on commercial monkey pellets. Tooth abcesses are common and, if untreated, can result in a draining fistula from the maxillary sinus beneath the eye. Correction involves removal of the canine teeth and antibiotic treatment.

Nutrition

The native diet of the squirrel monkey consists of fruits, cereals, vegetables and some insects. Modern laboratory practice normally consists of a commercial primate diet with 20-25% protein and 6-7% fat. Such diets are then supplemented with a variety of foodstuffs including many fruits, unsalted peanuts, cereal grains, carrots, milk, eggs and even orange juice. Some laboratories also supplement the diet with meal worms. Squirrel monkeys have a requirement for vitamine D_3 rather than D_2 and either this vitamine must be provided in the diet or the animals must have access to ultraviolet light (with protective quartz filters over the lamps to protect the eyes of the animals and handlers). At times special research diets demand a chemically defined or liquid diet. These are more expensive to prepare and may result in some digestive problems but they can be fed for limited periods of time[28,29].

There is limited data available on the nutritional requirements[20]. Folic acid deficiency can occur with squirrel monkeys and has been shown (when supplemented) to be beneficial during pregnancy[30]. Similarly, ascorbic acid deficiency is sometimes observed in colonies, probably as a result of the fact that this vitamine is normally dusted on commercial pellets and removed if the pellets are soaked prior to feeding[31]. Maintenance of protein levels is crucial for successful reproduction and high abortion rates can be attributed to protein deficiency[32].

Hand rearing techniques have been developed for the bottle raising of infant squirrel monkeys and the composition of squirrel monkey milk is known[33,34].

Frequency of feeding is also important with squirrel monkeys. They should be fed at least twice a day and more frequent feedings result in less stress and less feed wastage among the animals. Newly arrived animals should be fed more frequently and, with such animals, it is common to soak the pellets in water or milk to enhance their acceptance.

Squirrel monkeys (males) reach adult stage at 550 to 1135 g dependent on subspecies. Females reach adult size at 365 to 750 g. Captivity lifespan is less than 22 years but survival to 8 to 12 years is not unusual[35]. Fertility is usually maintained until death.

Basic pulmonary, cardiovascular and temperature values, as well as serum chemistries, have been determined for the squirrel monkey and readers are referred to a recent summary[20].

<u>Chromosomal identification of subspecies</u>

Squirrel monkeys have a diploid number of chromosomes of 44. Early work indicated discrepancies with regard to the number of chromosomes which were acrocentric in morphological appearance[36,37]. From work carried out in the mid-1970's it is now known that these differences represent different subspecies of squirrel monkeys which have different geographical points of origin[38-41]. It is now recognized that animals with five acrocentric pairs of chromosomes are of Peruvian origin, those with six pairs from Bolivia, Brazil or Colombia, and those with seven acrocentric pairs are from Guyana. Differences in C and G banding patterns have also been noted for monkeys from different regions[42]. Similar differences have been observed with owl monkeys (<u>Aotus</u>) and this characteristic has been used to enhance breeding efficiency in captivity. Similar studies are presently underway with squirrel monkeys.

REPRODUCTIVE PHYSIOLOGY

<u>Seasonality and adaptation to captivity</u>

As has already been noted, the squirrel monkey living in the wild experiences a distinct seasonality of cycling response and this seems to be correlated with the dry period of the year coinciding with the initiation of the mating season. The gestation period, with very rapid foetal growth during the last third of pregnancy, (and lactation) seems to correlate with the flush of forest growth[43-45]. Births occur over an 8-12 week period with a definite peak in the middle of this time. The exact cause of the seasonal response is not known but it is not believed to be correlated with photoperiod changes since semiannual changes in the photoperiod of the Amazon region is only about eleven minutes. Mating in the wild is from June to September with births occurring from December to February. Under captive conditions in the northern hemisphere the seasonality is maintained for at least five years[46] but there is a gradual shift of the mating and birth seasons so that births occur in July and August[1,45]. This response is also observed in captivity when using a standard ovulation-induction regimen[47] and is manifested with a 79.5% decrease in the ovulatory response during the summer season[4,48]. This latter response has been attributed to a decrease in follicle stimulating hormone (FSH) or a decreased responsiveness to that hormone, since administration of a higher dose results in increased ovulation[49]. Oocytes produced from this treatment are normal and capable of fertilisation out of season[50]. In northern climates the squirrel monkey can be expected to adapt to captivity in about nine months but will continue to show seasonal patterns even in environmentally controlled conditions.

Follicular development, ovulation and endocrinology

Laparoscopy[51,52] has been extensively used to study follicular morphology in the squirrel monkey. Based on over 600 such observations it is evident that prior to ovulation the upper portion of the follicle becomes very transparent and that at times a vascular pattern is observed on the surface of the follicle (as in Old World species). More frequently, however, ovulation is accompanied by hemorrhaging with the distinct appearance of a classic corpus hemorrhagicum within four hours. Luteinisation follows ovulation[53,54].

Examination of the circulating serum oestrogens and progesterone during the cycle reveal levels that are strikingly higher than with Old World species or humans. A similar phenomenon has been observed in other New World species. Peak and nadir concentrations of oestradiol have been found to be 503 $\pm$ 57.5 and 81. $\pm$ 8.2 pg/ml respectively. Serum progestins reached peak concentrations of 399 $\pm$ 27.7 ng/ml, usually three to four days after the oestradiol peak[55,56].

High serum levels are not restricted to just the gonadal steroids in the squirrel monkey. Resting levels of cortisol approach 405 μg/100 ml[57]. This high adrenal output is confirmed by very high concentrations of urinary free cortisol[58].

The oestrogen stimulation near the time of ovulation has other effects on the reproductive tract as well. Ovariectomized animals undergo cervical changes in histology and in the localization of glycogen, phosphorylases, glycogen synthetase and branching enzyme which can be renewed with the administration of low doses of oestrogen[59-61]. If diethylstilboestrol implants are placed in adult female squirrel monkeys about 30% of the resultant follicles contain more than one oocyte. This raises the possibility of neogenesis of oocytes in this species[62].

Immunofluorescence techniques have been used to study the hypothalamo-infundibular LRH tract in the squirrel monkey through the cycle[63,64]. Preliminary data from these studies show serum FSH and luteinizing hormone (LH) levels progressively decrease from the luteal phase to the late follicular phase. In the case of FSH the decrease is from an average of 16 mIU/ml to about 5 mIU/ml in the late follicular phase.

Detection of oestrus and pregnancy

Traditional mating behaviour, as a sign of oestrus, is difficult to detect in squirrel monkeys. For routine examination of the cycle, vaginal cytology is used. Although not as accurate as in other laboratory species, this procedure allows one to approximate the stage of the cycle[18,65-68]. Vaginal smears are taken with a cotton swab or by aspiration of a small quantity of water placed in the vagina with an eye dropper. The smeared slides are then air-dried and can be stained by the Papanicolaou procedure. There is a sharp drop in the percentage of acidophilic nucleated cells at the peak of oestrus. At times, after ovulation, there is a white discharge of desquamated cells from the vagina and some have attempted to equate this to the post-oestrus condition in the hamster. This phenomenon, however, is quite variable in both its incidence and time of occurrence.

It is uncertain if all cycles are ovulatory in the squirrel monkey. One worker found histological evidence of ovulation in only one of 20 animals examined[67]. The short natural cycle of the squirrel monkey could indicate a higher incidence of anovulatory cycles. In contrast, laparoscopic examination of ovaries at seven to nine day intervals in the author's laboratory has indicated that some squirrel monkeys have quite regular ovulatory cycles.

Table 1 shows various techniques that have been used to diagnose pregnancy in the squirrel monkey.

Table 1. Pregnancy detection in the squirrel monkey

Characteristic	Days after conception	References
Uterine size increase (by laparotomy)	20 to 25	69
Chorionic gonadotropin:		
(a) plasma	20 to 105	70
(b) urine	40 to 60	71
Uterine size increase	42 to 56	72
(by palpation)	61	70
Diabetes insipidus	60	73
	60 to 135	68
Maternal weight gain	60 to 95	74
	67 to 147	68
Visual abdominal enlargement	74 to 102	74
Fetal skeleton by x-ray	81	70

Of the methods listed, uterine size increase and chorionic gonadotropic concentration occur early in the first trimester at the time that the embryo is in the primitive streak stage. Recently a pregnancy test kit has been developed at the U.S. National Institutes of Health[71] which can be used with squirrel monkeys between 40 and 60 days of pregnancy. This has an inherent risk of 10% for false negative responses.

Any increase of uterine width (detected by laparotomy, laparoscopy or palpation) to greater than 20 mm will indicate pregnancy. The infant can be palpated by 70 days.

Gamete physiology and fertilisation

Despite the lack of extensive research in many areas of squirrel monkey physiology, reproduction has been studied for a number of years. Techniques of ovulation induction and semen collection, as well as artificial insemination, have been described [75-77].

Semen collection is normally accomplished utilizing a small rectal probe with the animal, anaesthetized, in a restraining device[78]. The handler should use a minimum of force to place the male in the restrainer. The rectal probe should be 12-13 cm in length with a diameter of 0.6 cm[75]. Longitudinal electrode plates (copper or silver) along the probe then deliver a circular pattern of current to the male accessory glands. A rhythmic electric pulse from 0 to a maximum of ten volts, at three to four second intervals,should yield a semen sample approximately 125 mg in weight. Squirrel monkey semen coagulates almost immediately upon collection but will subsequently liquify if held at $37^{\circ}C$ for 10 to 15 minutes. The sperm concentration of ejaculates will range from 80 to 300 x 10^6 per ml of liquified semen. From 40 to 80% of the sperm will show motility but the species has a relatively high incidence of morphologically abnormal sperm ranging from 35 to 51%[79]. The sperm-rich fraction of the semen has the following concentrations (mg%) of lactic acid, citric acid and fructose: 41.9, 2.7 and 0.4. Comparable values for the seminal plasma are 151.0, 48.0 and 110.4 respectively.

The dimensions of the squirrel monkey sperm (μm $\pm$ S.E. of the mean) are as follows: head length, 5.11 $\pm$ 0.02; head width, 3.51 $\pm$ 0.01; midpiece length, 9.03 $\pm$ 0.12; principle piece length, 55.34 $\pm$ 0.13; total length, 69.24 $\pm$ 0.15. The morphology of the squirrel monkey sperm has been extensively studied using transmission and scanning electron microscopic techniques[80-83]. Dorsoventral differences are not noted and if a thick swelling of the midpiece is found it usually reflects immaturity of the sperm rather than a characteristic of the squirrel monkey sperm. The sperm head is thicker than that observed in lower forms such as the tupaia, and has less surface area. There is evidence of an apical swelling or ridge and the posterior margin of the acrosome has a serrated appearance. Examination of freeze-etched samples indicate that this structural arrangement exists within the head as a series of tube-like structures ending further towards the posterior margin than is evident from the surface. This distinctive appearance of the posterior acrosomal margin has not been seen in Old World monkeys and may be unique to the cebids. There is an eccentric insertion of the midpiece into the posterior aspect of the sperm head. The mitochondria are very fine in cross section and make multiple turns around the midpiece. The number of gyres approximates 53. Mitochondria on the midpiece are very regularly arranged.

Ovulation induction can occur with a variety of regimens. Original procedures involved the use of nine days of 200 IU of pregnant mares serum (PMS) with 250-500 IU of human chorionic gonadotropin (HCG) given on the last four days[76]. This results in superovulation (release of more than the normal single ovum) and the timing of ovulation is difficult to control. In later work, the luteal phase of the normal cycle was mimiced with five days treatment with progesterone (5 mg per day) prior to the start of the ovulation induction regimen[47]. Domestic animal pituitary FSH (1 mg per day for four days) was found to be superior for controlling follicular growth and, coupled with HCG, for controlling ovulation to single or double ovulations. This was compared with PMS and human menopausal gonadotropin (HMG). The latter serves as an FSH source and is effective in inducing follicular growth but control of the number of developing follicles is difficult and often this treatment results in cystic conditions with the ovaries. The PMS-HCG regimen is still the preferred treatment where multiple ovulations are desired. Varying doses of HCG have been used (following four days treatment of FSH, 1 mg) to determine the minimal effective dose[84]. The ovulatory response is shown in Figure 1.

Contrary to the experience with some other animals, ovulation induction schemes can be repeated within squirrel monkeys over several years with no refractoriness to the gonadotropins. Using the FSH-HCG regimen described above, squirrel monkeys have been ovulated twenty or more times (at intervals of three weeks or more) with no significant effect on the percent of animals ovulating or the number of ovulations per animal. There was an increase in the percent of animals responding with follicular growth after the fifth induction[85]. The reason for the lack of refractoriness (antigonadotropic antibodies?) perhaps reflects the low doses used or the lack of a suitable adjuvant to enhance antibody response.

During the anovulatory season of the squirrel monkey (July to September in northern climates) the effectiveness of the above FSH-HCG regimen decreases (Fig. 2.). The decrease is believed due to a decreased sensitivity of the monkey to the level of FSH because increasing the daily dose of FSH to 2 mg, or giving 1 mg per day for five rather than four days, enhances ovulation[49]. This suggests that the normal season level of FSH is near the minimum threshold dose required for follicular stimulation. Oocytes recovered as a result of ovulation induction during the off-season are capable of fertilization both in vivo and in vitro and pregnancies resulting from such induction have gone to term with delivery of normal offspring.

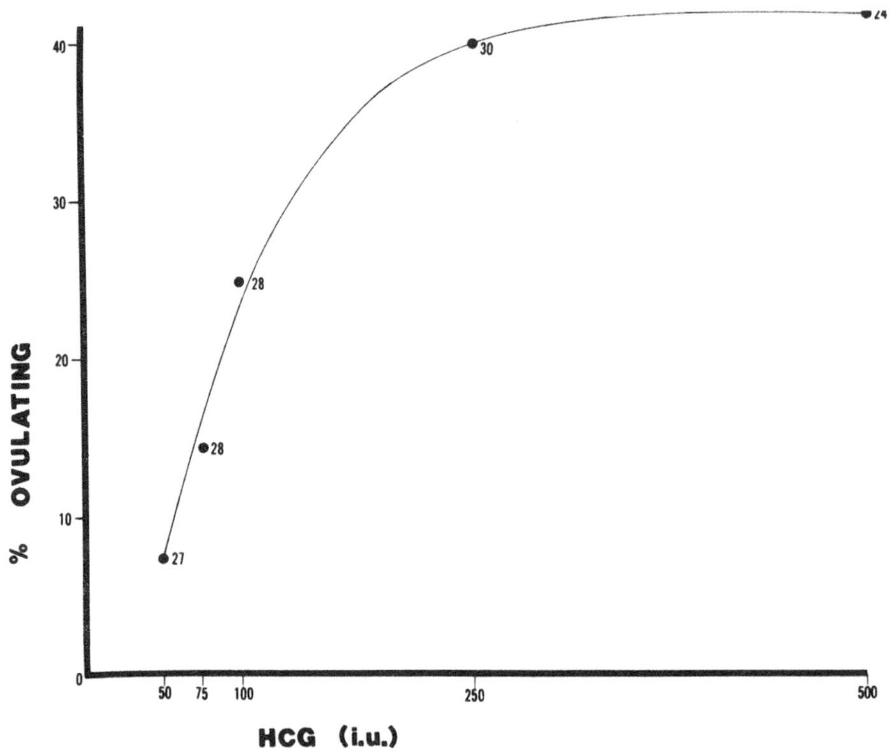

Figure 1. Minimal effective dose of HCG to induce ovulation in squirrel monkeys following treatment with FSH (1 mg) for five days. Values at each point indicate numbers of animals tested.

There are only limited reports of artificial insemination in the squirrel monkey. In early studies[77] five animals were inseminated vaginally with semen collected by electroejaculation. Inseminations followed an PMS-HCG induction regimen and occurred on the first or second day following cessation of the regimen. Fertilised ova were recovered from the oviducts and uteri of animals sacrificed 72 hr later (three monkeys). Two animals were not sacrificed. They did not go to term but may have been pregnant. There was an indication that the gonadotropin treatment may have speeded ovum transport through the female reproductive tract, a phenomenon observed in other primates and laboratory species.

Although not used in artificial insemination, studies have been conducted on the freezing and storage of squirrel monkey sperm[86]. The procedure involved preincubation at 37°C and then a two-step dilution with an extender consisting of 11% lactose, 4% glycerol and 20% egg yolk. A 45 minute total glycerol equilibration time was used. Post-thaw motility was above 50% using this procedure. To the knowledge of this author, no squirrel monkeys have been inseminated with frozen semen and examined for evidence of fertilisation.

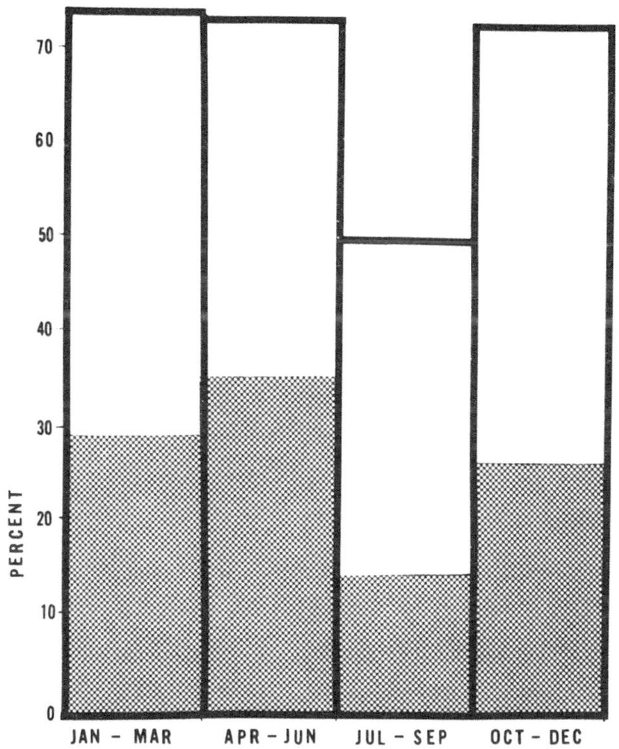

Figure 2. Seasonal response in follicular growth and ovulation following a gonadotropin regimen (in the northern hemisphere). Open bars: percent of animals showing follicular growth. Hatched bars: percent of animal ovulating.

Studies have been carried out on the fertilisation and preimplantation development of the embryo. _In vitro_ fertilisation has been achieved and will be discussed later in this chapter. The time required for sperm capacitation has been determined to be 4.7 $\pm$ 2.6 hr with the earliest possible penetration after mixing of sperm and ova (_in vitro_) at 2.0 hr[87]. These values are comparable with values obtained for other primate species including humans. Laparoscopic procedures have been used to recover _in vivo_ fertilised blastocysts from the squirrel monkey uterus[88,89]. From such data, and the results of timed development studies following _in vitro_ fertilisation, it is possible to construct the temporal relationships of the sequence of events between fertilisation and implantation. These are shown in Table 2 and compared with similar events in other primate species[90].

Implantation, Uterine Development and Parturition

Little is known of implantation and placentation in the squirrel monkey. In his classic study of placental development Luckett[91] does not mention the squirrel monkey but devotes extensive review to the Callithricidae. At this time extrapolation from that information must be made to the squirrel monkey and this area is in need of more extensive research emphasis. It is known that *in vitro* profusion of squirrel monkey placentae results in the recovery of a wide variety of progesterone metabolites, a condition also found with baboons, macaques, chimpanzees and orang-utans. In contrast in the human, hepatic or another peripheral metabolic mechanism is responsible for pregnanediol and reduced progesterone metabolites found in the blood and urine[92].

Table 2. Time course of early embryonic development in primates (hr post fertilisation)

	Squirrel Monkey	Rhesus Monkey	Baboon	Human
First Cleavage	16-40	24-36	-	30-38
Second Cleavage	46-52	36-48	48	38-46
Third Cleavage	52-73	48-72	48-72	51-72
Morula	96	-	120-148	96-135
Blastocyst	96-120	-	<120	123-147

Pregnancy associated plasma proteins (PAPPs) have been studied in several species of nonhuman primates and in chimpanzees and orang-utans these appear to be immunologically identical to human PAPPs[93]. In macaques, equivalent partially cross reactive PAPPs are found but in the squirrel monkey only faint traces of these proteins, unique to the pregnant female, are observed.

A summary of 512 squirrel monkey pregnancies over nine years has recently been reported.[94] The majority (84%) of pregnancies resulted in live births. Of those born alive, 4% died within 24 hours and an additional 7% died within the first week of life. Of those not delivered alive, 26% were aborted and 74% were stillborn. During the nine year period 30 of 63 female deaths were reproduction related. Hemorrhage at delivery was the most common death cause (9 cases) with an additional seven deaths due to dystocia or poor fetal presentation. Six died as a result of complications following a retained placenta. There was a significant correlation between birth weight and infant survival and mortality was especially high with infants weighing less than 80 g at birth. This factor emphasises the earlier statement that initial indices of genetic selection for establishment of squirrel monkey lines will probably relate to birth and weaning weights.

One case of an ectopic pregnancy in the squirrel monkey has been reported[95].

There is increased water consumption by the mother during the last two months of pregnancy. Just prior to birth there may be changes in the eating and sleeping habits and the mother often will become withdrawn and inactive. If housed with an 'aunt' the interaction between the two will become less. Most births occur at night. Infants emerge from the birth canal and once their head and arms are free they grasp the mothers abdominal hair and aid in delivery. Once born they move to the back of the mother and begin the behavioural postures previously mentioned.

After the first seven days their weight gain should be at a steady pace. By six weeks of age the offspring should approximate 150 g (either sex). By 14 weeks females will be nearly 200 g and males about 250 g. By 30 weeks the weights for females and males should be 350 and 400 g respectively. A comprehensive study of reflexes and behavioural characteristics of developing squirrel monkeys has recently been published[96].

APPLIED STUDIES

Historical

Early research on the squirrel monkey was almost entirely based on their small size and low cost[97]. The first formal reports of research were in 1957 and related to the sensory and motor areas of the cerebral cortex. These early studies and subsequent work in the early 1960's have been reviewed[98]. This was the time that represented the beginnings of space exploration and preliminary work was done with squirrel monkeys to study the effects of unusual atmospheric conditions. Squirrel monkeys were found to be more resistant to high oxygen pressures but they did not tolerate low oxygen pressures as well as man. Some work was done on maintaining squirrel monkeys in pressurised chambers and no immediate or delayed adverse physiological effects were noted even when the animals were exposed to seven atmospheres of a 97% helium, 3% oxygen mixture. The effect of gravitation force with rotational speeds of from two to ten RPMs were studied. Squirrel monkeys were found to tolerate unusually high force-time profiles. Most animals survived exposure to 400 G at onset rates of 36 G per second. This remarkable tolerance of the squirrel monkey to gravitational forces lead to recommendation of the squirrel monkey for space flight. These early studies also provided strong profiles of baseline data that are still used in research today[20,98].

Space flight experimentation

On Friday, December 13, 1958 at 0338:44 Eastern Standard Time, a military Jupiter missile was launched on a ballistic trajectory which would carry it to a height of 300 miles and over a 1500 mile distance. In the nosecone of the rocket was a 30 pound, 750 in^3 biocapsule containing an adult squirrel monkey named 'Old Reliable'. The capsule was equipped for protection against shock and temperature extremes and to allow 24 hr survival of the animal. Electronic monitoring of the EKG, body temperature and respiration was also provided. Since the military Jupiter missiles were not designed for biological experiments, the animal had to tolerate an acceleration force of up to 15 G and a deceleration force of up to 45 G. The animal survived the flight until loss of the signal upon re-entry indicated a mishap. The nosecone was not recovered. Despite this loss, a great deal of basic information was obtained and on May 28, 1959 a second Jupiter missile carrying two monkeys (one squirrel monkey, 'Baker', and a captive-born rhesus) was launched under similar circumstances. Telemetered information showed that the animals survived the stresses of launch, free flight and re-entry with no harm. Both monkeys and the nosecone were recovered. By these two flights, man entered the space age and for the first time, the reactions of a primate to launch acceleration, weightlessness for over ten minutes and deceleration were monitored and found to be within the tolerance of man. Electrocardiograms indicated tachycardia during acceleration, return to normal during the period of weightlessness and a reoccurrence of the tachycardia during re-entry. These conditions provided positive clues to possible problems that were later evaluated before sending humans into space[99,100].

Reproductive Physiology

The squirrel monkey has served as an important model for studying seasonality and the effect of transport between hemispheres on reproduction. This work has previously been discussed in this chapter.

A second major area of research has related to ovulation induction using the squirrel monkey as a model for man. It has been found that hyperstimulation of the ovaries following human menopausal gonadotropin administration occurs in squirrel monkeys as in humans. Controlling mechanisms of seasonality, specifically relating to threshold doses of FSH, have already been monitored. Human chorionic gonadotropin (HCG) has long been used for ovulation induction in many species of animals and is a common therapeutic treatment for women who are anovulatory. Dose levels used in many domestic species approach 3 to 5000 IU and doses as high as 20,000 IU have been reported for use in women. Rabbits can be ovulated with as little as 25 IU and if that level is increased four fold, a chromosomal abnormality rate of 9.7% has been reported in six-day blastocysts [101]. Doses of HCG used with nonhuman primates are generally of the magnitude of 1000 to 2000 IU. Because of the adverse effects in rabbits and a general assumption that dose levels being used were exceedingly high, the squirrel monkey was used to determine the minimum effective dose to induce ovulation. This was found to be between 100 and 250 IU (This data is shown in Figure 1 earlier in this chapter).

Perhaps the most intensive use of the squirrel monkey in reproductive studies has been relative to the fertilisation process and, particularly, *in vitro* fertilisation. For decades scientists have been fascinated with the possibility of mixing sperm and eggs in a tube or dish and causing fertilisation to occur. Despite sporadic and often unconfirmed reports of success, it was not until 1951 that consistent success was achieved with *in vitro* fertilisation of rabbit ova. This major event was preceded, in the same year, by the discovery of the need for capacitation (i.e., a period of uterine incubation of the sperm before they could achieve the 'capacity' to fertilise). Today, a sizable number of laboratory species can be used in successful in vitro fertilisation studies. At least four laboratory species have produced living young as a result of in vitro fertilisation and subsequent embryo transfer. In primates, in vitro fertilisation has been reported in humans, baboons and the squirrel monkey[90]. In 1972 two reports appeared simultaneously which described preliminary positive results for the in vitro fertilisation of squirrel monkey oocytes[102,103]. In an expanded report of one of these studies, 22 mature oocytes were recovered and 11 of these had sperm in the perivitelline space, extrusion of the second polar body or pronuclear formation. Six ova cleaved to the two-cell stage[104]. From the second original report (from the laboratory of this author) expanded reports appeared in 1975 and 1979 summarising the studies[90,105-107]. To 1979 a level of 35% in vitro fertilisation had been achieved and embryos had developed to the eight cell stage. The optimal medium for fertilisation was found to be composed of TC-199 with 20% agamma newborn calf serum and 72 μg pyruvate per ml. The technique has been used to determine the fertility of captive males and it has been determined that the fatted male condition is not necessary for the production of fertile sperm. Although the sperm concentration and motility do fluctuate with the seasonal condition of the squirrel monkey, sperm can be obtained throughout the year and that sperm is capable of fertilising squirrel monkey ova in vitro.

The method of ovum recovery from the female also has little effect on in vitro fertilisation. Successful recovery occurred with 35.2% of the follicles when laparoscopic recovery was used and at a rate of 34.0% using laparotomy. The fertilisation rates of ova by these two methods of recovery were 43.3 and 35.7% respectively.

Interestingly, the size of the follicle had little effect of fertilisability. The fertilisation rates (in vitro) of oocytes recovered from 1, 2, 3 and 4 mm follicles (which contain 1.8, 5.0, 11.7 and 26.0 μl volume respectively) were 16.7, 50.0, 40.4 and 57.1% respectively. One of the very small follicles showed a significant difference in fertilisation rate probably reflecting the fact that some were early follicles and others may have been follicles undergoing atresia. The addition of insulin (10 and 100 mIU/ml) to the medium had, interestingly, a depressing effect on both ovum maturation and in vitro fertilisation rate.

In 1976 and 1977 laparoscopic transfers of in vitro fertilised squirrel monkey embryos were made to the infundibular end of the oviduct of synchronized recipient females. This procedure is illustrated in Figure 3.

None of these transfers resulted in pregnancy. These transfers were of one to four-cell embryos transferred to the oviduct. Subsequent success in England and Australia with human embryo transfers involved eight-cell embryos transferred to the uterine lumen which may lead to subsequent success with the squirrel monkey but such studies have not been made to date.

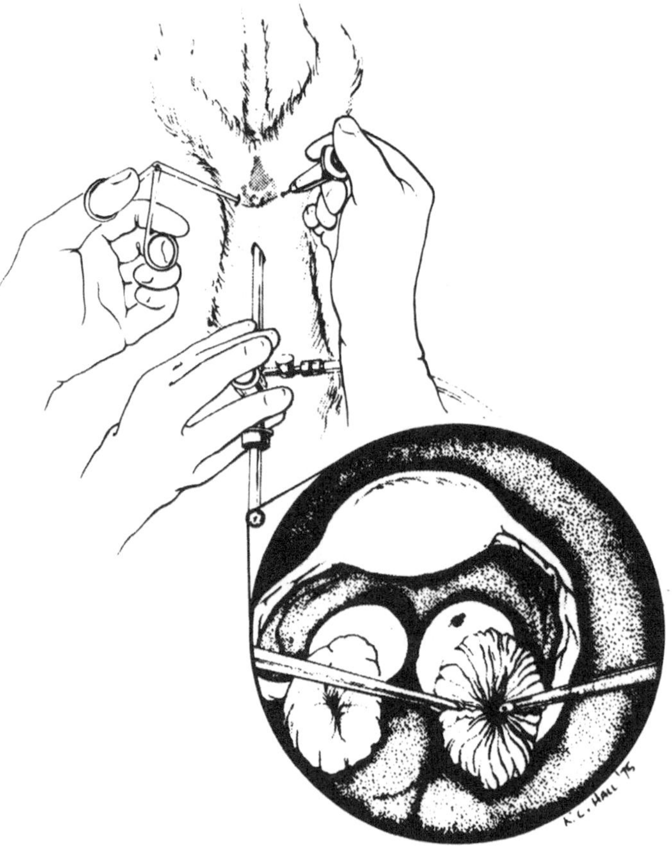

Figure 3. Diagrammatic representation of the technique for laparoscopic oviductal transfer in the squirrel monkey (Ref.51)

It is now possible to use squirrel monkey in vitro fertilisation procedures to examine the basic reproductive parameters of the species and to use this model for related studies in man. Sperm capacitation in vitro has been determined to be 4.7 hr with the earliest possible ovum penetration at 2.0 hr after addition of ejaculated sperm to the medium[87]. Recently, the effect of addition of cyclic nucleotides to the in vitro fertilisation culture medium has been studied and addition of dbcAMP at levels of 1 and 10 μM resulted in fertilisation rates of 90.2 and 90.0% compared with control levels of 60.0%. These additions had no effect on the percentage of embryos developing to the two-cell stage, however, suggesting that the cAMP effect is directed towards the sperm role in fertilisation. This is in accord with similar studies with other laboratory animals which show a role for cAMP in the acrosome reaction that occurs after capacitation but prior to sperm penetration through the zona pellucida. Interestingly, while the earliest sperm penetration of the ovum has been found to be two hours after insemination, if those sperm are treated with dbcAMP this time is reduced to 45 minutes. Addition of 10 μM dbcGMP to the culture system had no effect on fertilisation rate but did enhance the percentage of embryos developing to the two-cell stage (31.8 vs 23.1% for controls) indicating a possible sequential effect of these cyclic nucleotides on the fertilisation process.

The squirrel monkey is also the only primate species where successful laparoscopic recovery of in vivo fertilised uterine blastocysts has been accomplished[88,89]. This procedure is shown in Figure 4.

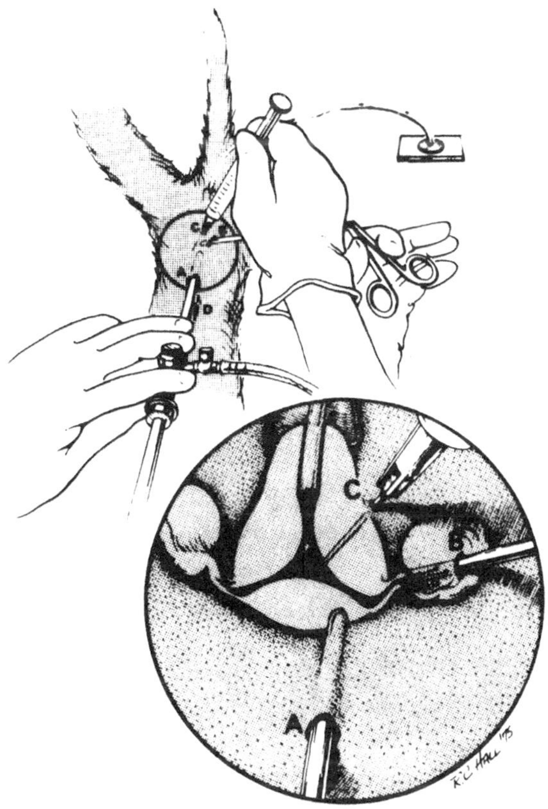

Figure 4. Diagrammatic representation of uterine fluid and blastocyst recovery technique from the squirrel monkey. A = incision for laparoscopy; B = alligator forceps inserted; C = needle inserted; D = umbilicus (Ref. 51).

Figure 5 illustrates one of the recovered uterine blastocysts at 93 to 109 hr after fertilisation.

Since the 1950's scientists have known that the pseudopregnant rabbit oviduct can be used for the temporary incubation and early development of embryos of various species. This procedure has been used, by shipment of the rabbit, to transport embryos of both domestic and laboratory species. In this author's laboratory, eight cell in vitro fertilised embryos have been transferred to the oviduct of a pseudopregnant rabbit and proceeded to develop to the 16 cell stage. These types of studies suggested the possibility that it might be possible to fertilise the ova from another species (with sperm of that same species) in the oviduct of the pseudopregnant rabbit (xenogenous fertilisation) and, indeed, that has been accomplished [108-111]. Squirrel monkey oocytes were recovered laparoscopically and surgically deposited (in 5 µl aliquots) into the infundibular end of the rabbit oviduct. Sperm suspension (0.05 ml) in medium was then added and the utero-tubal junction ligated. The ova were recovered 24 to 48 hr later and examined for evidence of fertilisation. The recovery rates for days 1, 2 and 3 of pseudopregnancy were found to range from 24 to 36% and were not significantly different. The fertilisation rates ranged from 21 to 35% with, also, no significant differences. No attempts have yet been made to transfer xenogenous fertilised squirrel monkey embryos and obtain a pregnancy.

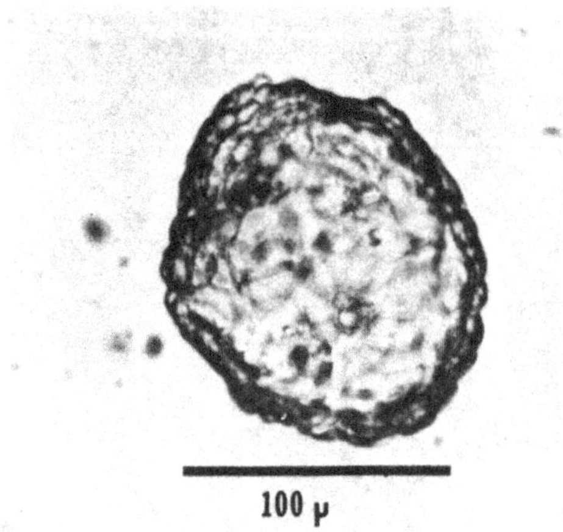

Figure 5. Uterine blastocyst recovered laparoscopically from a squirrel monkey 93 to 109 hr after fertilisation.

It is essential in fertilisation studies that proof of fertilisation occur. Ideally this results from successful transfer and birth of an offspring. In the absence of such proof, one must demonstrate the presence of the sperm midpiece and tail in the cytoplasm or use karyotypic procedures to show a 2N chromosome number[112].

Temperature Regulation

Squirrel monkeys have been utilised in behavioural studies relating to body temperature regulation [113-114]. These studies allow monkeys, maintained in restraint chairs at varying cool temperatures, to regulate temperature by pulling on a chain to allow a 30°C air draft to enter their chamber. To date these studies have demonstrated that even if behavioural thermoregulation is inefficient, it can be sustained with maximum vigor over long time periods. This behaviour is then supplemented by various autonomic adjustments when necessary, to fully regulate body temperature.

Atherosclerosis and Cardiovascular Studies

The squirrel monkey is readily susceptible to nutritionally induced atheroslerosis and naturally occurring atheroslerosis has been described[115-118]. Squirrel monkeys (and cebus monkeys) are very prone to saturated fat-induced hypercholesterolemia whereas the Old World species are not. These differences have been documented[119].

It is of interest that the diets inducing atherosclerosis can also be used to induce gallstones in squirrel monkeys for scientific study[120]. Monkeys fed in this way had an incidence of 83% gallstones with their first appearance at about three months.

Drug Evaluation and Virus Research

Combinations of behavioural tests and drug administration have been studied with squirrel monkeys over the past ten years. Initially monkeys were trained in a modified Wisconsin General Test Apparatus to discriminate between discs of different sizes and they were then injected with varying compounds and given the behavioural test[121]. Similar studies utilised tail-shocking on four minute periodic schedules and measurement of jaw clenching on a rubber bite hose to measure the effects of chlorpromazine, chlordiazepoxide and nicotine[122].

Drug evaluation can also be combined with studies of the normal physiological response of the monkey. An example of this would be tests of synthetic TPAL, a polypeptide reported to occur naturally in the hamster and capable of blocking ovulation. This compound was tested at two levels for antiovulatory activity in squirrel monkeys induced to ovulate[123].

Finally, recent emphasis in the area of virology has identified various oncornavirus particles in several primate species including the squirrel monkey [124]. This isolation was originally done by isolation from a lung tissue culture and more recently electron microscopy has been used to verify the occurrence of oncornavirus-like particles (similar to type D particles) in the squirrel monkey placenta[125].

REFERENCES

1. DuMond, F. V. (1968). The squirrel monkey in a seminatural environment. In: L. A. Rosenblum and R. W. Cooper (eds.) The Squirrel Monkey, p. 87. (New York: Academic Press)
2. Coe, C. L. and Rosenblum, L. A. (1978). Annual reproductive strategy of the squirrel monkey (*Saimiri sciureus*). Folia Primatol., 29, 19
3. Baldwin, J. D. (1970). Reproductive synchronization in squirrel monkeys (*Saimiri*). Primates, 11, 317
4. Harrison, R. M. and Dukelow, W. R. (1973). Seasonal adaptation of laboratory maintained squirrel monkeys (*Saimiri sciureus*). J. med. Primatol. 2, 277
5. Coe, C. L. and Rosemblum, L. A. (1974). Sexual segregation and its ontogemy in squirrel monkey social structure. J. Human Evolution 3, 551
6. Anderson, C. O. and Mason, W. A. (1977). Hormones and social behavior of squirrel monkeys (*Saimiri sciureus*). Hormones and Behavior 8, 100
7. Tarantino, S. J. (1970). Effect of cage confinement on social behavior in squirrel monkeys. Psychon.Sci. 20, 294

8. Latta, J., Hopf, S. and Ploog, D. (1967). Observation on mating behavior and sexual play in the squirrel monkey (*Saimiri sciureus*). *Primates* *8*, 229

9. Roy, M. A., Wolf, R. H., Martin, L. N., Rangan, S. R. S. and Allen, W. P. (1978). Social and reproductive behaviors in surrogate-reared squirrel monkeys (*Saimiri sciureus*). *Laboratory Animal Science* *28*, 417

10. Mendoza, S. P., Smotherman, W. P., Miner, M. T., Kaplan, J. and Levine, S. (1978). Pituitary-adrenal response to separation in mother and infant squirrel monkeys. *Developmental Psychology* *11*, 169

11. Levine, S., Coe, C. L. and Smotherman, W. P. (1978). Prolonged cortisol elevation in the infant squirrel monkey after reunion with mother. *Physiology and Behavior* *20*, 7

12. Hennessy, M. B., Kaplan, J. N., Mendoza, S. P., Lowe, E. L. and Levine, S. (1979). Separation distress and attachment in surrogate-reared squirrel monkeys. *Physiology and Behavior* *23*, 1017

13. Mendoza, S. P., Lowe, E. L. and Levine, S. (1978). Social organization and social behavior in two subspecies of squirrel monkeys (*Saimiri sciureus*). *Folia Primatol.* *30*, 126

14. Fairbanks, L. (1974). An analysis of subgroup structure and process in a captive squirrel monkey (*Saimiri sciureus*) colony. *Folia Primatol.* *21*, 209

15. DuMond, F. V. (1967). Squirrel monkey reproduction: The "fatted" male phenomenon and seasonal spermatogenesis. *Science* *24*, 1467

16. Nader, R. D. and Rosemblum, L. A. (1972). Hormonal regulation of the "fatted" phenomenon in squirrel monkeys. *Anat. Rec.* *173*, 181

17. Strayer, F. F., Taylor, M. and Yanciw, P. (1975). Group composition effects on social behavior of captive squirrel monkeys (*Saimiri sciureus*). *Primates* *16*, 253

18. Jarosz, S. J., Kuehl, T. J. and Dukelow, W. R. (1977). Vaginal cytology, induced ovulation and gestation in the squirrel monkey (*Saimiri sciureus*). *Biology of Reproduction* *16*, 97

19. Kerber, W. T., Conaway, C. H. and Moore Smith, D. (1977). The duration of gestation in the squirrel monkey (Saimiri sciureus). *Laboratory Animal Science* *27*, 700

20. Dukelow, W. R. (198). The squirrel monkey. In: Remfry, J. (ed.) *Universities Federation for Animal Welfare* (in press)

21. Kaplan, J. N. (1977). Breeding and rearing squirrel monkeys (*Saimiri sciureus*) in captivity. *Laboratory Animal Science* *27*, 557

22. Stolzenberg, S. J., Jones, D. C. L., Kaplan, J. N., Barth, R. A., Hodgen, G. D. and Madan, S. M. (1979). Studies with timed-pregnant squirrel monkeys (*Saimiri sciureus*). *J. med. Primatol.* *8*, 29

23. Patrick, R. L., Kaplan, C. M., Margetis, P. M. and Pani, K. C. (1968). Non-surgical extraction of teeth in small primates. *Laboratory Animal Care* *18*, 442

24. Johnson, P. T. and Chadwick, D. G. (1977). Canine tooth clipping by animal trappers as a suspected cause of dental abscess in the squirrel monkey (Saimiri sciureus). Laboratory Animal Science 27, 525

25. Hearn, J. P.(1977). Restraining device for small monkeys. Laboratory Animals 11, 261

26. Greenstein, E. T. (1975). Ketamine HCl, a dissociative anesthetic for squirrel monkeys (Saimiri sciureus). Laboratory Animal Science 25, 774

27. Foelsch, D. W. and Somazzi, E. (1973). Convenient sites for venipuncture in smaller primates. J. med. Prim. 2, 44

28. Newberne, P. M. and Hayes, K. C. (1979). Semipurified diets for nonhuman primates. In: Hayes, K. C. (ed.) Primates in Nutritional Research, p. 99 (New York: Academic Press)

29. Lang, C. M. (1968). The laboratory care and clinical management of Saimiri (Squirrel monkeys). In: Rosemblum, L. A. and Cooper, R. W. (eds.) The Squirrel Monkey, p. 193 (New York: Academic Press)

30. Rasmussen, K. M., Thenen, S. W. and Hayes, K. C. (1979). Folacin deficiency and requirement in the squirrel monkey (Saimiri sciureus). Am. J. Clin. Nutr. 32, 2508

31. Demaray, S. Y., Altman, N. H. and Ferrell, T. L. (1978). Suspected ascorbic acid deficiency in a colony of squirrel monkeys (Saimiri sciureus). Laboratory Animal Science 28, 457

32. Manocha, S. L. and Long, J. (1977). Experimental protein malnutrition during gestation and breeding performance of squirrel monkeys (Saimiri sciureus). Primates 18, 923

33. Hinkle, D. K. and Session, H. L. (1972). A method for hand rearing of Saimiri sciureus. Laboratory Animal Science 22, 207

34. Buss, D. H. and Cooper, R. W. (1972). Composition of squirrel monkey milk. Folia Primatol. 17, 285

35. Hopf, S. and Ploog, D. (1979). Life span in captive squirrel monkeys (Saimiri) with pathological and reproductive records. Primates 20, 213

36. Singh, D. N. and Garlick, N. L.(1972). Chromosomal studies in the squirrel monkey. J. Heredity 63, 379

37. Srivastava, P. K., Srivastava, A. K. and Lucas, F. V. (1969). Somatic chromosomes of squirrel monkey (Saimiri sciureus). Primates 10, 171

38. Jones, T. C., Thorington, R. W., Hu, M. M., Adams, E. and Cooper R. W. (1973). Karyotypes of squirrel monkeys (Saimiri sciureus) from different geographic regions. Amer. J. Physical Anthropol. 38, 269

39. Ardito, G. (1973). Numerical data on the chromosomes of the New World primates. J. Human Evolution 3, 319

40. Jones, T. C. and Ma, N. S. F. (1975). Cytogenetics of the squirrel monkey (Saimiri sciureus). Fed. Proc. 34, 1646

41. Ariga, S., Dukelow, W. R., Emley, G. S. and Hutchinson, R. R. (1978). Possible errors in identification of squirrel monkeys (Saimiri sciureus) from different South American points of export. J. med. Primatol. 7, 129

42. Ma, N. S. F., Jones, T. C., Thorington, R. W. and Cooper, R. W. (1974). Chromosome banding patterns in squirrel monkeys (Saimiri sciureus). J. med. Primatol. 3, 120

43. Dukelow, W. R. (1980). Captive breeding and laparoscopy in nonhuman primates. In: Morrow, D. A. (ed.) Current Therapy in Theriogenology, pp.1142-1150 (Philadelphia: W. B. Saunders Co.)

44. Wolf, R. H., Harrison, R. M. and Martin, T. W. (1975). A review of reproductive patterns in New World monkeys. Laboratory Animal Science 25, 816

45. Butler, H. (1974). Evolutionary trends in primate sex cycles. Contrib. Primat. 3, 2

46. Taub, D. M., Adams, M. R. and Auerbach, K. G. (1978). Reproductive performance in a breeding colony of Brazilian squirrel monkeys (Saimiri sciureus). Laboratory Animal Science 28, 562

47. Dukelow, W. R. (1970). Induction and timing of single and multiple ovulations in the squirrel monkey (Saimiri sciureus). J. Reprod. Fert. 22, 303

48. Dukelow, W. R. (1978). Reproduction in the squirrel monkey (Saimiri sciureus). Recent Advances in Primatology 2, 195

49. Kuehl, T. J. and Dukelow, W. R. (1975). Ovulation induction during the anovulatory season in Saimiri sciureus. J. med. Primatol. 4, 23

50. Jarosz, S. J. and Dukelow, W. R. (1976). Temperate season outdoor housing of Saimiri sciureus in the Northern United States. J. med. Primatol. 5, 176

51. Dukelow, W. R. and Ariga, S. (1976). Laparoscopic techniques for biomedical research. J. med. Primatol. 5, 82

52. Dukelow, W. R. (1978). Laparoscopic research techniques in mammalian embryology. In: Daniel, J. C. (ed.) Methods in Mammalian Reproduction, pp. 437-460. (New York: Academic Press)

53. Harrison, R. M. and Dukelow, W. R. (1974). Morphological changes in the Saimiri sciureus ovarian follicles as detected by laparoscopy. Primates 15, 305

54. Dukelow, W. R., Jewett, D. A. and Rawson, J. M. R. (1973). Follicular development and ovulation in Macaca fascicularis, Saimiri sciureus and Galago senegalensis. Amer. J. Physiol. Anthropol. 38, 207

55. Wolf, R. C., O'Connor, R. F. and Robinson, J. A. (1977). Cyclic changes in plasma progestins and estrogens in squirrel monkeys. Bio. Reprod. 17, 228

56. Wilson, M. I. (1977). Characterization of the oestrous cycle and mating season of squirrel monkeys from copulatory behaviour. J. Reprod. Fert. 51, 57

57. Brown, G. M., Grota, L. J., Penney, D. P. and Reichlin, S. (1970). Pituitary-adrenal function in the squirrel monkey. Endocrinol. 86, 519

58. Setchell, K. D. R., Chua, K. S. and Himsworth, R. L. (1977). Urinary steroid excretion by the squirrel monkey (Saimiri sciureus). J. Endocrinol. 73, 365

59. Graham, C. E. (1969). Estrogen-induced changes at the cervical squamocolumnar junction of the squirrel monkey. Amer. J. of Obstet.Gynecol. 104, 839

60. Graham, C. E. (1969). Glycogen and glycogen-metabolizing enzymes in the squirrel monkey uterine cervix. Amer. J. of Obstet. Gynecol. 102, 989

61. Graham, C. E. and Manocha, S. L. (1971). The effect of chronic estrogenic stimulation on the squirrel monkey cervical epithelium. Virchows Arch. Abt. B. Zellpath. 7, 147

62. Graham, C. E. and Bradley, C. F. (1971). Polyovular follicles in squirrel monkeys after prolonged diethylstilboestrol treatment. J. Reprod. Fert. 27, 181

63. Barry, J. and Croix, D. (1978). Immunofluorescence study of the hypothalamo-infundibular LRH tract and serum gonadotropin levels in the female squirrel monkey during the estrous cycle. Cell Tiss. Res. 192, 215

64. Barry, J. (1979). Immunofluorescence study of the preoptico-terminal LRH tract in the female squirrel monkey during the estrous cycle. Cell Tiss. Res. 198, 1

65. Rosenblum, L. A., Nathan, T., Nelson, J. and Kaufman, I. C. (1967). Vaginal cornification cycles in the squirrel monkey (Saimiri sciureus). Folia Primat. 6, 83

66. Hutchinson, T. C. (1970). Vaginal cytology and reproduction in the squirrel monkey (Saimiri sciureus). Folia Primat. 12, 212

67. Lang, C. M. (1967). The estrous cycle of the squirrel monkey (Saimiri sciureus). Laboratory Animal Care 17, 442

68. Travis, J. C. and Holmes, W. N. (1974). Some physiological and behavioural changes associated with oestrus and pregnancy in the squirrel monkey (Saimiri sciureus). J. Zool., Lond. 174, 41

69. Goss, C. M., Popjoy, L. T., Fusiler, J. L. and Smith, T. M. (1968). Observations on the relationship between embryological development, time of conception and gestation. In: L. A. Rosemblum and R. W. Cooper (eds.) The Squirrel Monkey, p. 171 (New York:Academic Press)

70. Nathan, T. S., Rosenblum, L. A., Limson, G. and Nelson, J. H. (1966). Diagnosis of pregnancy in the squirrel monkey. Anat. Rec. 155, 531

71. Hodgen, G. D., Stolzenberg, S. J., Jones, D. C. L., Hilderbrand, D. F. and Turner, C. K. (1978). Pregnancy diagnosis in squirrel monkeys: Hemagglutination test, radioimmunoassay, and bioassay of chorionic gonadotropin. J. med. Primatol. 7, 59

72. Rosenblum, L. A. (1968). Some aspects of female reproductive physiology in the squirrel monkey. In: L. A. Rosemblum and R. W. Cooper (eds.) The Squirrel Monkey, p. 147 (New York:Academic Press)

73. Clewe, T. H. (1969). Observations on reproduction of squirrel monkeys in captivity. J. Reprod. Fert. Suppl. 6, 151

74. Hopf, S. (1967). Notes on pregnancy, delivery, and infant survival in captive squirrel monkeys. Primates 8, 323

75. Bennett, J. P. (1967). Semen collection in the squirrel monkey. J. Reprod. Fert. 13, 353

76. Bennett, J. P. (1967). The induction of ovulation in the squirrel monkey (Saimiri sciureus) with pregnant mares serum (PMS) and human chorionic gonadotrophin (HCG). J. Reprod. Fert. 13, 357

77. Bennett, J. P. (1967). Artificial insemination of the squirrel monkey. J. Endocrinol. 37, 473

78. Kuehl, T. J. and Dukelow, W. R. (1974). A restraint device for electro-ejaculation of squirrel monkeys (Saimiri sciureus). Laboratory Animal Science 24, 364

79. Ackerman, D. R. and Roussel, J. D. (1968). Fructose, lactic acid and citric acid content of the semen of eleven subhuman primate species and of man. J. Reprod. Fert. 17, 563

80. Bedford, J. M. (1974). Biology of primate spermatozoa. Contri. Primat. 3, 97

81. Gould, K. G. (1980). Scanning electron microscopy of the primate sperm. Inter. Rev. Cytol. 63, 323

82. Martin, D. E. (1975). Comparative morphology of primate spermatozoa using scanning electron microscopy. I. Families Hominidae, Pongidae, Cercopithecidae and Cebidae. J. Human Evol. 4, 287

83. Matano, Y., Matsubayashi, K., Omichi, A. and Ohtomo, K. (1976). Scanning electron microscopy of mammalian spermatozoa. Gunma Symp. Endocrinol. 13, 27

84. Dukelow, W. R. (1979). Human chorionic gonadotropin:induction of ovulation in the squirrel monkey. Science 206, 234

85. Dukelow, W. R., Theodoran, C. G., Howe-Baughman, J. and Magee, W. T. (1981). Ovulatory patterns in the squirrel monkey (Saimiri sciureus). Animal Reprod. Science (in press)

86. Denis, L. T., Poindexter, A. N., Ritter, M. B., Seager, S. W. J. and Deter, R. L. (1976). Freeze preservation of squirrel monkey sperm for use in timed fertilization studies. Fertil.Steril. 27, 723

87. Kuehl, T. J. and Dukelow, W. R. (1981). Time relations of squirrel monkey sperm capacitation and ovum maturation in an in vitro fertilization system. J. Reprod.Fertil. (in press)

88. Ariga, S. and Dukelow, W. R. (1977). Nonsurgical (laparoscopic) uterine flushing and egg recovery techniques in the squirrel monkey (Saimiri sciureus). Primates 18, 453

89. Ariga, S. and Dukelow, W. R. (1977). Recovery of preimplantation blastocysts in the squirrel monkey by a laparoscopic technique. Fertil. Steril. 28, 577

90. Kuehl, T. J. and Dukelow, W. R. (1979). Maturation and in vitro fertilization of follicular oocytes of the squirrel monkey (Saimiri sciureus). Biol. Reprod. 21, 545

91. Luckett, W. P. (1974). Comparative development and evolution of the placenta in primates. Contri. Primat. 3, 142

92. Ryan, K. J. & Hopper, B. R. (1974). Placental biosynthesis and metabolism of steroid hormones in primates. Contri. Primat. 3, 258

93. Lin, T. M. and Halbert, P. (1978). Immunological relationships of human and subhuman primate pregnancy-associated plasma proteins. Int. Arch. Allergy appl. Immun. 56, 207

94. Rasmussen, K. M., Ausman, L. M. and Hayes, K. C. (1980). Vital statistics from a laboratory breeding colony of squirrel monkeys (Saimiri sciureus). Laboratory Animal Science 30, 99

95. McClure, H. M. and Chang, J. (1975). Ectopic pregnancy in a squirrel monkey. J. Amer. Vet. Med. Assoc. 167, 654

96. Kaack, B., Walker, L. and Brizzee, K. R. (1979). The growth and development of the squirrel monkey (Saimiri sciureus). Growth 43, 116

97. Cooper, R. W. (1968). Small species of primates in biomedical research. Laboratory Animal Care 18, 267

98. Beischer, D. E. and Furry, D. E. (1964) Saimiri sciureus as an experimental animal. Anat. Record 148, 615

99. Graybiel, A., Holmes, R. H., Beischer, D. E., Champlin, G. E., Pedigo, G. P., Hixson, W. C., Davis, T. R., Barr, N. L., Kistler, W. G., Niven, J. I., Wilbarger, E., Stullken, D. E., Augerson, W. S., Clark, R. and Berrian, J. H. (1959). An account of experiments in which two monkeys were recovered unharmed after ballistic space flight. Aerospace Medicine 30, 871

100. Beischer, D. E. (1968). The squirrel monkey in aerospace medical research. In: L. A. Rosenblum and R. W. Cooper (eds.) The Squirrel Monkey, p.347 (New York:Academic Press)

101. Fujimoto, S., Pahlavan, N. and Dukelow, W. R. (1974). Chromosome abnormalities in rabbit preimplantation blastocysts induced by superovulation. J. Reprod. Fert. 40, 177

102. Johnson, M. P., Harrison, R. M. and Dukelow, W. R. (1972). Studies on oviductal fluid and in vitro fertilization in rabbits and nonhuman primates. Fed. Proc. 31, 369

103. Cline, E. M., Gould, K. G. and Foley, C. W. (1972). Regulation of ovulation, recovery of mature ova of the squirrel monkey (*Saimiri sciureus*). *Fed. Proc.* *31*, 360

104. Gould, K. G., Cline, E. M. and Williams, W. L. (1973). Observations on the induction of ovulation and fertilization *in vitro* in the squirrel monkey (*Saimiri sciureus*). *Fertil.Steril.* *24*, 260

105. Kuehl, T. J. and Dukelow, W. R. (1975). Fertilization *in vitro* of *Saimiri sciureus* follicular oocytes. *J. med. Primatol.* *4*, 209

106. Dukelow, W. R. and Kuehl, T. J. (1975). *In vitro* fertilization of nonhuman primates. *La Fécondation; Colloque de la Société Nationale pour L'Étude de la Stérilité et de la Fécondité*, pp. 67-80

107. Dukelow, W. R. (1975). The morphology of follicular development and ovulation in nonhuman primates. *J. Reprod. Fertil. Suppl.* *22*, 23

108. Chan, P. J. and Dukelow, W. R. (1981). Cyclic nucleotide effects on preimplantation development of the squirrel monkey (*Saimiri sciureus*) embryo fertilized *in vitro*. *J. Expt. Zoology* (submitted)

109. DeMayo, F. J., Miziguchi, H. and Dukelow, W. R. (1980). Fertilization of squirrel monkey and hamster ova in the rabbit oviduct (xenogenous fertilization). *Science* *208*, 1468

110. Hirst, P. J., DeMayo, F. J. and Dukelow, W. R. (1981). Xenogenous fertilization of laboratory and domestic animals in the oviduct of the pseudopregnant rabbit. *Theriogenology* *15*, 67

111. DeMayo, F. J. (1981). Xenogenous Fertilization of Squirrel Monkey and Hamster Oocytes. M.S. Thesis, Endocrine Research Unit, Michigan State University, East Lansing, MI

112. Mizoguchi, H. and Dukelow, W. R. (1981). Gradual fixation method for chromosomal studies of squirrel monkey oocytes after gonadotropin treatment. *J. med. Primatol.* (in press)

113. Adair, E. R. (1970). Behavioral temperature regulation in the squirrel monkey: some limits of hypothalamic control. Proc. 2nd Conf. Exp. Med. Surg. Primates, pp.462-470. (New York:Karger,Basel)

114. Adair, E. R. (1976). Autonomic thermoregulation in squirrel monkey when behavioral regulation is limited. *J. Applied Physiol.* *40*, 694

115. Portman, O. W. and Andrus, S. B. (1965). Comparative evaluation of three species of New World monkeys for studies of dietary factors, tissue lipids and atherogenesis. *J. Nutr.* *87*, 429

116. Andrus, S. B. and Portman, O. W. (1966). Comparative studies of spontaneous and experimental atherosclerosis in primates. In: *Some Recent Developments in Comparative Medicine*, p.161. (London:Academic Press)

117. Middleton, C. D., Clarkson, T. B., Lofland, H. B. and Pritchard, R. W. (1964). Atherosclerosis in the squirrel monkey:naturally occurring lesions of the aorta and coronary arteries. Arch. Path. 78, 16

118. Portman, O. W., Alexander, M. and Maruffo, C. A. (1967). Nutritional control of arterial lipid composition in squirrel monkeys: Major ester classes and types of phospholipids. J. Nutri. 91, 35

119. Hayes, K. C. (1979). Diet and atherosclerosis in nonhuman primates. In: K. C. Hayes (ed.) Primates in Nutritional Research, p.181 (New York:Academic Press)

120. Osuga, T. and Portman, O. W. (1971). Experimental formation of gallstones in the squirrel monkey. Proc. Soc. Exp. Biol. Med. 136, 722

121. Uyeno, E. T. and Newton, H. (1972). Effects of chloridiazepoxide, reserpine and imipromine on the squirrel monkey (Saimiri sciureus). In: E. Goldsmith and J. Moor-Jankowski (eds.) Medical Primatology, p.328 (Basel:Karger)

122. Emley, G. S. and Hutchinson, R. R. (1971). Similar and selective actions of chlorpromazine, chlordiazepoxide, and nicotine on shock-produced aggressive and anticipatory motor responses in the squirrel monkey. Proc. 79th Ann. Conv., Amer. Psychological Assoc., p.759

123. Kuehl, T. J. and Dukelow, W. R. (1978). The effect of a synthetic polypeptide, threonyl-prolyl-arginyl-lysine, on ovulation in the squirrel monkey (Saimiri sciureus) and hamster. J. Reprod. Fertil. 52, 25

124. Heberling, R. L., Barker, S. T., Kalter, S. S., Smith, G. C. and Helmke, R. J. (1977). Isolation of an oncornavirus from a squirrel monkey (Saimiri sciureus) lung culture. Science 195, 289

125. Smith, G. C., Heberling, R. L., Helmke, R. J., Barker, S. T. and Kalter, S. S. (1977). Oncornavirus-like particles in squirrel monkey (Saimiri sciureus) placenta and placenta culture. J. Natl. Cancer Inst. 59, 975

Chapter 6

The Common Marmoset *(Callithrix jacchus)*

J. P. Hearn

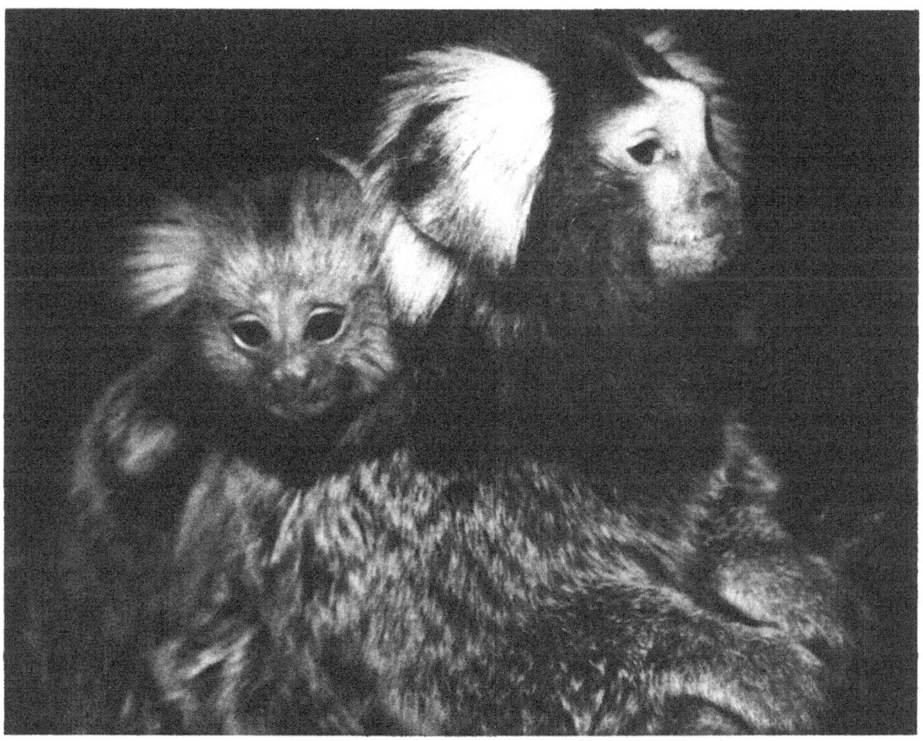

Callithrix jacchus

THE COMMON MARMOSET (Callithrix jacchus)

John P. Hearn

The Institute of Zoology
The Zoological Society of London
Regent's Park
London NW1 4RY
England

INTRODUCTION

The Common marmoset monkey, Callithrix jacchus jacchus, breeds more rapidly in captivity than any other primate. Because of its small size (adult body weight 400 g) it is easy to maintain in family groups in captivity, so eliminating the boredom and neuroses sometimes seen in the larger macaques and baboons that are often caged singly. Marmosets adapt well to captive conditions, to handling, sampling and experimental procedures, particularly if a system of rewards is used. They are economical to keep, normally produce twins, and because of their short generation interval, with sexual maturity at about 18 months of age, they can be established in captive, self-sustaining breeding colonies at a fraction of the time and cost taken for the larger, more conventional, laboratory primates.

There are disadvantages to the marmoset as a laboratory primate. Because of its small size, frequent blood sampling is not possible beyond a sample size of about 3 ml each week. If sampling has to be carried out over a period of weeks, then a sample size of 0.3 ml blood each day is a maximum without inducing anaemia. Its small size also precludes use of the marmosets in aspects of experimental surgery. There are undoubtedly metabolic differences between marmosets and man, as there are between any major groups of primates. However, these disadvantages are outweighed by the considerable advantages of the marmoset in many fields of scientific enquiry.

Background

A detailed account of the past breeding, usage and study of marmosets is not relevant here and references before 1970 are therefore restricted. While there are several reports of small breeding colonies during that time, successful breeding and application of Common marmosets in biomedical science developed mainly in the past ten years.

On the other hand, reports of the use of marmosets for other purposes go back a long way. Ladies at the French Court, including Madame Pompadour, considered it fashionable to carry a tame marmoset or tamarin in the décolletage. To those who know the distinctive smell of marmosets, and the mess they can make, that line of imagination is best not pursued.

Early reports on the captive breeding of marmosets[1,2] showed them to be highly fecund. Many attempts at establishing colonies failed, as animals imported from the wild were often in poor condition on arrival, with heavy parasite loads and susceptible to infections because of their debilitated state. The first few weeks required intensive care if animals were to survive but once adequate procedures were established, the trauma and loss over the period of adaption to captivity were greatly reduced[3].

It is interesting that the Common marmoset was 'adopted' as the New World primate of choice by investigators in the United Kingdom. The early evaluation of the species by Bill Kingston at the Pfizer Laboratories near Nottingham and by Bill Hiddleston at the ICI Laboratories near Manchester led to a development of basic breeding procedures. In the course of these studies the essential requirements for nutrition and veterinary care were evolved, but unfortunately little was published and the disastrous attempts by many zoos to keep and breed marmosets were largely unsuccessful. However, 10 years ago the essential procedures had been worked out, a few second generation captive born animals were produced, and a rapid expansion in the numbers of centres breeding and studying marmosets followed. They âre now important animals for scientific questions related to many aspects of reproductive and developmental biology as well as, for example, in immunology, teratology, cancer, dentistry, perception and cognition, behaviour, and neuroendocrinology. In other fields they have been found to be of limited value, for example as a 'screen' in pharmacology and toxicology, where their small size apparently makes them unsuitable[4]. Ironically, it was for this purpose that they were first evaluated.

Over the same period in the United States, the 'marmosets' also received a great deal of attention, but the species adopted were in fact not marmosets but tamarins. The major species studied were *Saguinus fuscicollis*, *Saguinus mystax*, *Saguinus oedipus* and *Saguinus labiatus*. With the exception of *S. labiatus*, most *Saguinus* species proved to be highly strung, difficult to breed and slow to adapt to captive conditions. However, the work of Dienhardt[5,6], Epple[7,8] and Gengozian[9,10] overcame many of the difficulties. It remains true, nevertheless, that even second generation captive born tamarins are more difficult to handle and breed than the Common marmoset, which under the correct conditions of management becomes almost blasé to life in the laboratory.

Status in the Wild

While the laboratory studies proceeded, a greater appreciation of the status of these animals in the wild was being achieved through the work of Coimbra Filho[11-13], Mittermeier[14-16], Soini[17] and others. It became apparent, as indicated in the laboratory, that while many species of New World primates were threatened or endangered by forest clearance, the Common marmoset was an exception in that it was spreading, with successful introduction in recent times as far south as Rio de Janeiro, although the original distribution was concentrated in the eastern

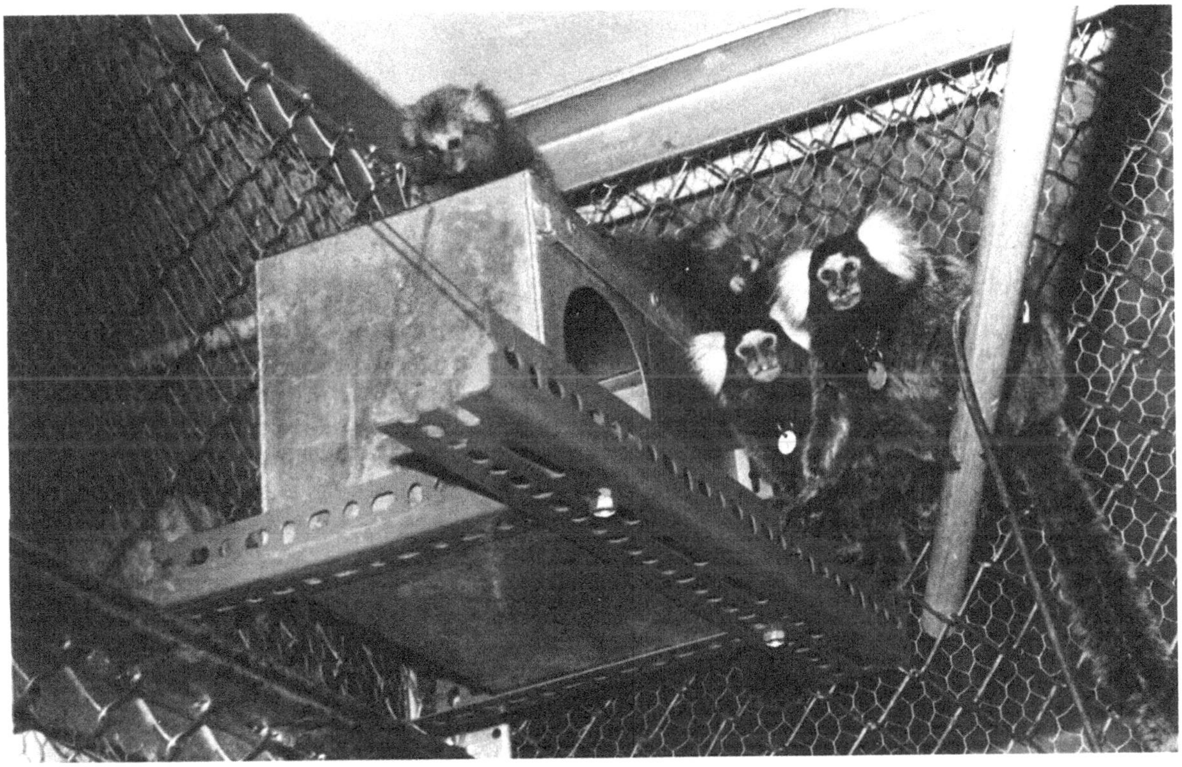

Figure 1. A family group of marmosets in the laboratory

equatorial forests up to 1000 miles from the Brazilian seaboard. However, the reports of social behaviour and organisation of marmosets and tamarins in the wild are still few and far between[18-20]. A number of other workers have carried out studies that have not appeared in print. Yet it is important that our captive management of primate species aims at an optimal balance of factors based on their habits and requirements in the wild. We have developed our captive management of the Common marmoset with this in mind, and according to their reproductive physiology as we discovered it; although the field data were usually gleaned from sources that were at best anecdotal and often owed more to imagination than fact.

The Scope of this Chapter

In this chapter a few aspects of the management of marmosets are given, followed by a summary of the reproductive physiology of the Common marmoset and a mention of some areas of biomedical science in which they have proved valuable. Many of the questions posed relate, due to the interests of the author, to the field of primate (including human) reproduction. It was for its rapid reproductive rate that we first selected the marmoset as our animal analogue for studies relevant to human reproduction. If you are working on reproduction in primates it helps to have a primate that reproduces well. Primate work is frustratingly slow at best when compared with similar work in rodents, but the closer physiological and endocrinological similarities between primates and the human primate make the effort worth while. The work we have managed to carry out over the past eight years on the marmoset has profited enormously from the advantages attached to these small primates; only a fraction of the work could have been completed in the same length of time (and at ten times the cost) in the larger, more conventional laboratory monkeys.

No single non-human primate is going to be an ideal animal analogue for studies related to human reproduction. One has to achieve a balance. The Great Apes, such as the chimpanzee, orang-utan and gorilla, are the best 'models', but they are endangered and widespread exploitation of wild stocks for biomedical research is unethical. Every attempt must be made to conserve these and other endangered primates, both in captivity and in the wild. The macaques and baboons are in many ways suitable for laboratory studies, but their reproductive rate in captivity makes the establishment of captive colonies long-term and costly. The Common marmoset is not a competitor with the rhesus and baboon, but it is fast becoming a generalised laboratory primate with considerable advantages for particular fields of science. It is the scientific question that counts and the appropriate species in which the question is asked then follows.

Primate research, and the colonies on which it is sustained, is of necessity long-term and expensive. It is unfortunate when one finds colonies that have outlived the scientific aims of their original founding and become private zoos or status symbols. The planning of such research requires careful thought and development over a period of at least three years ahead of the present. These days, successful primate breeding colonies are irreplaceable national assets. They are potentially too important and costly for their longer term future to be left to accident or chance.

MANAGEMENT

Animals and Availability

Common marmosets originate from eastern equatorial Brazil. In the wild they are reported as travelling in extended family groups or in large groups of up to 30 animals. The reports are anecdotal and unsubstantiated by publication in any detail. The same reports, obtained by the author from Brazilian and European workers who have observed such groups, indicate that in any group of marmosets there is only one female in breeding condition. Births occur throughout the year and all members of the group will assist in carrying the young, but the other females do not breed and are apparently inhibited in some way by the dominant pair.

In captivity marmosets are best maintained in male-female pairs. When compatible, they breed extremely well and additional space is then necessary for the expanding family as suggested below. If the animals are being imported from the wild, they often arrive in debilitated condition and great care is necessary over the first few weeks while they adapt to captive conditions. Full details of such procedures were published earlier[3]. However, if at all possible, it is now better to obtain the foundation stock for a new colony from a successful centre with excess captive born young. There is, rightly, a ban on export of Common marmosets from Brazil, the only country in which they are found, although some dealers claim to import them as native fauna from other South American countries. There are now enough successful colonies in Europe, the USA and elsewhere to make it almost unnecessary to import from the wild. Indeed, the price of captive bred marmosets has recently been declining as success in breeding becomes more widespread.

In the early 1970s it was possible to obtain wild caught Common marmosets for as little as US $15 each. When interest in the species increased, conditions of breeding worked out and their attributes of economy and fecundity appreciated, the price climbed, to $200 by the mid 1970s and to $500-600 each in the late 1970s, for either captive bred or wild caught animals. The trend is happily now downwards, with captive bred animals often available for $400-500 and sometimes as low as $300 each. The marmoset is the first of the primates where the price of captive bred is similar to that of wild caught animals, making it economically illogical to import from the wild.

Caging and Conditions

After considerable modification and development, the caging system (North Kent Plastic Cages Ltd, Home Gardens, Dartford, Kent, England) now used in the author's colony is shown in Figure 2. Cage racks contain four cages, each of dimension 60 x 60 x 90 cm, with provision for a small side-attached nest box (28 x 18 x 18 cm) that can be removed with the animals inside when they are to be held for blood sampling, pregnancy diagnosis, etc. Single cages, each with two perches and a shelf, are adequate in size for a pair of adults and one pair of twin young. Once the family expands to six, with a second set of twins born, an adjacent cage is added with a connection as shown between the lower pair of cages in Figure 2. Each cage has a base grid and a tray of wood shavings, changed once weekly.

The family cages as shown can be ranged round the walls of each animal room. An exercise cage (2 x 1 x 2m) is placed in the centre of each room (seen to the left in Figure 2) and this can be connected to any of the family cages by means of a length of flexible ducting (Flexible Ducting Ltd, Cloberfield, Milngavie, Glasgow, Scotland). The animals quickly learn to run through the ducting into the exercise cage and can move back and forth between home cage and exercise cage throughout the exercise period. In our colony, the ducting is rotated between the family cages once a day, each group of animals therefore receiving a 24 h period of exercise.

The purpose of the exercise cage, in addition to the obvious one of providing exercise and improving physical condition for all the animals, is two-fold.

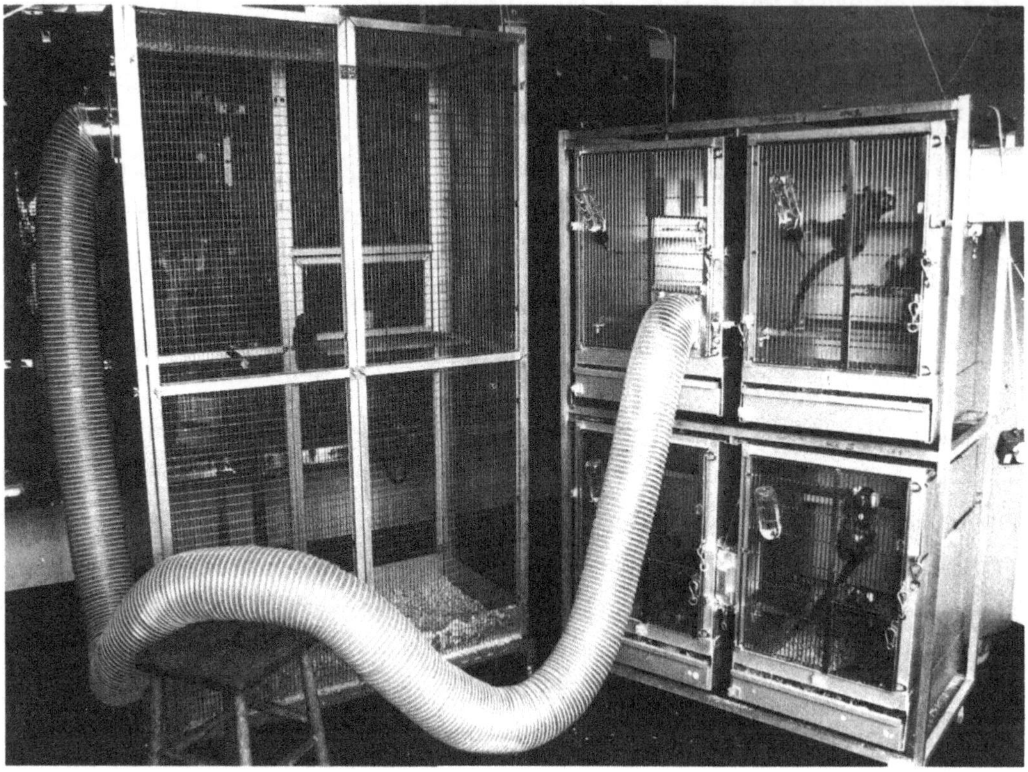

Figure 2. The system of caging (home cage and exercise cage) used in the author's laboratory

Firstly, for the family groups, a change in environment afforded once a week does a great deal to eliminate boredom. Secondly, for all the animals in the room, a different family in the central exercise cage each day provides a constant stimulant, source of interaction and entertainment, that transforms the environment in each room as a whole. To any who have seen the boredom and depression evident in many laboratory primates that are maintained in single cages over long periods of time, the ability to maintain marmosets in family groups and the provision of an exercise facility as described provides a marked contrast. With this system in operation, marmosets settle rapidly to laboratory conditions and the system retains the option of rapid capture of the animals, as required in most laboratories where physiological studies are in progress. The provision of these conditions, although thought unnecessary by some, has convinced us many times over of their effectiveness in improving health and alleviating boredom.

The temperature of the animal rooms is maintained at 20-25°C and the humidity between 50-70%. While both temperature and humidity are critical for recently wild caught marmosets, they are resilient when adapted to captivity and once second generation breeding is achieved, they can tolerate more extreme variations although they do best at the above levels.

The sense of smell is important to marmosets and they scent-mark their surroundings frequently, so a liberal supply of wooden perches or branches is advisable. In addition, they enjoy gnawing wood and in the wild they spend considerable time in feeding on the saps of certain trees[21]. Consequently, perches should be changed weekly, but cleaning of cages, other than the base trays, may be less frequent. Ideally, cages should be washed monthly as should the nest boxes, but not at the same time, so that the animals retain a familiar area in the cleaned cage.

It is necessary in any primate colony to institute an effective barrier system. Only staff who are directly involved in animal management and research are allowed access and they wear protective clothing: caps, masks, gloves, boots and overalls. A footbath of suitable disinfectant is placed at the door of each room and the floors are washed daily. No one who has been in recent contact with mumps, measles or other infectious diseases is allowed access. If a good barrier system is employed, then there can be more freedom within each room, such as the system of shared exercise caging described above.

Feeding

In the wild, marmosets eat fruits, insects and saps from particular trees, a difficult diet to match in captivity. However, they adapt rapidly to a pelleted diet (eg 'Mazuri' New World Diet: Scientific Diet Services Ltd, Stepfield, Essex, England) which can be dipped briefly in flavoured milk to vary the taste if necessary. About 15-20 g/day pelleted diet per animal is sufficient. In addition, cereals such as 'Farex' (Farley Baby Products, Plymouth, Devon, England), vegetables (carrots, lettuce), fruits (apple, orange, tomato, banana, grape), seeds (sunflower, nuts) and insects (locusts, mealworms) all prove acceptable and provide variety. Additional vitamin D_3 (approx. 1200 i.u./animal/ week) is necessary on a weekly basis to prevent rickets.

Handling Marmosets

If it is necessary to handle marmosets for palpation, blood sampling, measurement etc, then every animal should be trained to accept these procedures as routine. When Steve Lunn and I started to establish our first colony we were told by many "experts" that marmosets should be handled as little as possible as they were very easily stressed and the females would abort at the drop of a hat. With the few animals then available, five pairs were put aside as 'breeding pairs' and the remaining four pairs were treated as 'experimental'. On the latter group the routine procedures detailed below were developed, through daily catching and handling. Within a few weeks it was clear that the 'experimental' animals were thriving and all the females were pregnant, whereas the 'breeding' animals were nervous and showed no signs of pregnancy. From then on all animals were accustomed to frequent capture and handling and the colonies succeeded well beyond our initial expectations.

Of course the animals must always be treated with care and respect. New staff are carefully instructed in all procedures and asked to familiarise themselves with the animals. The animals are trained to enter nest boxes before they are caught up and they receive a reward, such as a piece of date or grape, after each procedure. They quickly become far more interested in looking around for the reward than in the procedure. There should on no account be attempts to capture animals by flailing around the insides of their cages with nets, as they will never adapt to such treatment. Talking to the animal in a calm voice, and ensuring that movements are unhurried and deliberate, also helps a great deal. Undoubtedly, if the animals are trained to co-operate with the handler, neither they nor the handler will be stressed and the quality of the research is vastly improved.

Sampling of Blood

The restraint device shown in Figure 3 allows the routine collection of blood

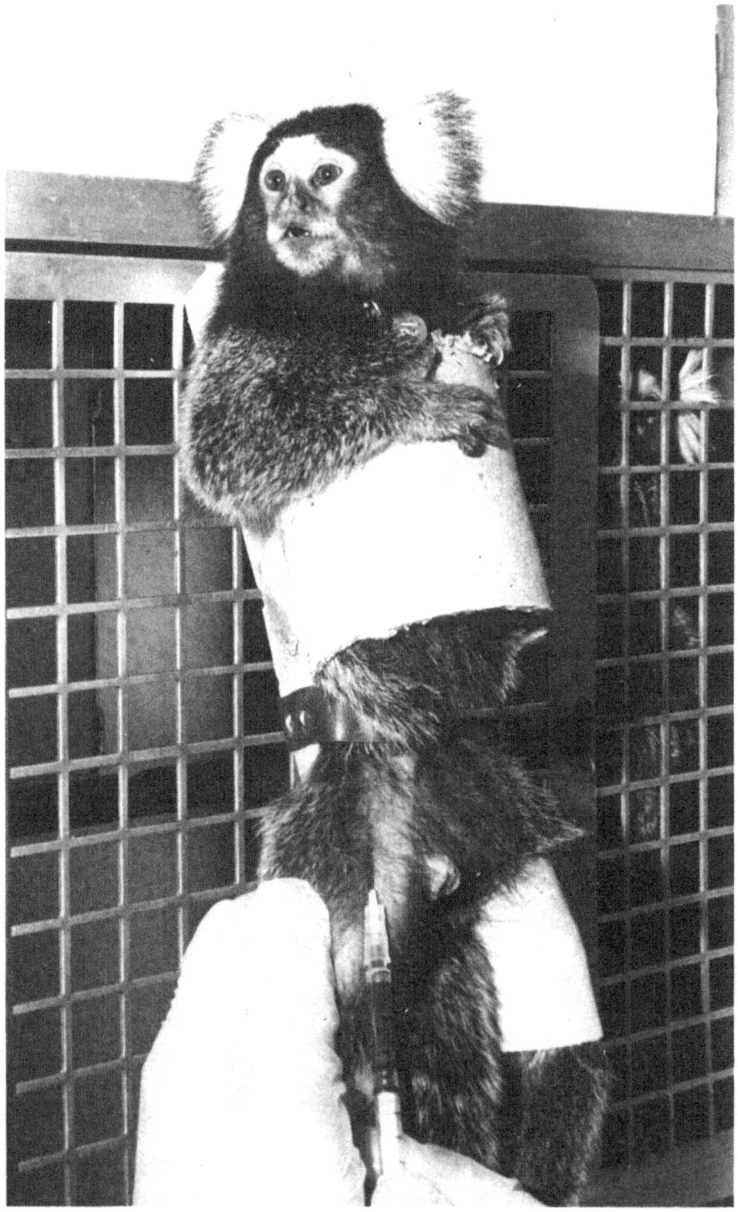

Figure 3. A restraint device for small primates, which can be attached to the side of a cage if necessary

with no stress to the trained, rewarded animal. One handler can capture, pick up, place the animal in the device and obtain the blood specimen with ease[22]. The device is constructed from plastic piping, Velcro straps and wood. It allows the monkey to be held securely without discomfort and marmosets (and other small monkeys) adapt to it with ease. Blood samples are routinely drawn from the upper region of the femoral vein as shown, using a 27 g needle and a 1 ml heparinised syringe. If a gentle approach is used, the procedure is rapid and haematomas are avoided by compressing the vein with a forefinger for a few seconds after removing the needle. The restraint device also allows the routine collection of vaginal lavage, transabdominal palpation for diagnosing and monitoring pregnancy, and any other simple inspection or dosing procedures.

Sampling of Urine

A simple system for collection of urine samples is shown in Figure 4. The cages used are rat metabolism cages (North Kent Cages Ltd) surrounded by a bucket which cuts down draughts. The urine passes into the polystyrene container beneath the cage, allowing the urine to be collected in a vial placed in an ice bath[3]. Marmosets suffer no ill effects from 24 h urine samples collected in this way over alternate days. However, with recent improvements in methods of measuring urinary hormones, collection of samples over a short period each day is sufficient to monitor reproductive function[23,24]. The volume of urine produced by marmosets (± s.e.m.) in 24 h is 17 ± 0.34 ml (n = 488; range = 3.0 - 47.0 ml).

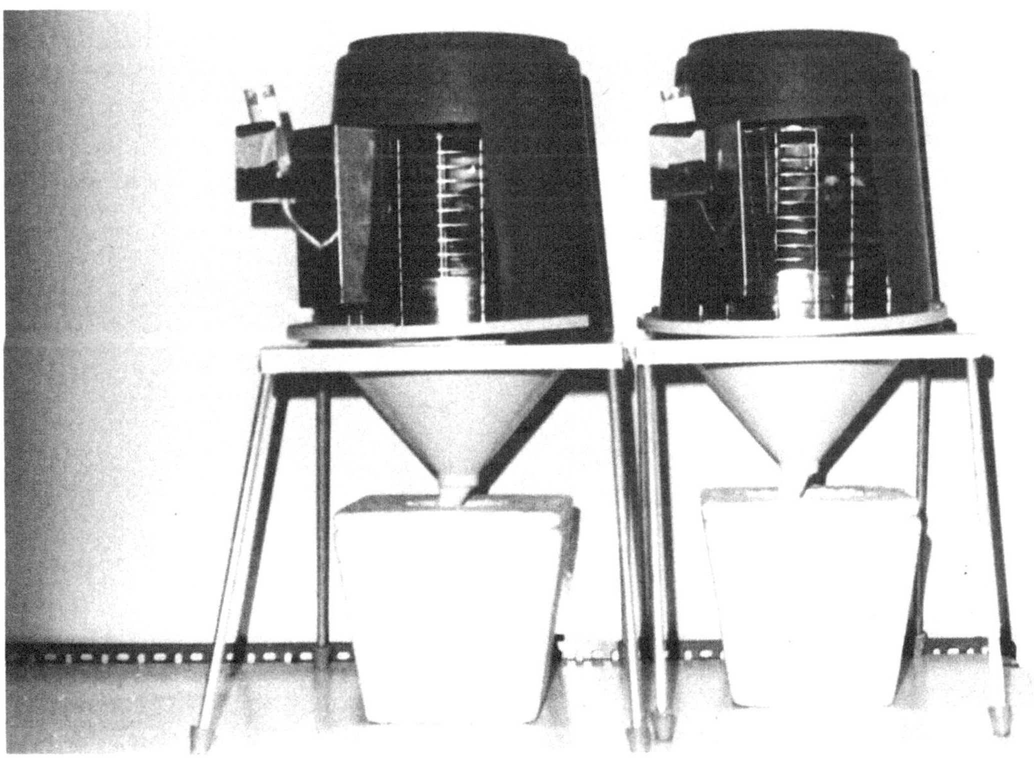

Figure 4. Collection of urine samples from marmoset monkeys

Detection of Pregnancy

Pregnancy may be diagnosed and monitored by analysis of hormones in plasma or urine, or by transabdominal uterine palpation. Details of analysis of hormones in urine and a comparison between different methods are reported elsewhere[25]. Profiles of hormones in plasma during early pregnancy are shown later in this chapter. Figure 5 shows the size of the uterus as measured by transabdominal palpation, using thumb and forefinger, for pregnancies that produced single, twin or triplet young. The size of foetal heads (width) during the last six weeks of pregnancy is also shown. Using this simple non-invasive system, pregnancy can be detected by the skilled operator between 21-28 days after ovulation. The presence of single, twin or triplet young can be determined after the 15th week, as can the size of the foetal heads. It is emphasised that palpation procedures should be carried out gently.

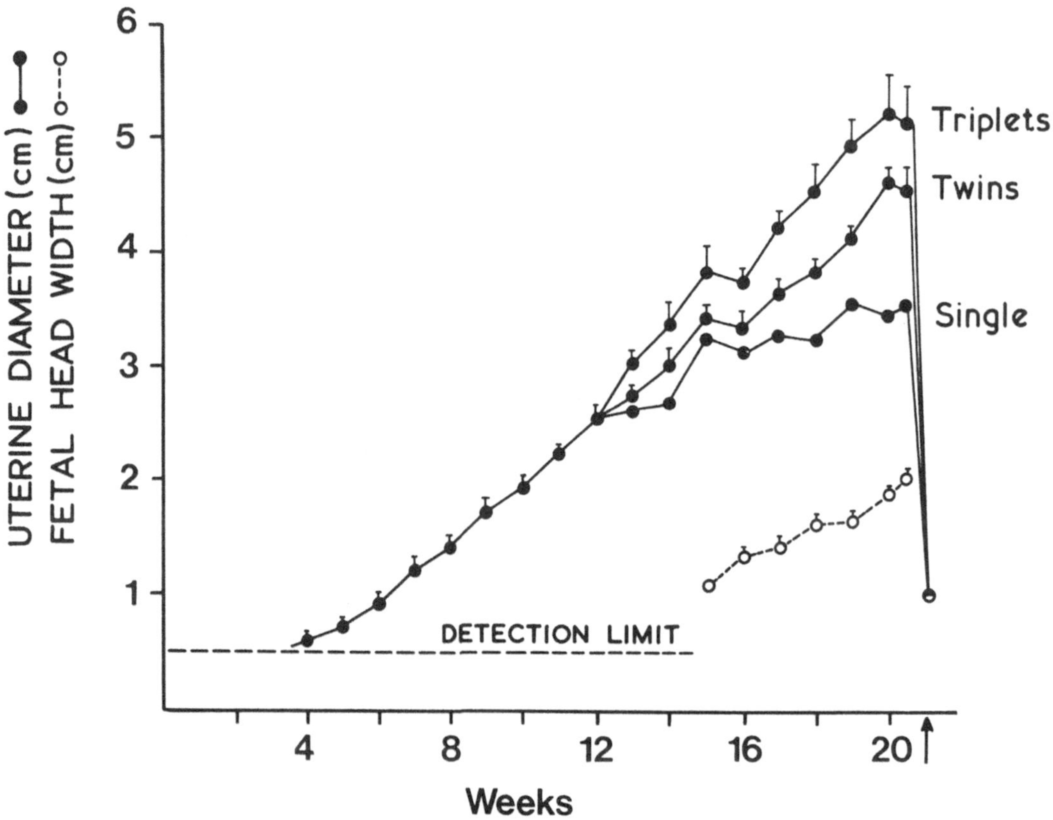

Figure 5. The diameter (± s.d.) of the uterine fundus (•) and the width of the foetal heads (o), measured by transabdominal palpation, in marmosets bearing single, twin and triplet young. The horizontal line represents the detection limit

Rearing of Young

As mentioned earlier, marmosets usually give birth to twins (70% of births) with triplets and single births not uncommon (20% and 10% respectively). The ratios of singles, twins and triplets vary considerably from year to year. Table 1 shows the ratios over the first few years of establishment of our colony from wild stock. The ratio of triplets has now returned to the level noted above. There is at present no explanation for these changes in ratio. The sex ratio at birth is 1:1 as expected and the twins are usually dizygotic.

Table 1. The incidence of triplet births in a marmoset colony (as a % of all births in the colony).

Year	% triplet births
1974	11.5
1975	17.8
1976	27.6
1977	43.3

Young marmosets are carried by all older members of the family, although they usually spend the night carried by their mother. It is important to leave young marmosets with their families, at least until the next set of young are born and reared. The young will then participate in the rearing of their younger siblings, who may be only 150 days younger than themselves. This is a necessary experience for the young to learn the complex requirements and behaviour for successful births and rearing their own young later on.

As noted above, marmosets frequently give birth to triplets. Except in very rare cases, the weakest triplet will die within a few days. This unnecessary loss to a colony can be avoided by instituting a suitable hand rearing regimen but separation of young from the family environment may cause abnormal development and behaviour. A successful compromise can be achieved if each triplet is removed in rotation for a 24 h period, maintained in an incubator and hand-fed, before being returned to its mother. In this way a "collaborative" rearing is possible (for details of diets, feeding rates, etc see Hearn and Burden[26]). At any time the mother has two infants while the third is in the incubator, preferably on a furry toy (Figure 6) which serves well as a surrogate mother. Marmosets are usually weaned between 40-60 days old. Using the system described, it is often possible to leave all three infants with the mother full time after about 25 days of age. The family group does not reject young removed in rotation for 24 h each in this way.

Fostering

A further option for dealing with the triplet 'problem' is to foster the third infant into another marmoset family that has only one infant. An age difference in the infants of up to one month can be tolerated. The necessary trick is to leave both the infant to be fostered and the infant from its new family in a nest box for half an hour. They will cling together and the new infant will thus

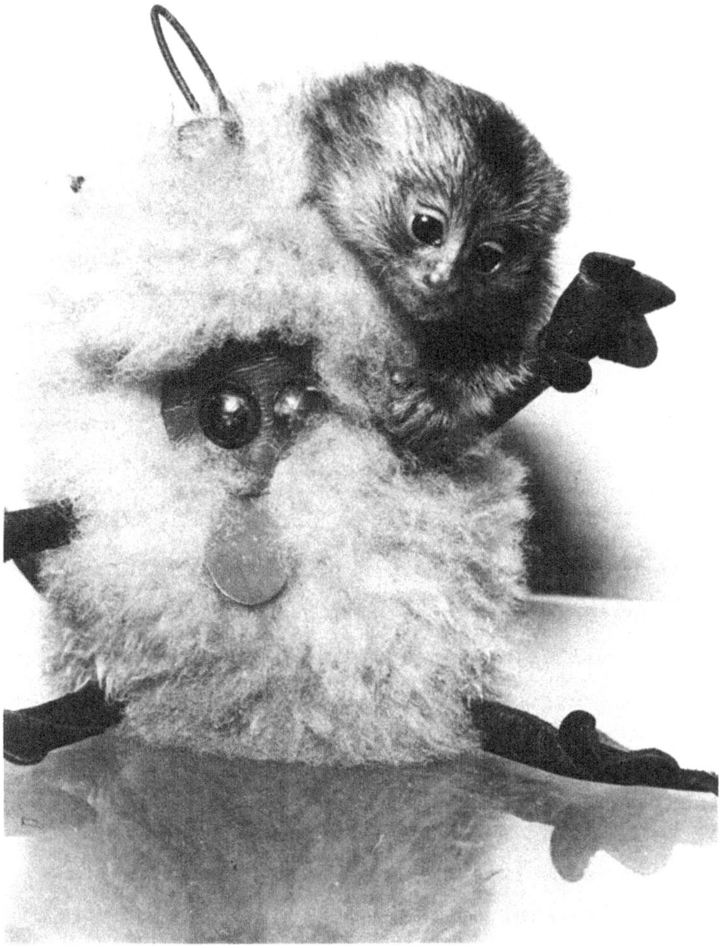

Figure 6. A 3-day old marmoset in a paediatric incubator clings to a surrogate mother

acquire some of the smell of the family. Both infants can then be carefully rubbed against the lower abdomen and inguinal regions of the foster parents, again helping to give the new infant a familiar smell. On their return to the family, the two infants should preferably be introduced to different family members who will carry them. If the trick is not discovered within an hour, the chances of successful fostering are high.

Author's Comment

On concluding this section, I can imagine wry smiles on the faces of some readers. Much of the above is common sense and, for a scientist, may be construed as either overstated, oversensitive or both. To which criticism, if it exists, I respond by emphasising the obvious again. You will not get any valid research work done with a stressed primate. If the results of the research are to be good, without unnecessary variation within experimental groups, interpretable and publishable, then priority must be given to the simple details outlined above. Primates are relatively intelligent animals and are seldom available in sufficient numbers to allow large experimental groups in which variation due to stress can be lost. Marmosets are most attractive animals, but only when they co-operate. The more attention given to the reduction of stress, the better the ensuing research.

REPRODUCTIVE PHYSIOLOGY

The Ovarian Cycle

In common with most New World primates, the female marmoset does not menstruate. There is no externally obvious change that allows prediction or detection of ovulation or menstruation[27]. However, the levels of ovarian steroids secreted during the cycle are high, in comparison with Old World primates and humans. The Common marmoset shows continual cycles throughout the year and there is no seasonal breeding as in the rhesus monkey, nor 'birth peaks' at certain times of the year as seen in many other primates.

The ovarian cycle in the Common marmoset is 28.6 ± 1.0 days (n = 19). The cycle may be divided into a follicular phase of 8.3 ± 0.3 days (n = 56) and a luteal phase of 19.2 ± 0.6 (n = 48). The levels of peripheral plasma progesterone found during the cycle are shown in Figure 7[28]. There is some discrepancy in the

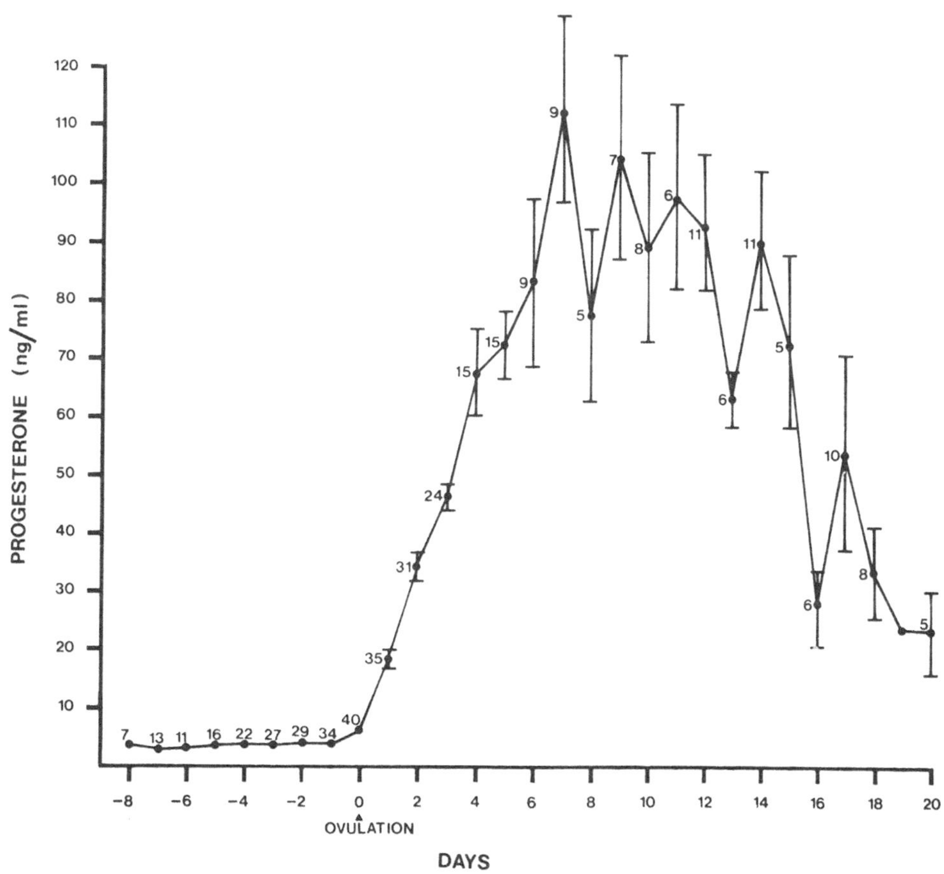

Figure 7. The amounts of progesterone (± s.e.m.) in the peripheral plasma of marmosets sampled either daily or three times each week throughout the ovarian cycle. The numbers at each point indicate the numbers of animals sampled on that day of the cycle

length of the cycle, since earlier reports indicated a 17 day cycle[29,30]. The length of the cycle reported here is calculated from analysis of over 100 cycles from 2nd to 5th generation captive born marmosets. It is possible that the earlier reports of cycle length in the Common marmoset were confused due to the studies being performed on wild caught animals within the first two years of their adaption to captivity. However, reports of most other New World primates, for example in other chapters of this volume, indicate an ovarian cycle length of 9 days (squirrel monkey) to approximately 17 days (tamarin) to approximately 22 days (Cebus); cycles that are usually shorter than the 28-33 days reported for many Old World primates. Marmosets mate frequently throughout the cycle and early pregnancy, although recent studies suggest an increase in female proceptive behaviour during the period of ovulation (Dixson and Kendrick: personal communication, 1982).

Pregnancy

The gestation period in the marmoset is 144 ± 2 days (n = 9) with a range from 141-146 days, from the day of ovulation to the day of birth. Figure 8 shows the levels of LH/CG, progesterone, oestradiol-17β and oestrone throughout pregnancy.

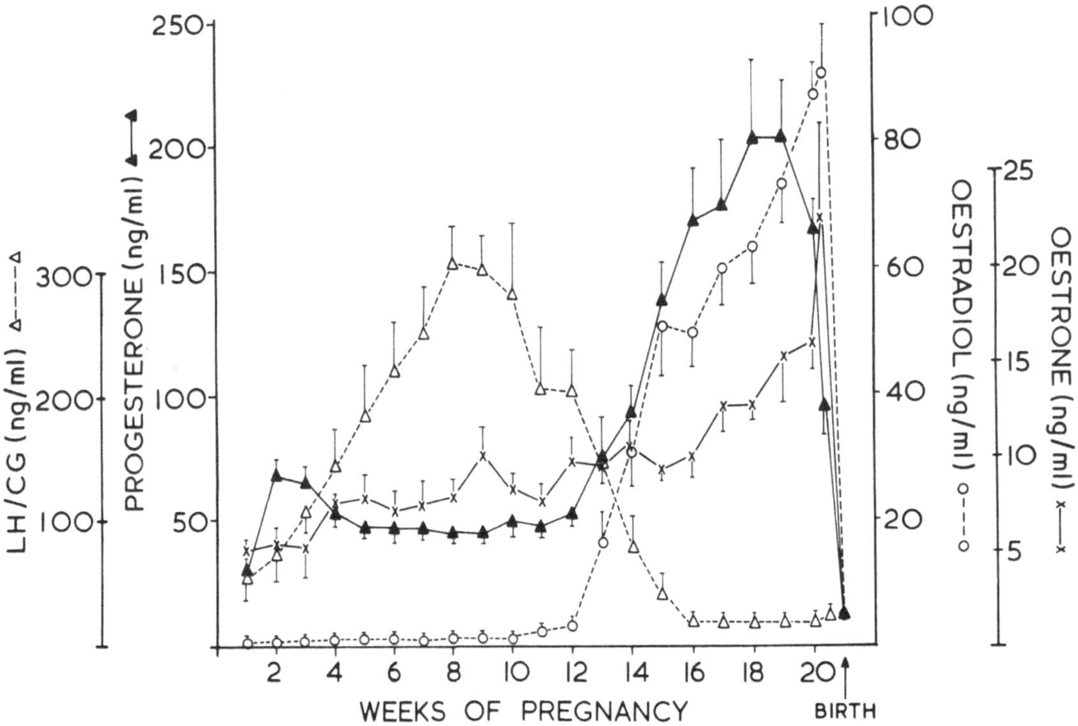

Figure 8. The peripheral plasma levels (± s.e.m.) of progesterone (▲), oestradiol-17β (o), oestrone (x) and LH/CG (Δ) during pregnancy in the marmoset monkey

Although the levels of oestradiol-17β appear low during the first 12 weeks of pregnancy, this is because of the scale used, as the levels rise gradually over this period from 2-10 ng/ml in peripheral plasma. Two further points may be made here. Firstly, the levels of chorionic gonadotrophin rise rapidly from day 10-15 in early pregnancy, reaching a peak between weeks 6-8. Secondly, there is a marked rise in the levels of steroids during the second half of pregnancy, in parallel with development of the feto-placental unit. This rise is similar in profile and level to that seen during the third trimester in women, while in rhesus monkeys and baboons such a rise does not occur. However, there are also differences in the metabolism of the three species that make such comparisons superficial.

Figure 9 shows the levels of androstenedione and testosterone throughout pregnancy in the marmoset. There is a similarity between these profiles and that of chorionic gonadotrophin shown in Figure 8, but this may be an association rather than cause and effect.

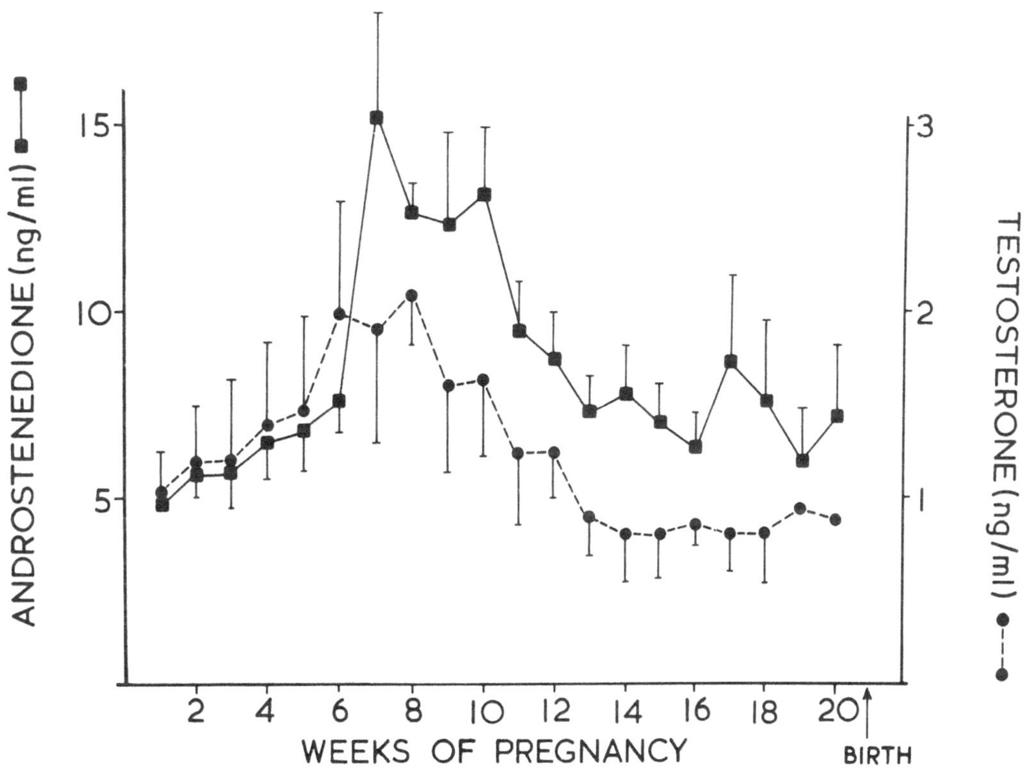

Figure 9. The peripheral plasma levels (± s.e.m.) of androstenedione (■) and testosterone (●) during pregnancy in the marmoset monkey

Figure 10 shows the levels of LH/CG, progesterone and oestradiol-17β during the first 30 days of pregnancy in two marmosets. The profiles show that chorionic gonadotrophin can be measured in the peripheral plasma from day 10-15 of pregnancy onwards, rising very rapidly to its peak between 6-8 weeks as shown in Figure 8. Figure 10 shows also that there is a marked secretion of oestradiol-17β during the luteal phase of the cycle. In this feature the marmoset once again resembles the human rather than the rhesus monkey or baboon.

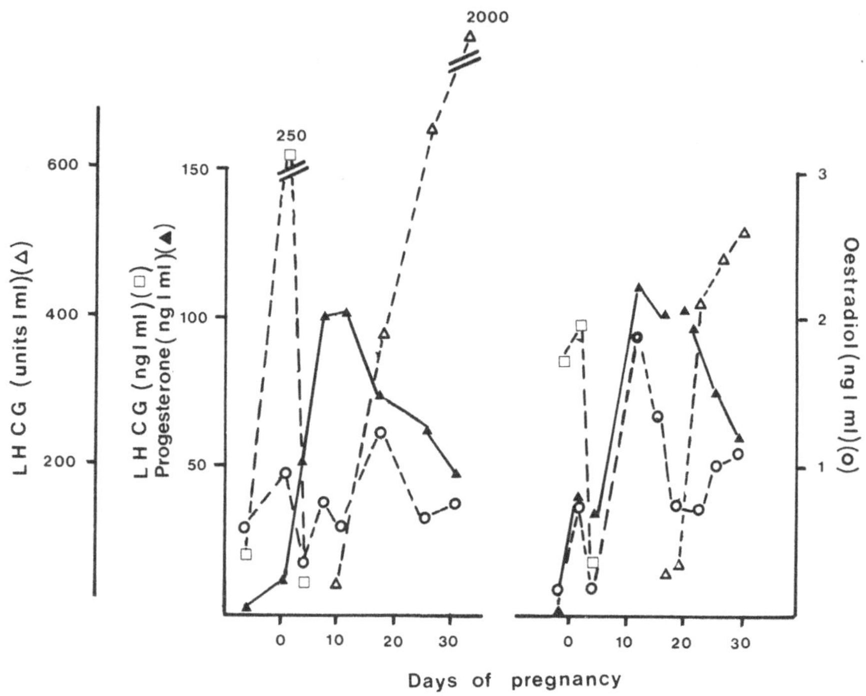

Figure 10. The peripheral plasma levels of progesterone (▲), oestradiol-17β (o and LH/CG (Δ) during the cycle of conception and the first 30 days of pregnancy in two marmoset monkeys. Day 0 = day of ovulation

The levels of progesterone measured throughout pregnancy in the peripheral circulation and in the utero-ovarian vein before and after removal of the feto-placental unit are shown in Figure 11. The results show that the levels of

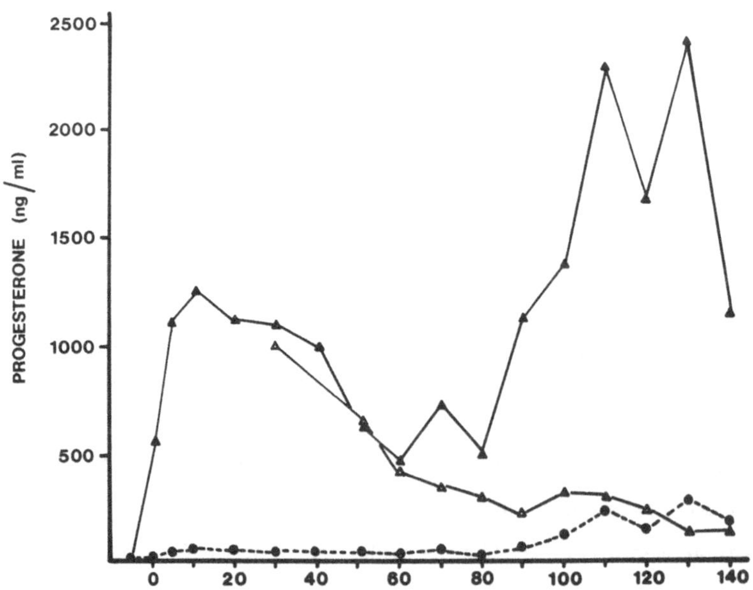

Figure 11. The levels of progesterone in the peripheral plasma (•) and in the utero-ovarian vein plasma before (▲) and after (Δ) removal of the feto-placental unit in marmoset monkeys

progesterone are very much higher in the utero-ovarian vein than in the peripheral circulation, and the profile of the latter reflects changes in the former only poorly. If one compares the levels before and after removal of the feto-placental unit, it becomes apparent that the corpus luteum is contributing the major proportion of progesterone up to day 60 of pregnancy, but after day 60 the placenta provides the major share throughout the second half of pregnancy while the amount secreted from the corpus luteum continues to decline.

Figure 12 shows the uterus of a Common marmoset, during the 15th week of pregnancy, exteriorised at laparotomy for recovery of utero-ovarian vein samples. Using a 27 g needle and a 1 ml heparinised syringe it is possible to draw these samples with ease. Indeed, the utero-ovarian vein in the marmoset is surprisingly easier to sample from than that of the rhesus monkey or baboon, where it is not much larger and seems prone to haematomas. The corpus luteum is very evident during early pregnancy in the marmoset, but after day 40 it is difficult to distinguish as it sinks back into the body of the ovary, much of which appears composed of luteinised interstitial tissue.

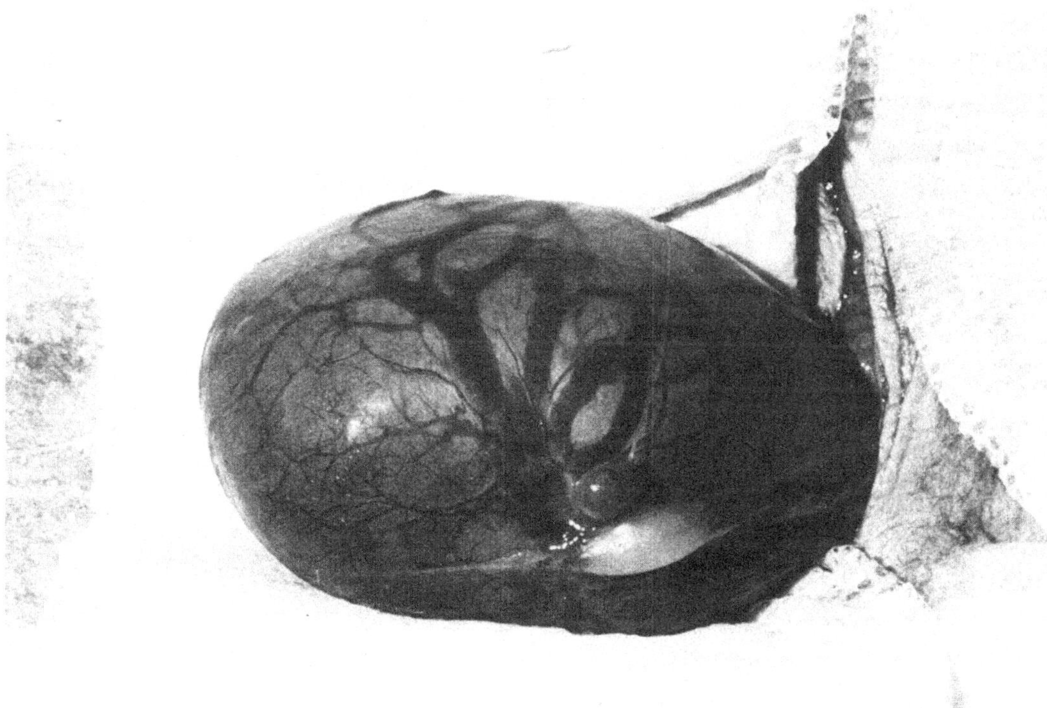

Figure 12. The uterus of a marmoset monkey, exteriorised at laparotomy, to show the ovary and the utero-ovarian vein

Post Partum Ovulation

In contrast to all other primates so far investigated, lactation does not inhibit follicular growth and ovulation in the marmoset. Seventyfour percent of 31 animals studied ovulated within 21 days of giving birth. The mean day of ovulation was 10.5 ± 0.7 (s.d.) with a range of 5-17 days[28]. This feature of reproduction in the marmoset adds significantly to its fecundity. Under optimal conditions of management, breeding females will rear twins or triplets (with help as detailed above) at 4½-5 month intervals for many years. In our colony there are several females now over 12 years of age still breeding in this way. Records from other colonies indicate that breeding will continue beyond 16 years of age (Gengozian: personal communication). However, our breeding programme is designed to provide replacement of the entire colony every 5-7 years. Table 2 shows a comparison of some factors affecting captive breeding of the baboon, marmoset and rhesus monkey.

Table 2. A comparison of some factors affecting the captive breeding, fecundity and economy of the baboon, marmoset and rhesus monkey in captivity

Factor	Baboon	Marmoset	Rhesus monkey
Size of females (kg)	8-15	0.3-0.4	3-7
Seasonal breeding in captivity	No	No	Yes
Average young born per female/year	0.8	5.0	1.0
Approximate generation interval (years)	5-7	1.5-2.0	4-6
Length of ovarian cycle	35	28	28
Gestation length (days)	185	144	165
Lactational anovulatory period	1-2 years	10 days	1 year

Lactation

The relationships between lactation, the suckling stimulus and return to ovulation were investigated recently[31]. During the ovarian cycle there were no consistent changes in plasma prolactin concentrations. During lactation those mothers suckling single or twin infants had higher prolactin levels than did non-suckling females and the levels were highest with twins. However, there was no statistically significant delay in the resumption of ovulation post partum in suckling compared with non-suckling females. The results showed that neither the suckling stimulus nor high levels of prolactin post partum delay the return of ovulation and fertility in the Common marmoset.

The young marmoset suckles for a period up to 100 days. Weaning commences by about 30 days when babies will take foods from the hands of their parents or siblings (but not usually if offered by anyone else). They are able to survive entirely on solid food and milk substitutes from 40 days of age, but will normally continue to suckle with varying frequency for a further 40-60 days. The mother's levels of plasma prolactin are usually indistinguishable from those of non-lactating animals by 70 days after giving birth[31].

The reasons for the differences in the pattern of return to fertility in lactating marmosets compared to other primates is uncertain. Those primates that show lengthy periods of infant dependency on the mother and who are immature at birth (eg. Great Apes and man) show long interbirth intervals that are induced by lactation[32], and usually produce single young. The marmoset has a long gestation and the young grow rapidly, becoming relatively independent of the mother before the next young are born, approximately 60 days later. The marmoset, therefore, may not need the more commonly seen lactation-induced delay in return to fertility.

The double physiological burden of simultaneous lactation and pregnancy is unusual in primates and may be related to two other factors in marmoset reproduction. Firstly, all members of the family or group carry the young of the fertile female, reducing the energy expended by her in rearing her own young. This is just as well since the young weigh about 28 g each at birth and grow rapidly. At birth a pair of twins represent 14-16% of adult body weight and by 50 days will total 37-42% of adult body weight. Secondly, our recent, and yet to be published, studies show that embryonic development during the first 70 days of gestation is slow in comparison with other primates, whereas after 70 days there is a rapid acceleration in foetal growth. The crown rump length of the marmoset foetus is a mere 1 cm at 70 days but is 4 cm at 100 days and nearly 8 cm at birth (144 days). These dimensions are very similar in single, twin and triplet pregnancies.

Chimaerism

The placenta of the marmoset is 'shared' by twin or triplet young and vascular anastomoses connect both placental discs. Figure 13 shows, for twins and triplets respectively, the anastomoses and the umbilical connections between each foetus and disc. The natural chimaerism displayed by the marmoset is an enigma in that it allows haemopoietic and bone marrow chimaerism yet does not result in freemartinism when male and female co-twins are present. Recent studies (Hearn and Chambers: in preparation) indicate that during late pregnancy male and female foetuses have similar levels of testosterone circulating in their blood yet the female is apparently not affected in its gonadal or behavioural development. In this regard the marmoset differs from the cow, where freemartins from twin births are frequent and infertile, and may be more similar to man where reproductive abnormalities have not been seen in the few cases studied. However, a discussion of chimaerism would merit a chapter by itself and is not appropriate here.

Growth and Development

Figure 14 shows the growth of marmosets from birth to 600 days of age. There is no difference in growth rates or adult body weight between male and female marmosets. It was found that the knee to heel length provided a good measurement with which to monitor the development of marmosets as this shows little variation between animals and gives an accurate method for ageing marmosets during the first 12 months of life. Adult skeletal size is reached at about 12 months, but

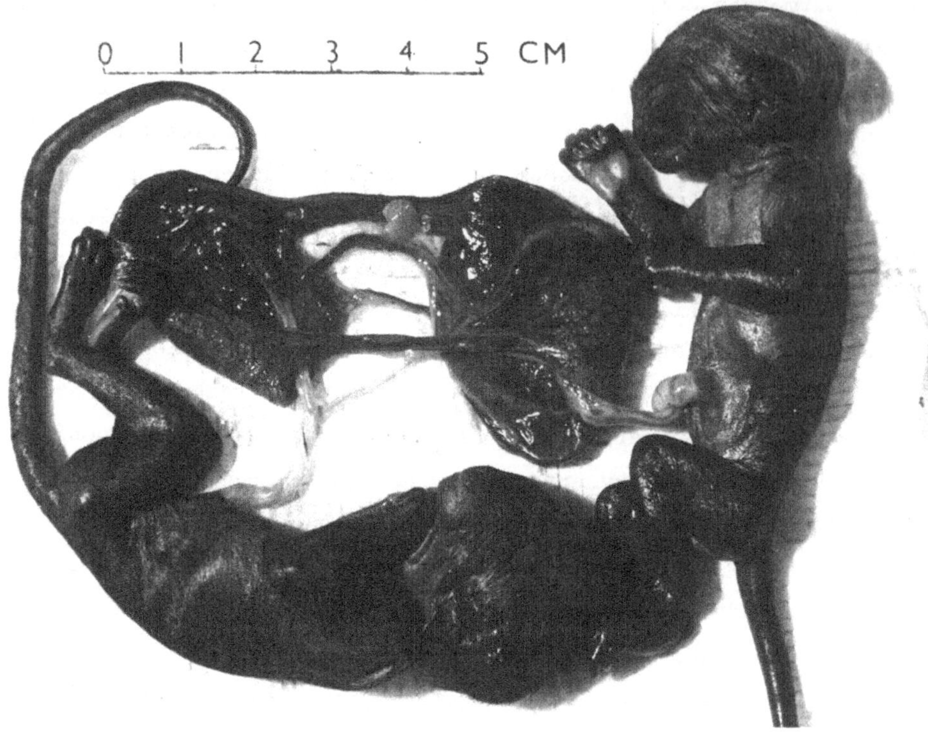

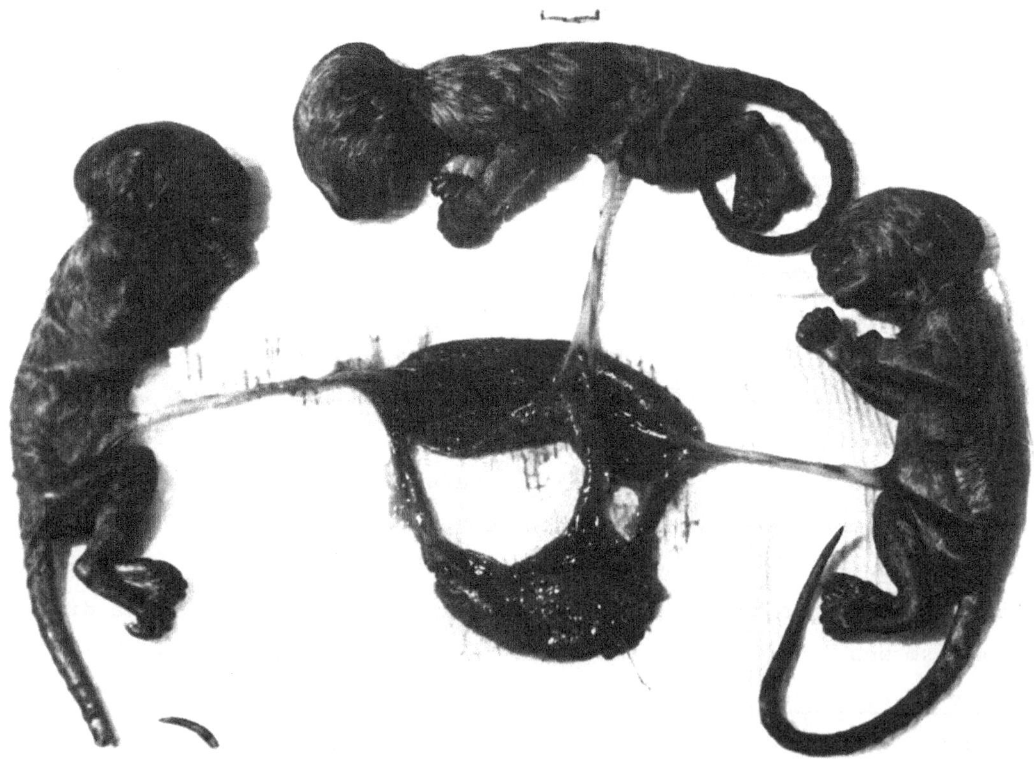

Figure 13. The anastomoses and vascular connections between foetuses and placental discs for twin and triplet births in the Common marmoset

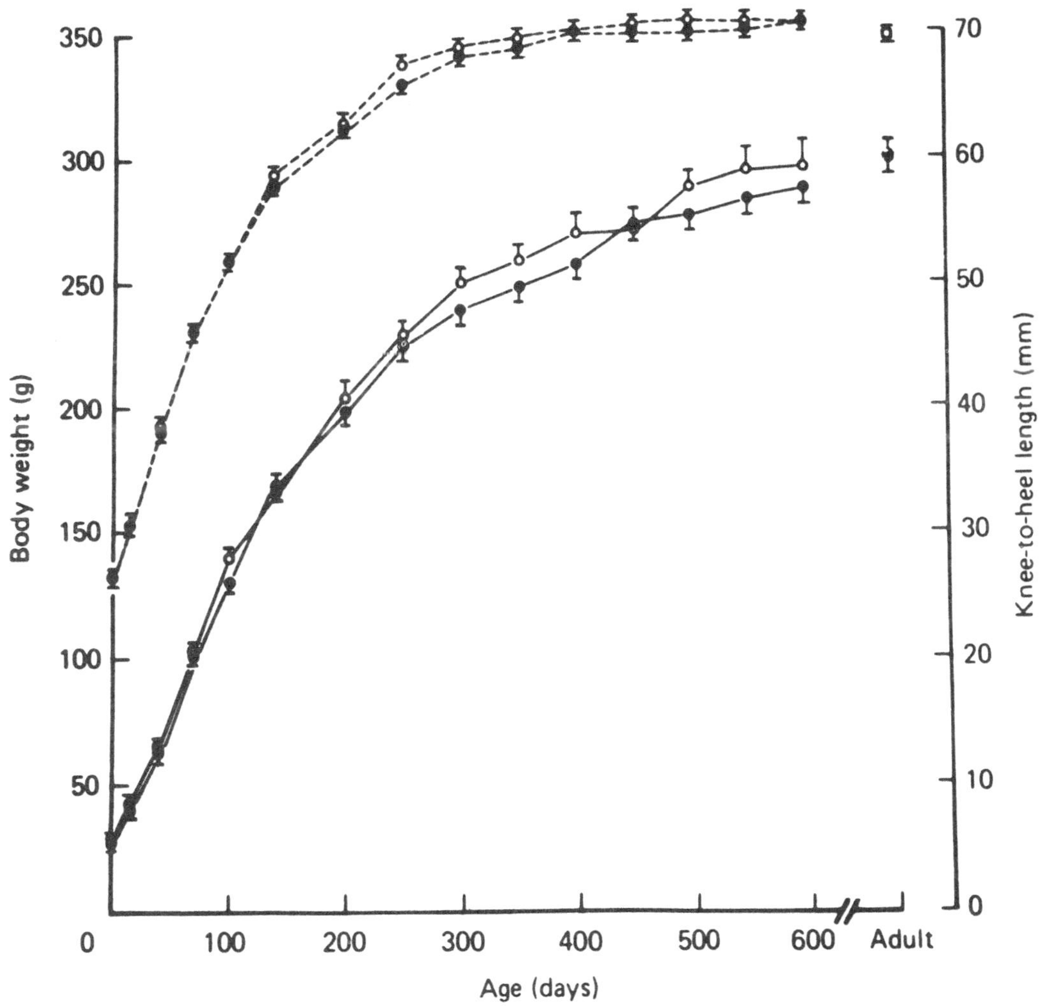

Figure 14. The growth of male (•) and female (o) marmosets in captivity, determined from measurements of body weight (——) and knee to heel length. Values are mean ± s.e.m. Each point represents a mean of 10-20 animals. The mean ± s.e.m. body weight (◘) and knee to heel length (■) of 20 adult males and 20 adult females are also shown

females do not commence regular ovarian cycles until 14-18 months and males do not become sexually mature until about 18 months although they are able to copulate by 14 months old. Full details of the growth and sexual development of the marmoset monkey were published earlier[33].

It is preferable to maintain young marmosets in family or peer groups until about 18 months old. The system we have evolved is to leave them with the family until approximately 1 year old, and then to place six unrelated animals (3 males, 3 females) together in a peer group until about 18 months old. By this time, a male and a female will have established a pair and may have produced young. All members of the peer group assist in rearing the young although only the dominant pair will breed. This system allows the most mature animals to form a breeding pair. Once the pair is established and young produced, the family can be removed to a separate breeding cage. By this stage the remaining animals in the group are mature enough to form pairs and will usually do so if separated. While it is possible to advance the breeding age of animals, especially by pairing an experienced adult of one sex with an inexperienced juvenile of the other, this may not lead to successful rearing of young[33]. It is undoubtedly better to wait a few months until the animals are fully sexually mature, when breeding and successful rearing of young becomes a routine matter.

Suppression of Fertility

As noted earlier, anecdotal reports of groups of wild marmosets indicate that only one female in a group breeds. The others will carry her young but are inhibited from breeding themselves. In the laboratory, it is possible to test this unusual phenomenon, but the mechanisms by which it is controlled are not understood. Figure 15 shows the effect on their ovarian cycles when three females are caged together. The 'dominant' female continues to cycle regularly, but the other two stop and will remain acyclic, and therefore infertile, as long

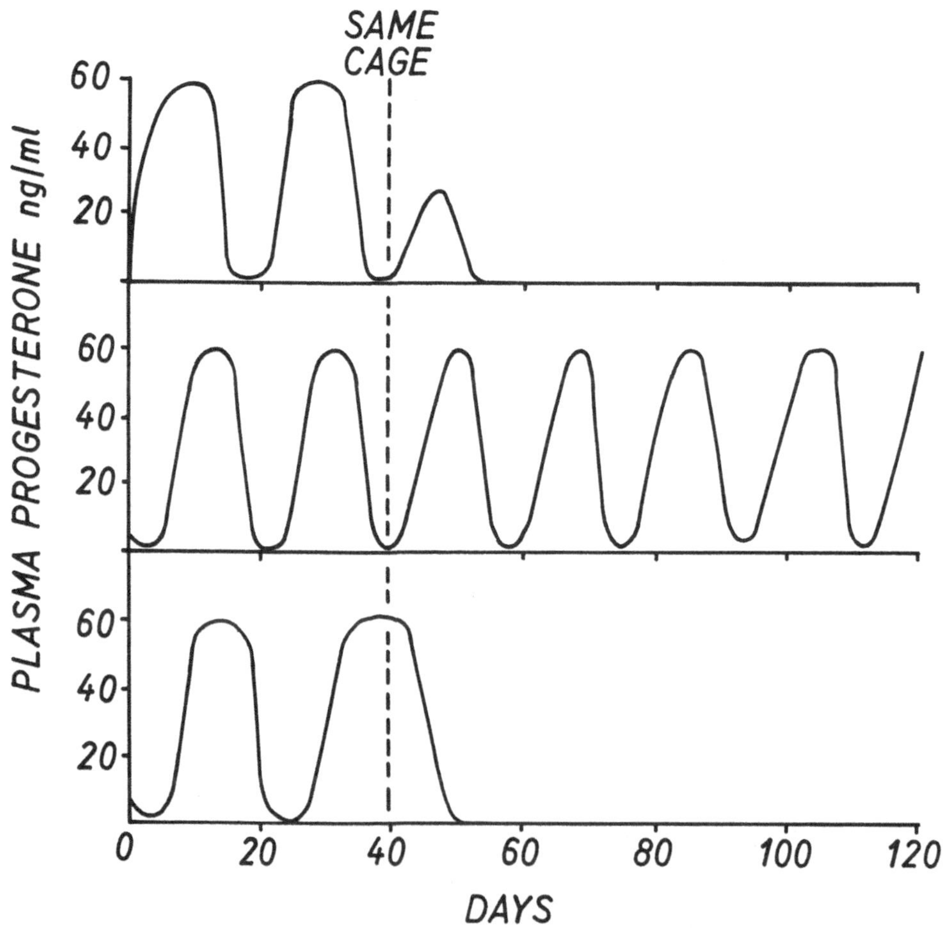

Figure 15. Diagrammatic representation of events when three cycling females are placed together in the same cage. The 'dominant' female continues to cycle while the subordinates cease ovarian cyclicity

as the dominant female is present. If the dominant female is removed from the group, then the next female in the heirarchy will start to cycle. In contrast to other primates studied to date, the marmoset appears to have a reproductive system with high fecundity, each female capable of producing on average up to 5 surviving young each year. The regular birth of twins, 144 day gestation, no lactation inhibition and no seasonal breeding lead to a reproductive rate that requires control in a novel way. The marmoset has developed such a novel mechanism. Ironically, marmosets therefore breed better in captivity than they do in the wild, for in captivity they may be kept in pairs whereas in the wild they move in families or groups where only the dominant female in a group will breed.

Although subordinate females in peer groups showed a complete inhibition of ovulation and fertility, no evidence was found to suggest similar suppression of fertility in subordinate males as these were not excluded from mating with the dominant female in any group[33].

In a coincidental experiment, presented in Figure 16, a young male with high testosterone levels was introduced to a dominant female who was placed in his home cage. The male showed an immediate fall in levels of circulating plasma testosterone, the levels remaining low for at least six weeks. It is not known in other primate species (including humans) whether dominant females exert similar inhibitory effects on males.

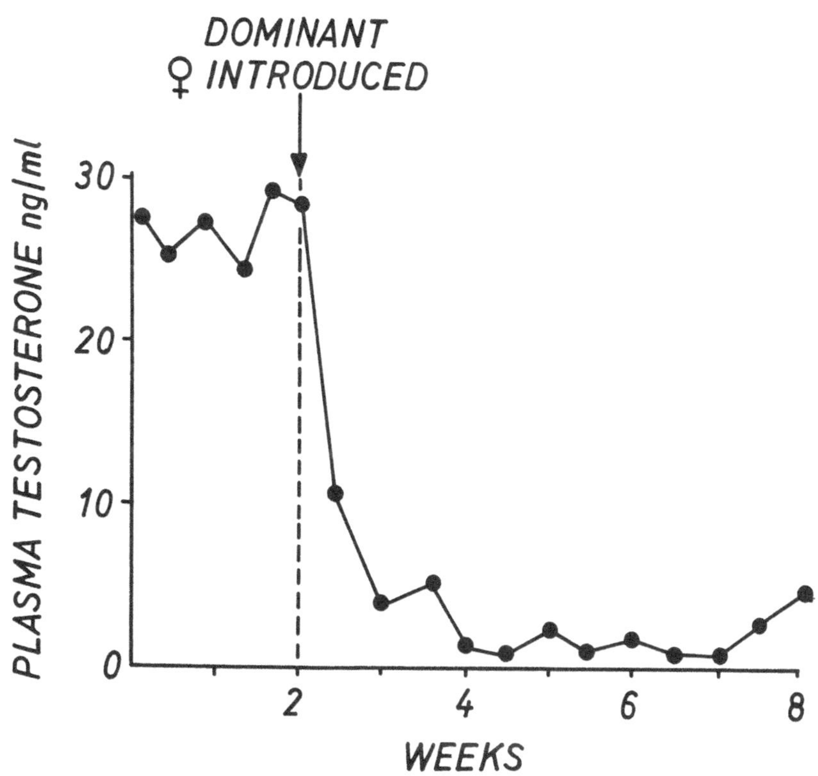

Figure 16. The effects on plasma testosterone in a young adult male marmoset when placed with a dominant female

A recent report in male talapoin monkeys suggested that elevated levels of plasma prolactin might be associated with inhibition of fertility in that species [34]. However, studies in the marmoset showed that prolactin is unlikely to be the causal effect of reproductive inhibition between females[35]. At present the mechanisms whereby the dominant female marmoset inhibits ovulation in her subordinates are unknown but they probably involve both pheromonal, physical and visual factors[36,8].

The Male Marmoset

In many species, studies on the reproductive physiology of the male tend to lag a long way behind those of the female, but there is now a fairly comprehensive knowledge of reproduction in the male marmoset, only a brief summary of which follows.

The growth and sexual development of the male marmoset was reported earlier, and related to female sexual development in the same captive colony[33]. Detailed studies of spermatogenesis and of sperm maturation have been completed by Dr Bill Holt and Dr Harry Moore at the Institute of Zoology and will appear shortly, as will studies of androgen binding protein and androgen receptors in the epididymis. In a further study, the ultrastructure of the epididymis in the human was compared with the talapoin, pig-tailed, patas, capuchin, spider and marmoset monkeys[37]. It was shown that the primate epididymis displayed several ultrastructural features not found in other mammals, but epididymal tissues in man were ultrastructurally more diverse than those of monkeys.

The fertilising ability of spermatozoa from different regions of the epididymis of the marmoset was assessed in the hamster denuded ova test _in vitro_[38]. The spermatozoa first acquired the ability to 'fertilise' in the distal caput and proximal corpus epididymis and the majority were fertile on reaching the proximal cauda region. Similar studies are currently in progress on the human.

In a recent paper[39], Alan Dixson showed for the first time in a male mammal that prolactin is elevated in males that carry their offspring. Although the levels of prolactin found in the male marmosets studied were five times those of control animals, there is no suppression of male fertility during the period when they are assisting in the rearing and weaning of their young.

The long term effects of immunising male marmosets against LHRH (luteinising hormone releasor hormone) were studied and found to present a relatively easy and reversible method of male sterilisation[40,41]. However, when antibody levels were high the effects resembled a physiological hypophysectomy with complete interruption of spermatogenesis and suppression of testosterone secretion. Interestingly, the males continued to mate with their female partners during this period. In a further study, the effects of 6chloro-6deoxy glucose on male libido and fertility were investigated in marmosets, again showing a reversible antifertility effect[42]. But when the doses of this compound were increased (x 5) in a preliminary safety test, results were obtained that precluded further development of this approach.

Undoubtedly, there are many questions in male reproductive physiology of primates that could be suitably investigated in the marmoset. The basic studies completed so far indicate the physiology to be not dissimilar to the human and the problem of managing, handling and taking blood samples from male marmosets are minor in comparison to those attached to studying male rhesus monkeys or baboons. Moreover, their lack of seasonal breeding and highly successful reproduction in captivity make them available for study throughout the year. With the development of new agents for regulating male fertility, such as gossypol and its analogues, a small male primate is essential for studying the mechanisms of action and aspects of safety. Many such agents are expensive and difficult to synthesise in bulk, so the small size of the marmoset allows highly efficient and economical studies to be carried out.

APPLIED STUDIES

The distinction between basic and applied studies in reproduction is not a real one. Much of the basic investigation immediately translates into practical aspects of management or application to various fields, while 'applied' approaches invariably serve as tools to increase basic knowledge. In this section, a few of the areas of reproduction in which the Common marmoset has proved a valuable species for advanced investigations are summarised and some recent work on the developmental physiology of marmosets in our laboratory is noted.

Control of Fertility

Studies of the control of fertility in primates are essentially long term. This is especially so if it requires a control period of normal fertility, followed by an experimental period of induced fertility and then an extended time while normal fertility is resumed. For such studies the marmoset has many advantages and its reproductive rate and economy in captivity enable the work to be completed in a small fraction of the time and cost required in any other currently available laboratory primate. Studies in the male were referred to above, but a series of studies in the female have been completed. These studies concentrate especially on the role of chorionic gonadotrophin in early pregnancy and the effects of immunising female marmosets against this hormone[43-45].

Chorionic gonadotrophin was shown to be an essential hormone for successful implantation and active or passive immunisation against its β subunit will prevent pregnancy from continuing. However, the reversibility of this system presents problems in that recurrent abortions were found to occur as the levels of antibodies declined. The mechanisms that allow implantation to proceed in presence of antibodies to hCG-β, and yet an abortion to occur later, were discussed elsewhere[46,47] but are not fully understood. It is likely that antibodies to hCG-β do not just block the luteotrophic support of the corpus luteum, but also may act directly on the developing embryo.

An account of research carried out on the marmoset monkey in relation to puberty, control of LH secretion and immunisation against pregnancy was published earlier[48].

Embryonic Development

The high fecundity of the marmoset and its normal production of twins allows

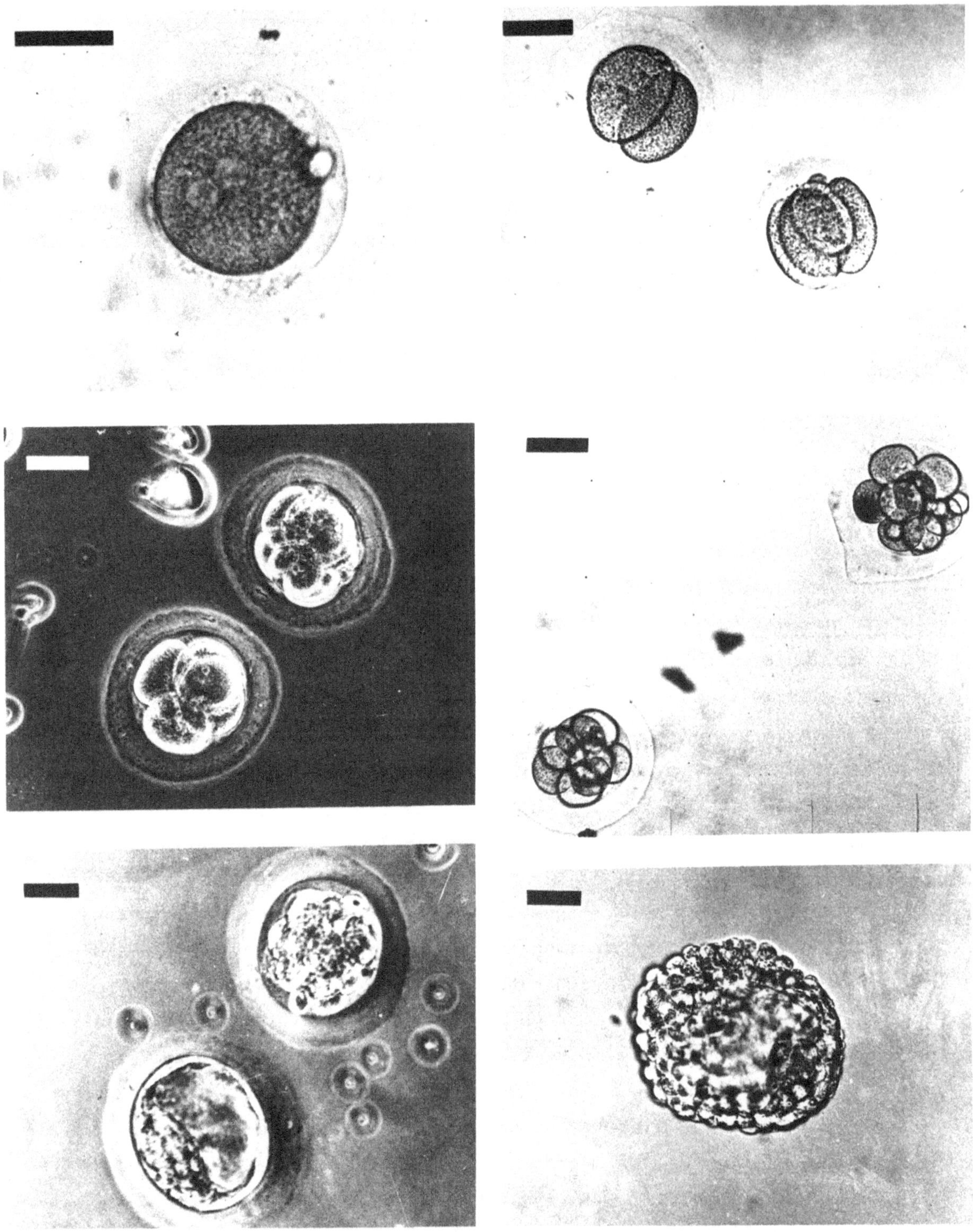

Figure 17. Stages of embryonic development, from 1 cell to hatched blastocyst, recovered during the first 10 days of pregnancy in marmoset monkeys. The measurement bar shown in each picture is 50μ

rapid progress in studying the endocrinology and timing of events during early pregnancy. There is little detailed knowledge of the first six weeks of pregnancy in primates with regard to the endocrinology and physiology of implantation and early embryonic development. Yet many aspects remain to be investigated, especially now with the development of in vitro fertilisation, embryo storage and transfer in humans. For reasons of ethics and availability, such studies cannot be carried out in humans or apes.

In the marmoset, the timing of ovulation can be determined by hormone assays. Implantation commences between days 10-12 after ovulation, at about the same time seen in the rhesus monkey and baboon, but a few days later than that reported for the human[49]. The marmoset is extremely resilient and the simple surgical procedures involved in laparotomy and recovery of embryos are tolerated with no apparent stress. Indeed, most animals are pregnant again within two weeks of the operation. Figure 17 shows embryos recovered from marmoset monkeys at timed intervals from ovulation during the first 11 days of pregnancy. Most embryos pass from the fallopian tube to the uterus on day 4 of pregnancy, 'hatch' from the zona pellucida on day 10 and attach to the endometrium on days 11-12 to commence the process of implantation. Figure 18 summarises the age and stage of

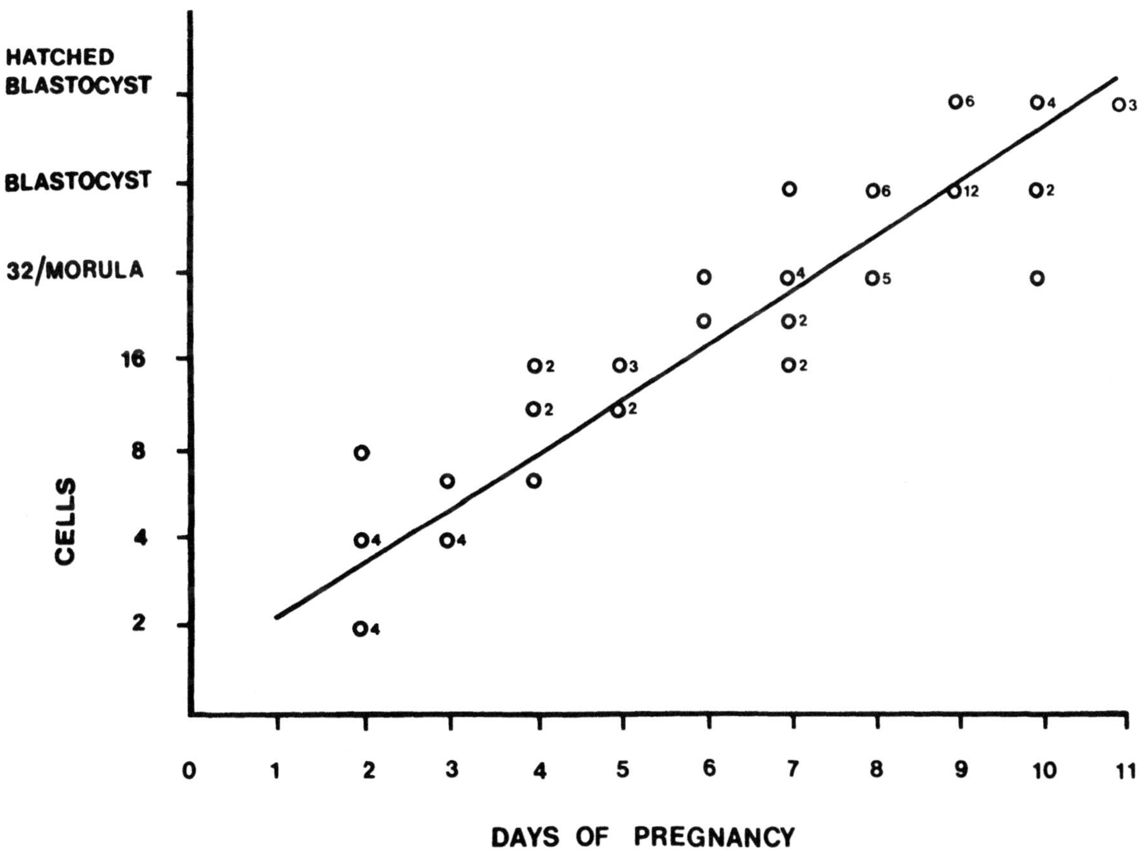

Figure 18. The stages of development of marmoset embryos recovered during the first 11 days of pregnancy. The numbers at points indicate the numbers of embryos recovered at that stage and time. The line is a line of 'best fit'. It is apparent that considerable variation in rates of embryonic development is tolerated in this primate

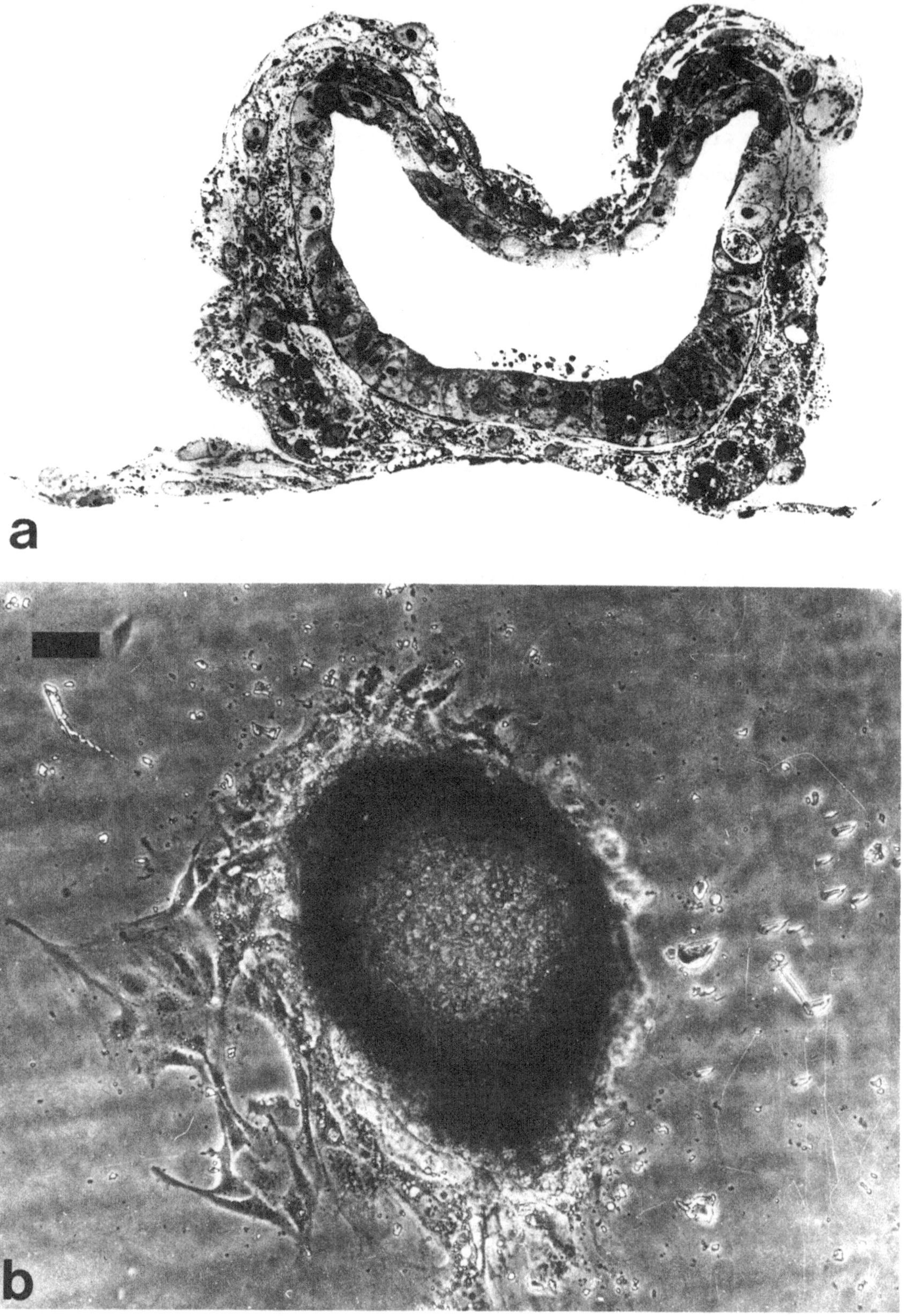

Figure 19. (a) Section through an embryo grown <u>in vitro</u> for an extended development to the equivalent of day 20 of pregnancy.

(b) The embryo before fixation and sectioning

development of embryos recovered during the first 11 days of pregnancy. It is apparent that there is some variation, even in the stages of development of twin embryos, during this period. The precise synchrony in rodents of embryonic development with endometrial changes is unlikely to be necessary for successful implantation in primates.

It is not intended here to go into detail of several inter-related studies currently nearing completion and being prepared for publication in our laboratory. The studies on *in vitro* fertilisation, freezing of embryos, transfer of embryos and the pre- and post-implantation development of embryos *in vivo* and *in vitro* show some novel features of primate developmental physiology. It has proved possible to grow embryos *in vitro* up to the 20th day of 'pregnancy', enabling, for the first time, detailed studies of development and differentiation over this period in a primate. Figure 19 shows a section through one such embryo and present research is validating *in vitro* with *in vivo* growth. These and other studies indicate a great potential for the study of developmental antigens, embryonic secretions, differentiation and micromanipulation, as well as more applied aspects of cell line culture, fertility regulation and teratology. These are exciting prospects for the years ahead.

CONCLUSIONS

1. The account given here emphasises the potential of the Common marmoset in investigations of reproductive physiology. Undoubtedly, this potential holds promise for many studies in reproduction and other fields. Yet one does not wish to promote 'use' of an animal, particularly a primate, in any research unless it is essential and that species is the only one in which the studies can be carried out appropriately. For such work, however, the marmoset is now the only laboratory primate generally established in self-sustaining, captive breeding colonies successful to the fifth generation in captivity.
2. In order to carry out research work that means anything, priority must be given to the conditions of management, especially with a primate species that is otherwise prone to stress and boredom. Under optimal conditions of care and management, marmosets breed very well and are amenable to handling and experimental procedures. They are resilient and hardy when subjected to experimental surgery, recovering quickly especially when returned immediately to their family groups.
3. The high fecundity of marmosets makes them particularly valuable in studies of reproductive physiology and the control of fertility. Their normal production of twins enables rapid progress in studies of embryonic development and feto-maternal relationships during pregnancy. Their relatively rapid attainment of sexual maturity assists in studies of neonatal and pubertal development.

ACKNOWLEDGEMENTS

I thank Sara Gems for her excellent assistance in all the recent studies reported here. My colleagues, Dr Keith Hodges, Dr Harry Moore and Mr Chris Harlow, are involved in several of the studies. In the earlier work reported, I thank Dr Stephen Lunn, with whom I started and developed our marmoset adventures, Dr David Abbott, Dr Pamela Chambers, Dr Keith Hodges and Mr Martin Hulme. I am grateful to Mrs Barbara Murrill, Mr Terry Noble, Mr Frank Burden and the animal management staff at the Institute of Zoology, London and the MRC Reproductive Biology Unit, Edinburgh for their care of the marmoset colonies as we built them.

The research work summarised above is supported by the Medical Research Council and Agricultural Research Council through programme grants, the World Health Organisation through project grants and by a core support grant to the Institute of Zoology from the ABRC.

REFERENCES

1. Kingston, W. R. (1973). Marmosets and tamarins. Lab. Anim. Handb., 4, 243-250
2. Hiddleston, W. A. (1976). Large scale production of a small laboratory primate, Callithrix jacchus. In: T. Antikatzides, S. Erichsen and A. Spiegel (eds.) The Laboratory Animal in the Study of Reproduction, pp. 51-57. (Stuttgart: Gustav Fischer Verlag)
3. Hearn, J. P., Lunn, S. F., Burden, F. J. and Pilcher, M. M. (1975). Management of marmosets for biomedical research. Lab. Animals, 9, 125-134
4. Heywood, R. and James, R. W. (1980). Toxicological models for testing chemical fertility regulating agents. In: T. C. Anand Kumar (ed.) Non Human Primate Models for Study of Human Reproduction, pp. 219-232. (Basel: Karger)
5. Deinhardt, F. (1970). Use of marmosets in biomedical research. In: E. I. Goldsmith and J. Moor-Jankowski (eds.) Medical Primatology, pp. 918-925. (Basel: Karger)
6. Wolfe, L. G., Ogden, J. D., Deinhardt, J. B., Fischer, L. and Deinhardt, F. (1972). Breeding and handrearing marmosets for viral oncogenesis studies. In: E. I. Goldsmith and J. Moor-Jankowski (eds.) Breeding Primates, pp. 145-157. (Basel: Karger)
7. Epple, G. (1970). Maintenance, breeding and development of marmoset monkeys (Callitrichidae) in captivity. Folia Primat., 12, 57-76
8. Epple, G. (1973). The role of pheromones in the social communication of marmoset monkeys (Callitrichidae). J. Reprod. Fert. (Suppl.), 19, 447-454
9. Gengozian, N. (1969). Marmosets: their potential in experimental medicine. Ann. N. Y. Acad. Sci., 162, 336-362
10. Gengozian, N. (1976). Characterisation of the antibody response of the marmoset to sheep red blood cells. Clin. Exp. Immunol., 23, 525-535

11. Coimbra Filho, A. F. and Mittermeier, R. A. (1978). The gouging, exudate eating and the 'short-tusked' condition in Callithrix and Cebuella. In: D. Kleiman (ed.) The Biology and Conservation of the Callitrichidae, pp. 105-117. (Washington: Smithsonian Institution Press)

12. Coimbra Filho, A. F. (1971). Os saguis do genero Callithrix da regiao oriental brasiliera e um caso de duplo-hibridismo entre tres de suas formas. Rev. Brasil. Biol., 31(3), 377-388

13. Coimbra Filho, A. F. (1972). Aspectos ineditos do compartamento de saguis do genero Callithrix. Rev. Brasil. Biol., 32(4), 505-512

14. Mittermeier, R. A., Bailey, R. C. and Coimbra Filho, A. F. (1978). Conservation status of the Callitrichidae in Brasilian Amazonia, Surinam and French Guiana. In: D. Kleiman (ed.) The Biology and Conservation of the Callitrichidae, pp. 137-146. (Washington: Smithsonian Institution Press)

15. Mittermeier, R. A., Coimbra Filho, A. F. and van Roosmalen, M. (1978). Conservation status of the Callitrichids. In: H. Rothe , H. J. Wolters and J. P. Hearn (eds.) Biology and Behaviour of Marmosets, pp. 17-40. (Gottingen: Eigenverlag Rothe)

16. Mittermeier, R. A., Bailey, R. C., Sponse, L. E. and Wolf, K. E. (1977). Primate ranching - results of an experiment. Oryx, 13(5), 449-453

17. Castro, R. and Soini, P. (1978). Field studies on Saguinus mystax and other Callitrichids in Amazonian Peru. In: D. Kleiman (ed.) The Biology and Conservation of the Callitrichidae, pp. 73-78. (Washington: Smithsonian Institution Press)

18. Dawson, G. A. (1978). Composition and stability of social groups of the tamarin, Saguinus oedipus oedipus. In: D. Kleiman (ed.) The Biology and Conservation of the Callitrichidae, pp. 23-38. (Washington: Smithsonian Institution Press)

19. Ramirez, M. F., Freese, C. H. and Revilla, J. (1978). Feeding ecology of the pygmy marmoset, Cebuella pygmaea, in Northeastern Peru. In: D. Kleiman (ed.) The Biology and Conservation of the Callitrichidae, pp. 91-104. (Washington: Smithsonian Institution Press)

20. Neyman, P. F. (1978). Aspects of the ecology and social organisation of free ranging cotton top tamarins (Saguinus oedipus) and the conservation status of the species. In: D. Kleiman (ed.) The Biology and Conservation of the Callitrichidae, pp. 39-72. (Washington: Smithsonian Institution Press)

21. Lacher, E., Fonseca, G. A., Alves, C. and Magalhaes-Castro, B. (1982) Observations on exudate-eating, scent marking and urination in free living Callithrix jacchus pennicilata. (In press)

22. Hearn, J. P. (1977). A device for restraining small monkeys. Lab. Animals, 11, 261-262

23. Hodges, J. K., Czekala, N. M. and Lasley, B. L. (1979). Estrogen and

luteinising hormone secretion in diverse primate species from simplified urinary analysis. J. Med. Primatol., 8, 349-364

24. Hodges, J. K., Gulick, B. A., Czekala, N. M. and Lasley, B. L. (1981). Comparison of urinary oestrogen excretion in South American primates. J. Reprod. Fert., 61, 83-90

25. Lunn, S. F., Hobson, B. M. and Hearn, J. P. (1979). Pregnancy diagnosis in the Common marmoset, Callithrix jacchus, using immunoprecipitation and transabdominal uterine palpation. Folia Primat., 32, 200-206

26. Hearn, J. P. and Burden, F. J. (1979). 'Collaborative' rearing of neonatal marmosets. Lab. Animals, 13, 131-133

27. Hearn, J. P. and Renfree, M. B. (1975). Prealbumin proteins in the vaginal flushings of the marmoset, Callithrix jacchus. J. Reprod. Fert., 43, 159-161

28. Chambers, P. L. and Hearn, J. P. (1979). Peripheral plasma levels of progesterone, oestradiol-17β, oestrone, testosterone, androstenedione and chorionic gonadotrophin during pregnancy in the marmoset monkey, Callithrix jacchus. J. Reprod. Fert., 56, 23-32

29. Hearn, J. P. and Lunn, S. F. (1974). The reproductive biology of the marmoset monkey, Callithrix jacchus. In: F. J. Perkins and P.N. O'Donoghue (eds.) Breeding Primates for Developmental Biology. Lab. Anim. Handb., 6, 191-202

30. Preslock, J. P., Hampton, S. H. and Hampton, J. K. (1973). Cyclic variations of semen progestins and immunoreactive estrogens in marmosets. Endocrinology, 92, 1096-1101

31. McNeilly, A. S., Abbott, D. H., Lunn, S. F., Chambers, P. L. and Hearn, J. P. (1981). Plasma prolactin concentrations during the ovarian cycle and lactation and their relationship to return of fertility post partum in the common marmoset, Callithrix jacchus. J. Reprod. Fert., 62, 353-360

32. Short, R. V. (1980). The great apes of Africa. J. Reprod. Fert. Fert. Suppl., 28, 3-11

33. Abbott, D. H. and Hearn, J. P. (1978). Physical, hormonal and behavioural aspects of sexual development in the marmoset monkey, Callithrix jacchus. J. Reprod. Fert., 53, 155-166

34. Keverne, E. B. (1979). Sexual and aggressive behaviour in social groups of talapoin monkeys. In: Sex, Hormones and Behaviour. Ciba Symp., 62, 271-297. (Amsterdam: Excerpta Medica)

35. Abbott, D. H., McNeilly, A. S., Lunn, S. F., Hulme, M. J. and Burden, F. J. (1981). Inhibition of ovarian function in subordinate female marmoset monkeys (Callithrix jacchus jacchus). J. Reprod. Fert., 63, 335-345

36. Abbott, D. H. (1979). The sexual development of the common marmoset monkey, Callithrix jacchus. PhD Thesis, University of Edinburgh

37. Moore, H. D. M. and Pryor, J. P. (1981). The comparative ultrastructure of the epididymis in monkeys and man : a search for a suitable animal model for studying epididymal physiology in primates. Am. J. Primatol., 1, 241-250

38. Moore, H. D. M. (1981). An assessment of the fertilising ability of spermatozoa in the epididymis of the marmoset monkey (Callithrix jacchus). Int. J. Androl., 4, 321-330

39. Dixson, A. F. and George, L. (1982). Prolactin and parental behaviour in a male New World primate. Nature, 299, 551-553

40. Hodges, J. K. and Hearn, J. P. (1977). Effects of immunisation against LHRH on reproduction of the marmoset monkey, Callithrix jacchus. Nature, 265, 746-747

41. Hodges, J. K. and Hearn, J. P. (1979) Long term suppression of fertility by immunisations against LHRH and its reversibility in female and male marmoset monkeys. In: G. P. Talwar (ed.) Recent Advances in Reproduction and Regulation of Fertility, pp. 87-96. (Amsterdam: Elsevier)

42. Hearn, J. P. (1980). The effects of 6C6D on the fertility and libido of male marmoset monkeys. In: A. Kumar (ed.) Non Human Primate Models for Study of Human Reproduction, pp. 207-213. (Amsterdam: Elsevier)

43. Hearn, J. P. (1976). Immunisation against pregnancy. Proc. R. Soc. B., 195, 149-160

44. Hearn, J. P. (1979). Immunological interference with the maternal recognition of pregnancy in primates. Ciba Symp., 64, 353-375

45. Thanavala, Y. M., Hearn, J. P., Hay, F. C. and Hulme, M. (1979). Characterisation of the immune response in marmoset monkeys immunised against hCG-β subunit and its relationship to their subsequent fertility. J. Reprod. Immunol., 1, 263-273

46. Hearn, J. P. (1979). Long term suppression of fertility by immunisation with hCG-β and its reversibility in female marmoset monkeys. In: G. P. Talwar (ed.) Recent Advances in Reproduction and Regulation of Fertility, pp. 427-438. (Amsterdam: Elsevier)

47. Hearn, J. P. (1980). The immunobiology of chorionic gonadotrophin. In: J. P. Hearn (ed.) Immunological Aspects of Reproduction and Fertility Control, pp. 229-245. (Lancaster: MTP Press)

48. Hearn, J. P., Abbott, D. H., Chambers, P. L., Hodges, J. K. and Lunn, S. F. (1978). Use of the common marmoset, Callithrix jacchus, in reproductive research. Prim. Med., 10, 40-49

49. Hearn, J. P. (1980). Endocrinology and timing of implantation in the marmoset monkey, Callithrix jacchus. Prog. Rep. Biol., 7, 262-269

Index